HUMAN VITAMIN B₆ REQUIREMENTS

Proceedings of a Workshop

Letterman Army Institute of Research
Presidio of San Francisco, California
June 11-12, 1976

Committee on Dietary Allowances
Food and Nutrition Board
National Research Council

NATIONAL ACADEMY OF SCIENCES
Washington, D.C.   1978

NOTICE: The project that is the subject of this report was approved by the Governing Board of the National Research Council, whose members are drawn from the Councils of the National Academy of Sciences, the National Academy of Engineering, and the Institute of Medicine. The members of the Committee responsible for the report were chosen for their special competences and with regard for appropriate balance.

This report has been reviewed by a group other than the authors according to procedures approved by a Report Review Committee consisting of members of the National Academy of Sciences, the National Academy of Engineering, and the Institute of Medicine.

This workshop conference was supported by NIAMD Grant No. 1 R13 AM17546–01.

Library of Congress Cataloging in Publication Data
Main entry under title:

Human vitamin B_6 requirements.

Includes bibliographies.
1. Vitamin B_6—Congresses. 2. Vitamin B_6 in human nutrition—Congresses. I. National Research Council. Committee on Dietary Allowances.
[DNLM: 1. Pyridoxine—Congresses. QU195 H918 1976]
QP772.P9H85   612.'399   77–16844
ISBN 0–309–02642–3

Available from:

Printing and Publishing Office
National Academy of Sciences
2101 Constitution Avenue, N.W.
Washington, D.C. 20418

Printed in the United States of America

Committee on
Dietary Allowances

H. N. MUNRO, *Chairman*

JOHN G. BIERI

GEORGE M. BRIGGS

CHARLES E. BUTTERWORTH, JR.

GILBERT A. LEVEILLE

WALTER MERTZ

GEORGE M. OWEN

ROY M. PITKIN

HOWERDE E. SAUBERLICH

Acknowledgments

The Food and Nutrition Board gratefully acknowledges the editorial contributions of Howerde E. Sauberlich, Department of Nutrition, Letterman Army Institute of Research, and Myrtle L. Brown, Food and Nutrition Board, National Academy of Sciences.

Contents

Contents

1

Vitamin B₆: Chemistry, Absorption, Metabolism, Catabolism, and Toxicity

M. BRIN

INTRODUCTION AND CHRONOLOGY

One cannot undertake to review the broad aspects of this subject without reflecting upon the important contributions of Esmond Snell and the late Paul Gyorgy toward the development of our understanding of the requirements for, and the model functions of, vitamin B_6. Vitamin B_6 was discovered during one of the most active decades for the identification of unidentified growth factors. This was accomplished with various methods of bioassay and biochemical detective work, long before the current era of sophisticated specific analytical and isolation techniques.

The chronology of the development of our understanding, isolation, and crystallization of vitamin B_6 is shown in Table 1-1 (Rosenberg, 1945). The first observations of acrodynia were made on a diet deficient in riboflavin (as carefully as such could be studied in 1926) by Goldberger and Lilly. In 1932, Ohdake isolated a compound with the formula of vitamin B_6 from rice polishings; however, he failed to recognize its vitamin function. It remained for the late Paul Gyorgy to differentiate the "rat pellagra preventative factor" from riboflavin and to name the new vitamin "B_6." Within the next few years, five dif-

1

TABLE 1-1   Chronology for Vitamin B_6 Discovery

1926	Goldberger and Lillie reported the occurrence of a characteristic dermatitis, called acrodynia, on rats fed a diet deficient in vitamin B_2.
1932	Ohdake in Japan isolated a compound of the formula $C_3H_{11}O_3N \cdot HCl$ from rice polishings but failed to recognize its vitamin character.
1934	Gyorgy established the difference of the "rat pellagra preventative factor" from vitamin B_2 (and vitamin B_1) and called the new vitamin "B_6."
1938	The isolation of the pure crystalline vitamin B_6 was announced independently by five different groups, namely, Lepkovsky, Keresztesy and Stevens, Gyorgy, Kuhn and Wendt, and Itiba and Miti.
1939	The chemical structure was elucidated and vitamin B_6 was synthesized independently by two groups of workers—by Kuhn, Westphal, Wendt and Westphal in Germany and by Keresztesy, Stevens, Harris, Stiller, and Folkers in the United States.

SOURCE: Rosenberg (1945).

ferent research groups of Lepkovsky, Keresztesy and Stevens, Gyorgy, Kuhn and Wendt, and Itiba and Miti characterized the structure. Subsequently, the vitamin itself was synthesized independently by two groups: Kuhn and coworkers in Germany and Keresztesy and associates in the United States.

The ubiquitous distribution of vitamin B_6 through the entire plant and animal kingdoms is now recognized. Some analytical data for its content in commonly consumed foodstuffs have been summarized in Research Report No. 36 of the USDA Home Economics Division (Orr, 1969). These were interpreted by Schroeder (1971) a few years later as revealing that a predominant portion of the vitamin B_6 is removed in food processing and/or preservation and storage. Schroeder recommended improved and broadened food enrichment to compensate for this. This recommendation has been reinforced by recent proposals of the NAS/NRC Food and Nutrition Board (1974).

The purpose of this report is to highlight the chemical and physical aspects of vitamin B_6, the biochemical interconversion of the three active forms, and the absorption and safety of the compounds. This paper will not dwell upon the enzymatic biochemical functions of vitamin B_6 in intermediary metabolism as they relate to human nutrition, since these subjects will be covered in other papers at this conference.

NOMENCLATURE

The IUPAC-IUB Commission on Biological Nomenclature (CBN) has recently published recommended nomenclature for vitamin B_6 and related compounds according to the numbering systems shown in Figure 1-1 (Mayes et al., 1974). The term "vitamin B_6" is recommended as the

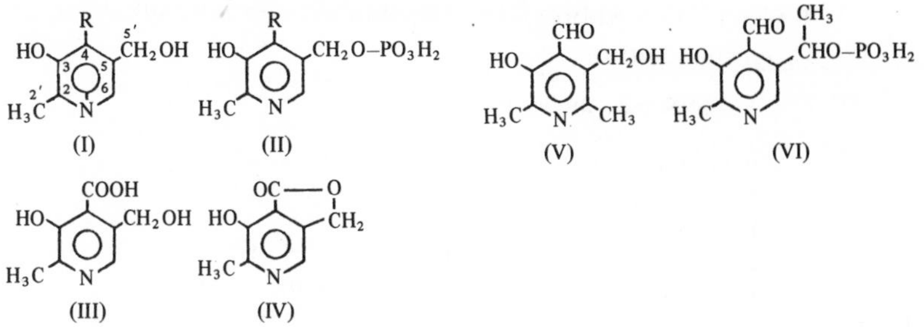

FIGURE 1-1 Structures for vitamin B_6 nomenclature.

generic descriptor for all 3-hydroxy-2-methylpyridine derivatives that exhibit the biological activity of pyridoxine in rats. Compound (I), R = $-CH_2OH$,3-hydroxy-4,5-bis(hydroxy methyl)-2-methylpyridine, is called pyridoxine. (The 4'-OH group, when removed, creates the pyridoxyl alkyl residue.) If R = $-CHO$ in compound (I), it is referred to as pyridoxal. If the oxygen atom is removed from the CHO group, the residue is referred to as pyridoxylidene. When R in compound (I) = $-CH_2NH_2$, the compound is referred to as pyridoxamine. The 5'-phosphoric esters of pyridoxine, pyridoxal, and pyridoxamine should be designated pyridoxine-5'-phosphate (or pyridoxine-5'-P) and so on for the other two forms. The generic form for the 5'-phosphate is shown in (II). The oxidized metabolites of pyridoxal such as 3-hydroxy-5-hydroxymethyl-2-methylpyridine-4-carboxylic acid (III) and the corresponding lactone, (IV), should be designated 4-pyridoxic acid and 4-pyridoxolactone, respectively. Three less commonly occurring metabolites are formed by oxidation at position-5'-, namely, the aldehyde (isopyridoxal), the carboxylic acid (5'-pyridoxic acid), and its lactone (5'-pyridoxal lactone). Two other derivatives are also shown: 6-methylpyridoxal, (V), and 5'-methylpyridoxal-5'-P, (VI), which are names that have been derived according to conventional rules of organic nomenclature.

Abbreviated designations have also been suggested by the CBN. These are shown in Table 1-2. The first P refers to the pyridoxine core structure, the L refers to the aldehyde, the M to the amine, and N to the alcohol form. The terminal P's are added when the compounds are in the 5'-phosphate form.

PHYSICAL AND CHEMICAL PROPERTIES OF VITAMIN B_6

Information on the physical properties of vitamin B_6 was obtained from various key references in the literature (Harris *et al.,* 1968; McDawson,

TABLE 1-2   Abbreviated Designations for Vitamin
B₆ Nomenclature

Trivial Name (Abridged)	Abbreviation
Pyridoxal	PL
Pyridoxamine	PM
Pyridoxine	PN
Pyridoxal-P	PLP
Pyridoxamine-P	PMP
Pyridoxine-P	PNP

SOURCE: Mayes *et al.* (1974).

1962; Snell, 1963b). In Table 1-3 (Harris *et al.*, 1968) it is noted that the
ultraviolet absorption spectra of the vitamers vary significantly with
the pH of the solution. This is because each is converted to a variety of
aqueous ionic forms depending upon pH and other physical factors
(Snell, 1963b). The pK values for vitamin B₆ are shown in Table 1-4
(Snell, 1963b).

TABLE 1-3   Ultraviolet Absorption Spectra of Vitamins B₆

Compound	0.1 N HCl λ max, nm	ε max liter/ (mole) (cm)	pH 7.0 λ max, nm	ε max liter/ (mole) (cm)	0.1 N NaOH λ max, nm	ε max liter/ (mole) (cm)
Pyridoxine hydrochloride	291	8,700	254 / 324	3,760 / 7,100	244 / 309	6,700 / 6,950
Pyridoxine 5-phosphate	290	8,700	253 / 325	3,700 / 7,400	245 / 310	6,500 / 7,300
Pyridoxal hydrochloride	288	9,100	317 / 390	8,800 / 200	240 / 300 / 390	8,300 / 6,100 / 1,700
Pyridoxal 5-phosphate monohydrate	293 / 334	7,200 / 1,300	388	5,500	389	6,600
Pyridoxamine dihydrochloride	293	8,500	253 / 325	4,600 / 7,700	245 / 308	5,900 / 7,300
Pyridoxamine 5-phosphate dihydrate	293	9,000	253 / 325	4,700 / 8,300	245 / 308	6,700 / 8,000

SOURCE: Harris *et al.* (1968).

TABLE 1-4   pK Values for Vitamins B_6

Compound	pK_1	pK_2	pK_3	pK_4
Pyridoxal	4.20–4.23	8.66–8.70	13	
Pyridoxamine	3.31–3.54	7.90–8.21	10.4–10.63	
Pyridoxine	5.00	8.96–8.97		
Pyridoxal-5-phosphate	<2.5	4.14	6.20	8.69
Pyridoxamine-5-phosphate	<2.5	3.25–3.69	5.76	8.61

SOURCE: Snell (1963).

Additional physical characteristics of vitamin B_6 are shown in Table 1-5 (Harris *et al.*, 1968; McDawson, 1962; Snell, 1963b; Windholz, 1976). Generally, the three forms and the phosphate occur as white crystals that are soluble in water, less so in alcohol, and often insoluble in ether. They melt, usually, with decomposition. In addition, aqueous solutions of the three forms are unstable in light and often destroyed by heating. Pyridoxine hydrochloride can form the dimer in hot aqueous solutions. While pyridoxamine and pyridoxine hydrochlorides are stable in hot dilute mineral acid and alkalies, aqueous solutions of pyridoxal hydrochloride are not stable in the latter.

METHODS OF DETECTION

Assays for vitamin B_6 comprise both chemical and combinations of chemical and biological methods. The chemical assays are more suitable for the pure materials such as may occur in pharmaceutical preparations. The biological (and/or microbiological) assays may be more suitable for the determination of vitamin B_6 in natural products.

Chemical assays have employed the phenolic nature of pyridoxine through coupling reactions with 2-6-dichloro-*p*-quinone chlorimide or N,2,6,trichloro-*p*-quinone imine (Lieck and Sondergaard, 1958), diazotized sulfanilic acid (Swaminathan, 1940), diazotized-*p*-amino-acetophenone (Brown *et al.*, 1945), or ferric chloride (Greene, 1939). Fluorometric methods are available for the lactone of 4-pyridoxic acid (Fujita and Fujino, 1955) and the cyanohydrins of pyridoxal and pyridoxal phosphate (Bonavita and Scardi, 1959).

In nature, most of the vitamin B_6 is in bound form, probably as enzyme-coenzyme complexes necessitating hydrolytic release before assay. Some of these problems have been reviewed (Storvick and Peters, 1964). The released forms of vitamin B_6 can either be oxidized to 4-pyridoxic acid and assayed fluorometrically as described above, or the hydrolysates could be assayed microbiologically as determined by

TABLE 1-5 Physical Characteristics of Vitamins B_6

Name and Source	Molecular Weight	Physical Form	Melting Point	Solubility
Pyridoxal hydrochloride Harris et al., 1968	203.6	White rhomboid crystals	126[a] (165)	50 H_2O 1.7 95% EtOH 1% AQ = pH 2.7
Pyridoxamine dihydrochloride Harris et al., 1968	241.1	Deliquescent white platelets	226-27[a]	50 H_2O 0.65 95% EtOH 1% AQ = pH 2.4
Pyridoxine hydrochloride Harris et al., 1968	205.7	White prisms	204-6[a]	22, H_2O 1.1 EtOH Insoluble ether 10% AQ = pH 3.2
Pyridoxal-5-phosphate Snell, 1963	265.15	White crystals	Oxime 229-30[a]	Oxime insoluble H_2O, EtOH, Ether Colorless in acid, yellow in alkaline

[a]Melts with decomposition.

turbidity, acid production, or dry weight of bacterial or yeast growth (Snell, 1950). An official method has been published by the Association of Vitamin Chemists, Inc. (1966), using *Saccharomyces carlsbergensis* 4228 as a test organism. More recently, a modification of an acid hydrolysis of animal tissue, followed by a chromatographic separation of the three forms, followed by a determination microbiologically of the three individual eluates against their own standard curves, has been shown to be successful for these assays (Brin, 1970). The differential response of various lactic acid bacilli to the multiple forms of vitamin B_6 has been used as the basis of a differential assay (Orr, 1969). This assay requires the use of *Streptococcus faecalis* (responding to both pyridoxamine and pyridoxal), *Lactobacillus casei* (responding only to pyridoxal), and *Saccharomyces carlsbergensis* (responding to all three forms). There is also an assay for total vitamin B_6 activity by a mutant of *Neurospora sitophila* (Stokes *et al.*, 1963).

More recently, the technique with N,N-diethyl-*p*-phenylenediamine (DEPA) was compared to the USP method (chloroimide reaction) in the assay of various types of multivitamin preparations. The three procedures gave comparable results whether done by manual or automated technology (Pelletier and Madere, 1974). Gel filtration also may be used (sephadex LH-20) to separate and determine the six types of vitamin B_6 (Abe *et al.*, 1974). High performance cation exchange chromatography has been applied for commercial vitamin preparations (Callmer and Davies, 1974). In studies concerning the vitamin B_6 content of chick embryo liver, preparative thin layer chromatography can be used to separate the various forms of vitamin B_6 in tissues (Smith and Dietrich, 1971). The fluorometric determination of pyridoxic acid lactone was employed to determine the concentration of the forms involved.

Biological assays for vitamin B_6 have as their advantage the measurement of the biologically available vitamin in the material being assayed. While pyridoxal and pyridoxamine are slightly less active when incorporated into the diet, these assays are so meaningful that suitable assays based upon growth response have been reported for rats and chicks (Sharma *et al.*, 1946; Briggs *et al.*, 1942). The biological assay, because of cost and length of assay time, has been largely replaced by the other methods previously described, however.

More recently, there has been interest in the determination of pyridoxal phosphate levels in blood as a means for evaluating nutritional status (Chabner and Livingston, 1970). The assay requires the preparation of a bacterial tyrosine apodecarboxyase, followed by the simultaneous incubation of the apoenzyme, ^{14}C-labeled substrate, and pyridoxal phosphate source, with the release of $^{14}CO_2$ as the final determinant.

THE BIOSYNTHESIS OF VITAMIN B₆

Strong evidence is available that there is synthesis of vitamin B_6 in the human gastrointestinal tract (Linkswiler and Reynolds, 1950). While the prime basis for this paper is chemical, nevertheless it is considered appropriate to include information on the biosynthesis of vitamin B_6. Perhaps biosynthesis is a nonfactor in human nutrition, since the vitamin is a mandatory micronutrient dietary requirement for man. Accordingly, it must be synthesized in the plant kingdom or by microorganisms or by other species not requiring it as a dietary essential.

In Figure 1-2 is shown the pathway by which pyridoxine is synthesized by a mutant of *E. coli* (which is blocked between pyridoxine and pyridoxal) from three discrete glycerol units (Hill and Spenser, 1970). (Note that these authors referred to pyridoxine as "pyridoxol.") One glycerol is incorporated by way of pyruvate as a two-carbon fragment probably at the oxidation level of acetaldehyde. The other two glycerol units are incorporated intact, possibly by way of triosphosphate. More recently, a biosynthetic pathway of vitamin B_6 has been studied with cell suspensions of the vitamin B_6 producing bacteria, *Achromobacter cycloclastes* [AMS 6201 (Ishida *et al.*, 1973)]. The summation of their work is shown in Figure 1-3. Here it is observed that the glycerol referred to previously is shown as an important component of the final vitamin B_6 molecule but that gammaaminobutyric acid carbon may also contribute significantly.

ABSORPTION OF VITAMIN B₆ IN THE INTESTINE
AND ACROSS THE HUMAN PLACENTA

In experimental animals, there appears to be a linear relationship between vitamin B_6 dosage and the excretion of 4-pyridoxic acid and/or

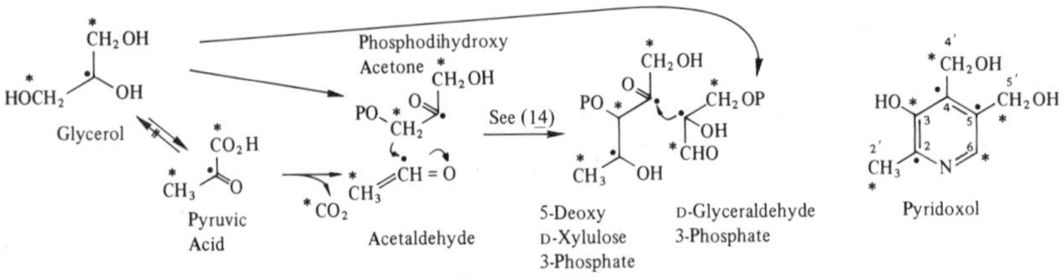

FIGURE 1-2   Incorporation of glycerol into vitamin B_6.

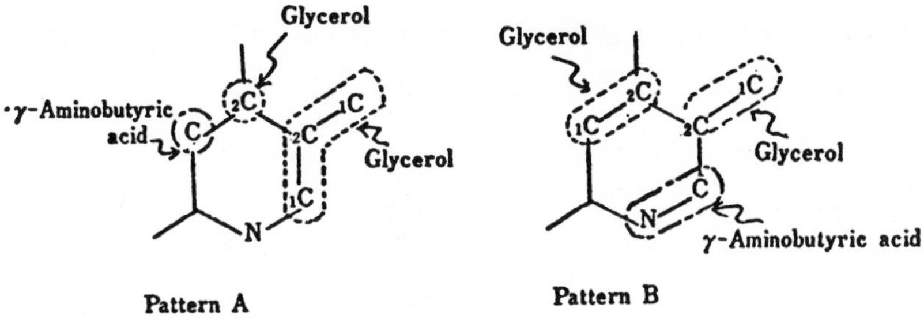

FIGURE 1-3   Distribution of ^{14}C in vitamin B_6.

radioactivity (from the labeled vitamin) in urine (Scudi *et al.*, 1940). Similar findings were obtained in man (Brain and Booth, 1964). The linear relationship between dosage and urinary excretion was taken to indicate absorption by diffusion. Absorption seems to occur in the jejunum and the ileum but primarily in the upper small intestine, since ileal resections had virtually no effect. Also, absorption from the colon was very slight (Booth and Brain, 1962). Similarly, passive transport was suggested by studies in the rat and the hamster small intestine *in vitro* (Serebro *et al.*, 1966; Spencer and Bow, 1964). It has also been reported that the feeding of D-sorbitol apparently increased vitamin B_6 absorption in rats on low vitamin B_6 diets (Okuda *et al.*, 1960). It was explained that this might have been attributed to an increase in the synthesis of the vitamin by intestinal microorganisms. Patients with idiopathic steatorrhea often showed reduced pyridoxine absorption although there was no specific correlation between malabsorption of pyridoxine and the histological appearance of intestinal biopsies (Brain and Booth, 1964). This information has been recently reviewed (Matthews, 1974).

Another aspect of vitamin B_6 absorption is the transplacental distribution of vitamin B_6 between mother and cord blood. It has been suggested that the intake of vitamin B_6 by the mother during the last trimester of pregnancy determines the nutritional state of the neonate with respect to this vitamin (Ziegler *et al.*, 1969). When plasma pyridoxal phosphate was measured at birth in premature infants, weighing approximately 2 kg, deficient levels were observed, again suggesting that transport becomes more active during the last trimester of pregnancy.

Two groups, at least, have demonstrated that there is a positive gradient of vitamin B_6 in cord blood over that of mother blood, ranging approximately 3 times as high for total vitamin B_6 to between 2.5 and 5

TABLE 1-6   Vitamin B_6-Vitamer Levels in Plasma Samples of Paired Cord and Maternal Bloods

Form of Vitamin B_6	Number of Samples	Levels [a] in Blood	
		Mother	Cord
Pyridoxine	20	193 ± 31.8	894[b] ± 190.8
Pyridoxal	20	309 ± 32.4	972[c] ± 152.6
Pyridoxamine	21	483 ± 70.1	636 ± 121.7
Total[d]	21	1,182 ± 152.8	2,531[b] ± 367.9

SOURCE: Brin (1971).
[a]Values are in millimicrograms per 100 ml plasma.
[b]Statistically significant difference (paired t-test) $p < 0.01$.
[c]$p < 0.001$.
[d]Total value is not sum and was determined without resin separation.

times as high for individual vitamers (Contractor and Shane, 1970; Brin, 1971) (Table 1-6). In Table 1-7 are shown the differences of erythrocyte aminotransferase activity of paired cord and maternal bloods. Cord erythrocytes had about twice the activity for the enzyme as that of the mother blood in both cases (Brin, 1971). These data suggest a very active mechanism for the transport of vitamin B_6 across the placental barrier. The measurement of erythrocyte enzymes has been found to be useful in the evaluation of nutritional status (Albert and Brin, 1960; Brin, 1964) and appears to be more practical than the use of plasma for this purpose (Brin et al., 1954; Brin et al., 1960).

While studies showing vitamin deficiency in mothers have failed to find associated neonatal clinical sequelae, evidence of biochemical aberrations in vitamin B_6 metabolism was found in 60 percent of women in one study (Heller et al., 1973).

TABLE 1-7   Erythrocyte Aminotransferase Activities of Paired Cord and Maternal Bloods

Erythrocyte Aminotransferase Enzyme	Number of Samples	Activity[a] of Enzyme in Blood	
		Mother	Cord
Oxalacetic (OAT)	21	1,252 ± 103.9	1,880[b] ± 83.9
Pyruvic (PAT)	21	195 ± 30.0	310[c] ± 32.7

SOURCE: Brin (1971).
[a]Activity is expressed as milligrams of pyruvic acid formed per 100 ml of hemolysate per hour.
[b]$p < 0.0001$.
[c]Statistically significant difference (paired t-test) $p < 0.01$.

METABOLISM OF VITAMIN B$_6$ VITAMERS

There are three aspects of vitamin B$_6$ metabolism that are of sufficient importance to be included in this section, namely, the interconversion of the vitamin B$_6$ forms, the biochemical degradation of vitamin B$_6$, and the chemical relationships of vitamin B$_6$.

The interconversions of various forms of vitamin B$_6$ have been studied intensively. While, as described previously, various microorganisms have specific needs for specific forms (Rabinowitz and Snell, 1947), it appears that the three forms are approximately equally active in supporting animal growth. This suggests that they are readily interconvertible as they are also converted to their respective phosphate coenzymes. An outline of the interconversions is shown in Figure 1-4 (Snell and Haskell, 1971). Phosphorylation is accomplished by

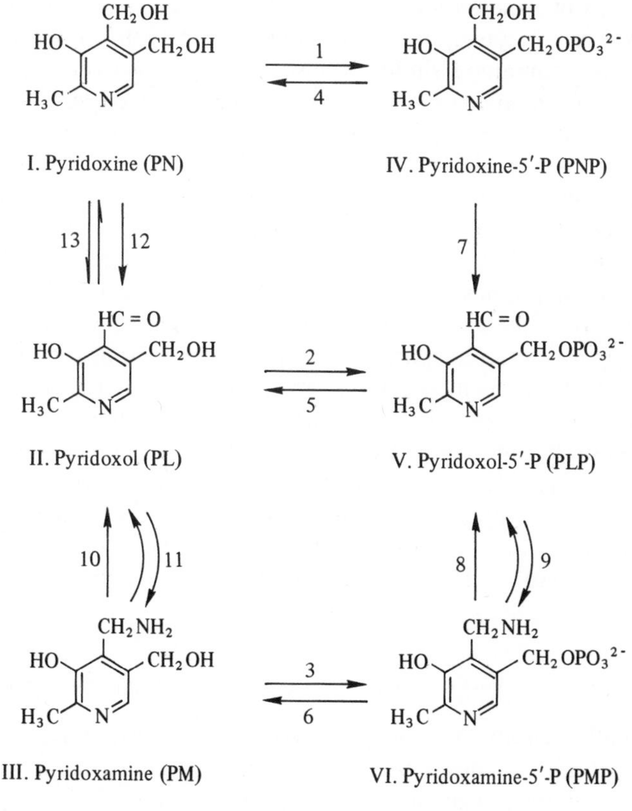

FIGURE 1-4   Interconversion of vitamins B$_6$.

pyridoxal kinase (EC 2.7.1.35) with the reverse reactions, 4, 5, and 6, by various phosphatases. Reactions 7, 8, and 10 by which the -ine, -al, and amine phosphates and/or the three amines are oxidized to pyridoxal, are accomplished by pyridoxal-P-oxidase. The conversion of pyridoxal 5-P to pyridoxamine-5-P and pyridoxal to pyridoxamine are carried out by transaminases and the conversions of pyridoxine to pyridoxal by pyridoxine dehydrogenases (EC 1.1.1.65). It is recognized that the unphosphorylated forms are generally transported across membranes more efficiently, thereby suggesting a mechanism by which the vitamin can be retained in the cell, probably in bound form to various apoenzymes (McCoy and Colombini, 1972). Purification procedures for the pyridoxine phosphate oxidase (Wada, 1970) and an acid phosphatase with pyridoxine phosphorylating activity (Tani and Ogata, 1970) have been described.

Pyridoxal kinase activity has been reported to be 50 percent lower in erythrocytes of American blacks than that of American whites. Lymphocytes, granulocytes, and cultured skin fibroblasts from black and white donors contained similar kinase activity, however (Chern and Beutler, 1975). *In vivo* studies in normal human subjects suggested that pyridoxine was taken up by red cells where it was converted to pyridoxal phosphate and then to free pyridoxal. This conversion was followed by gradual release of a proportion of pyridoxal into plasma (Anderson *et al.*, 1971). Pyridoxal phosphate was not released into the plasma of stored blood but remained in the red blood cells. By the use of tritiated compounds it was concluded that the different forms of vitamin B_6 fit a kinetic metabolic model that assumes an equilibration between pyridoxal-5-phosphate and pyridoxamine-5-phosphate but essentially unidirectional reactions in other metabolic conversions (Johansson *et al.*, 1974). Recent work on biogenic amine interactions with vitamin B_6 vitamers suggests that dopa, dopamine, norepinephrine, and serotonin inhibit brain pyridoxal kinase while tyrosine, tryptophan, and 5-hydroxytryptophan have no effect (Neary *et al.*, 1972). It is suggested that this interrelationship may represent a form of metabolic regulation. These data are illustrated in Table 1-8 (Neary *et al.*, 1972).

OXIDATIVE CONVERSION OF VITAMIN B_6 TO METABOLITES

While small amounts of pyridoxal, pyridoxamine, and pyridoxine and their phosphorylated derivatives are excreted into the urine of man and rats, the predominant metabolite is 4-pyridoxic acid (Rabinowitz and Snell, 1949; Huff and Perlzweig, 1944). The enzyme forming pyridoxic

TABLE 1-8   Activity of Pyridoxal Kinase in the
Presence of Tyrosine and Its Derivatives

Compound Added	Pyridoxal Phosphate Formed, nM	Decrease of Pyridoxal Phosphate, %
None	59 ± 4	0
Tyrosine	58 ± 4	0
Dopa	30 ± 5	49
Dopamine	8 ± 0	86
Norepinephrine	13 ± 2	78

SOURCE: Neary *et al.* (1972).

acid does not oxidize pyridoxal phosphate. It is a FAD-dependent general aldehyde oxidase (aldehyde: oxygen oxidoreductase, EC 1.2.3.1) of liver (Schwartz and Kjeldgaard, 1951). Xanthine oxidase, however, does not oxidize pyridoxal. Neither 4-pyridoxic acid nor its lactone has vitamin B_6 activity (Snell and Rannefeld, 1945). Subcutaneously administered 4-pyridoxic acid is recovered quantitatively from the urine of human subjects, suggesting that there is no further degradation of this compound (Reddy *et al.*, 1958). More recent studies have shown that in addition to the excretion of pyridoxine, pyridoxic acid, the lactone of pyridoxic acid, and pyridoxal in urine, there is the excretion of a ureido-pyridoxyl complex. In this case, one NH_2 group of urea has reacted with the OH group of the hemiacetal form of the aldehyde in position 4 of pyridoxal (Bernett and Pearson, 1969). When small amounts of tritiated pyridoxine were administered to human subjects, only about 15–20 percent of the isotope was excreted in urine within the first day. A half-life of between 18 and 38 days was calculated for the remainder of the dose (Johansson *et al.*, 1966).

VITAMIN B_6 FUNCTION IN TRANSAMINATION AND
DECARBOXYLATION REACTIONS

The functions of vitamin B_6 and the phosphorylated coenzyme forms in transamination and decarboxylation reactions have been reviewed (Guirard and Snell, 1964; Snell, 1963a). Included are descriptions of the enzymatic and the nonenzymatic model systems by which vitamin B_6 functions. The contributions of E. E. Snell and his colleagues in this area of chemical nutritional research are to be noted with admiration.

ANTAGONISTS OF VITAMIN B$_6$

In Table 1-9 some vitamin B$_6$ antagonists are presented. Those of natural origin include linatine, gyromitrin, methylhydrazine, agaritine, canavanine and canaline, and cycloserine (Klosterman, 1974). Linatine is obtained from linseed or the flax plant, while gyromitrin, agaratine, and methylhydrazine are found in wild and domestic mushrooms. In these cases, hydrazines are formed; these compounds, in turn, form complexes with pyridoxal or pyridoxal phosphate. Canaline from the jack bean is a substituted hydroxylamine and forms oximes with pyridoxal and pyridoxal phosphate. Cycloserine, formed by certain actinomyces, is the next lower homologue of canaline and reacts similarly. It is suggested that the overall effects of the hydrazines and hydroxylamines may also be strong inhibitors of pyridoxal phosphokinase, since they are often bound by the enzyme more firmly than

TABLE 1-9   Some Vitamin B$_6$ Antagonists

Natural origin[a]	Proposed mechanism
Linatine (linseed, flax plant)	Hydrolysis yields 1-amino-O-proline, a substituted secondary hydrazine
Gyromitrin, methylhydrazine (Helvella exculanta-wild mushroom)	Methyl-N-formyl hydrazine formed during cooking
Agaritine (Agaricus bisporus-commercial mushroom)	γ-glutamyl-4-OH methyl phenyl-hydrazine
Canavanine, canaline (jack bean)	Substituted hydroxylamine (forms oximes with PL, PLP)
Cycloserine (Actinomyces)	Next lower homolog of canaline (forms stable complex with PLP)
L-Dopa (velvet bean)	Binds PLP (also decarboxylase effect)
Mimosine (Mimosa) B-cyanoalanine (Vicia)	Inhibits PLP enzymes
Nonnatural antagonists	Proposed mechanism
Isonicotinic hydrazide[b]	Combines PL, PLP, competitive inhibition for PLP enzymes
Penicillamine[c]	Forms thiazolidine
Allylglycine,3-mercapto-propionic acid,4-deoxy-pyridoxine[d]	Inhibition of L-glutamate carboxylase relieved by PLP only after 4-deoxypridoxine

[a]Klosterman (1974).
[b]Vilter et al. (1954).
[c]Thier and Segal (1972).
[d]Horton and Meldrum (1973).

pyridoxal itself. L-dopa, the compound used therapeutically for Parkinsonism, is also found naturally in the legume *Mucuna deeringiana* (velvet bean) widely grown for forage in Asia, where it is often used in the treatment of nervous disorders. It has been shown to combine with PLP to form a complex which is inhibitory to liver L-dopa decarboxylase. The administration of vitamin B_6 unfortunately can both eliminate adverse reactions to L-dopa as well as promote its usefulness. Mimosine or 3-hydroxy-4-keto-1 (4H) pyridinealanine is toxic to animals probably by forming a complex with PLP. It is shown to inhibit a number of PLP-requiring enzymes. While the effects of betacyanoalanine, a neurotoxin obtained from vicia species, can be reversed in the rat by PL, this is probably due to a noncompetitive inhibition for L-aspartate betadecarboxylase.

Vitamin B_6 antagonists that do not occur naturally include isonicotinic hydrazide (INH), which has been used for tuberculosis therapy for many years. Its antagonism has been explained as the result of INH combining with pyridoxal and pyridoxal phosphate and subsequent excretion of these compounds in the urine (Vilter *et al.*, 1954). INH may also compete competitively with pyridoxal phosphate dependent enzymes (Krishnaswamy, 1974). Penicillamine is used often in the treatment of cystinuria or Wilson's disease. Its use may be accompanied by vitamin B_6 deficiency as manifested by peripheral polyneuropathy (Thier and Segal, 1972).

The administration of allylglycine, 3-mercaptopropionic acid, and 4-deoxypyridoxine to mice and baboons has been shown to result in convulsive seizures (Horton and Meldrum, 1973). It was observed that immediately before the seizure there was gross inhibition of glutamate decarboxylase. This inhibition was relieved by pyridoxal phosphate but only after the *in vivo* administration of 4-deoxypyridoxine. Pyridoxal phosphate had no effect following the administration of the other two compounds. This finding suggested that three different mechanisms were involved in the inhibition of L-glutamate decarboxylase as a consequence of the administration of the three compounds (Horton and Meldrum, 1973). Deoxypyridoxine has been used to initiate vitamin B_6 deficiency in human subjects (Mueller and Vilter, 1950). This antagonism can be corrected by administration of pyridoxine.

TOXICOLOGY OF VITAMIN B_6

As soon as pyridoxine became available in relatively pure form, it was tested for toxicity by the LD_{50} technique. It was shown that the LD_{50}

was 3,700 mg/kg body weight when pyridoxine was injected sub-cutaneously and 5,500 mg/kg on oral administration (Unna, 1940). The daily administration of vitamin B_6 over a period of 80 days to dogs (20 mg/kg) and rats (25 mg/day) failed to produce any toxic manifestations or histopathological changes. Rats receiving 2.5 mg daily were raised through three generations. Other studies have been recently reviewed (Zbinden, 1973) in which heroically high doses of vitamin B_6, of the order of 1,000 mg/kg (equivalent to 70 g/day for man) for several days, caused hind leg paralysis in rats and dogs associated with focal damage of peripheral nerves and degeneration of the dorsal tracts of the spinal cord, the dorsal roots, and the dorsal spinal ganglia. Paradoxically, the histopathological changes were not distinguishable from those induced by isoniazid. A satisfactory explanation has not been found, although in human therapy, vitamin B_6 is usually given in daily doses up to 50 mg and is rarely used even at several hundred milligrams per day except when vitamin B_6 antagonists are administered for therapeutic reasons. Data for the acute toxicity for vitamin B_6 are shown in Table 1–10. Included are LD_{50} data for oral, intravenous, and subcutaneous admin-istrations to the mouse and the rat. For oral administration, the toxicity of pyridoxine, pyridoxal-5-phosphate, or pyridoxamine is very low, being of the order of 2,000–6,000 mg/kg of body weight for the mouse or rat (Hoffmann-La Roche, unpublished observations). Parenteral administration results in an LD_{50} of 500 to 700 mg/kg body weight for these compounds, while the subcutaneous LD_{50} is of the same order of magnitude as that of oral administration. Additional work has been done in our laboratories on testing of pyridoxine hydrochloride by standard techniques for eye and skin irritation (2 percent in water). Pyridoxine hydrochloride was considered nonirritating to rabbit eyes and skin (Hoffmann-La Roche, unpublished observations).

It was reported that when vitamin B_6 deficiency was induced in pregnant rats by feeding a deficient diet plus 4-desoxypyridoxine in the drinking water, fetuses were small, appeared anemic, and showed teratogenic effects such as omphalocele, exencephaly, cleft palate,

TABLE 1-10   Acute Toxicity (LD_{50}) of Vitamins B_6, mg/kg

Form	Mouse		Rat	
	Oral	Intravenous	Oral	Subcutaneous
Pyridoxine HCl	6,000	700	6,000	3,700
Pyridoxal-5-P	2,000	580	–	–
Pyridoxamine	5,000	500	–	–

SOURCE: Hoffmann-La Roche, Inc., unpublished observations.

micrognathia, digital defects, and splenic hypoplasia (Davis *et al.,* 1970). Conversely, there was no teratogenesis as a consequence of giving high doses of up to 80 mg/kg body weight per day orally, on days 6 to 15 of gestation, to Wistar rats (Khera, 1975).

LITERATURE CITED

Abe, M., T. Nishimune, and R. Hayashi. 1974. Separative determination of the six types of vitamin B_6 by gel filtration. Vitamins (Japan) *48*:545–549.

Albert, D. J., and M. Brin. 1960. Comparison of serum and erythrocyte hemolysate transaminase systems. Fed. Proc. *19*:321.

Anderson, B. E., C. E. Fulford-Jones, J. A. Child, M. E. J. Beard, and C. J. T. Baetman. 1971. Conversion of vitamin B_6 compounds to active forms in the red blood cell. J. Clin. Invest. *50*:1901–1909.

Association of Vitamin Chemists, Inc. 1966. Vitamin B_6. *In* Methods of Vitamin Assay, 3rd ed., John Wiley & Sons, New York, pp. 209–221.

Bernett, G. E., and W. N. Pearson. 1969. Isolation and identification of a new urinary metabolite of ^{14}C-pyridoxine in the rat. Fed. Proc. *28*:559.

Bonavita, V. and V. Scardi. 1959. Studies on glutamic-oxalacetic transaminase. II. The properties of two derivatives of pyridoxal 5-phosphate. Arch. Biochem. Biophys. *82*:300–309.

Booth, C. C., and M. C. Brain. 1962. The absorption of tritium-labelled pyridoxine hydrochloride in the rat. J. Physiol. (London) *164*:282–294.

Brain, M. C., and C. C. Booth. 1964. The absorption of tritium-labelled pyridoxine HCl in control subjects and in patients with intestinal malabsorption. Gut *5*:241–247.

Briggs, G. M., Jr., R. C. Mills, D. M. Hegsted, C. A. Elvehjem, and E. B. Hart. 1942. The vitamin B_6 requirement of the chick. Poultry Sci. *21*:379–383.

Brin, M. 1964. Use of the erythrocyte in functional evaluation of vitamin adequacy. *In* D. Surgenon and C. F. Bishop (eds.), Red Cell. Academic Press, New York, pp. 451–478.

Brin, M. 1970. A simplified Toepfer-Lehmann assay for the three vitamin B_6 vitamers. *In* D. B. McCormick and L. D. Wright (eds.), Methods in Enzymology, Vitamins and Coenzymes, Vol. 18, Part A, Academic Press, New York/London, pp. 519–523.

Brin, M. 1971. Abnormal tryptophan metabolism in pregnancy and with the oral contraceptive pill. II. Relative levels of vitamin B_6-vitamers in cord and maternal blood. Am. J. Clin. Nutr. *24*:704–708.

Brin, M., R. E. Olson, and F. J. Stare. 1954. Metabolism of cardiac muscle. VIII. Pyridoxine deficiency. J. Biol. Chem. *210*:435–443.

Brin, M., M. Tai, A. S. Ostashever, and H. Kalinsky. 1960. The relative effects of pyridoxine deficiency on two plasma transaminases in the growing and in the adult rat. J. Nutr. *71*:416–420.

Brown, E. B., A. F. Bina, and J. M. Thomas. 1945. The use of diazotized *p*-aminoacetophenone in the determination of vitamin B_6 (pyridoxine). J. Biol. Chem. *158*:455–461.

Callmer, K., and L. Davies. 1974. Separation and determination of vitamin B_1, B_2, B_6 and nicotinamide in commercial vitamin preparations using high performance cation-exchange chromatography. Chromatographia *7*:644–650.

Chabner, B., and D. Livingston. 1970. A simple enzymic assay for pyridoxal phosphate. Anal. Biochem. *34*:413–423.

18   M. BRIN

Chern, C. J. and E. Beutler. 1975. Pyridoxal kinase. Decreased activity in red blood cells of Afro-Americans. Science *187*:1084–1086.

Contractor, S. F., and B. Shane. 1970. Blood and urine levels of vitamin B_6 in the mother and fetus before and after loading of the mother with vitamin B_6. Am. J. Obstet. Gynecol. *107*:635–640.

Davis, S. D., T. Nelson, and T. H. Shepard. 1970. Tetraogenicity of vitamin B_6 deficiency: Omphalocele, skeletal and neural defects, and splenic hypoplasia. Science *169*:1329–1330.

Food and Nutrition Board. 1974. Proposed Fortification Policy for Cereal Grain Products, National Academy of Sciences, Washington, D.C.

Fujita, A., and K. Fujino. 1955. Fluorometric determination of vitamin B_6. IV. Fractional determination of vitamin B_6 components and 4-pyridoxic acid in the urine. J. Vitaminol. *1*:290–296.

Greene, R. D. 1939. Preparation of vitamin B_6 from natural sources. J. Biol. Chem. *130*:513–518.

Guirard, B. M., and E. E. Snell. 1964. Vitamin B_6 function in transamination and decarboxylation reactions. Compr. Biochem. *15*:138–199.

Harris, S. A., E. E. Harris, and R. W. Burg. 1968. Pyridoxine. Kirk-Othmer Encycl. Chem. Tech. *16*:806–824.

Heller, S., R. M. Salkeld, and W. F. Koerner. 1973. Vitamin B_6 status in pregnancy. Am. J. Clin. Nutr. *26*:1339–1348.

Hill, R. E., and I. D. Spenser. 1970. Biosynthesis of vitamin B_6: Incorporation of three-carbon units. Science *169*:773–775.

Hoffmann-La Roche. Unpublished observations.

Horton, R. W., and B. S. Meldrum. 1973. Seizures induced by allylglycine, 3-mercaptopropionic acid and 4-deoxypyridoxine in mice and photosensitive baboons, and different modes of inhibition of cerebral glutamic acid decarboxylase. Br. J. Pharmacol. *49*:52–63.

Huff, J. W., and W. A. Perlzweig. 1944. A product of oxidative metabolism of pyridoxine, 2-methyl-3-hydroxy-4-carboxy-5-hydroxymethylpyridine (4-pyridoxic acid). I. Isolation from urine, structure, and synthesis. J. Biol. Chem. *155*:345–355.

Ishida, M., H. Nagayama, and K. Shimura. 1973. Distribution patterns of ^{14}C in the labelled vitamin B_6 prepared with the cell-suspension of *Achromobacter cycloclasters*. Agric. Biol. Chem. *37*:1881–1892.

Johansson, S., S. Lindstedt, U. Register, and L. Wadstrom. 1966. Studies on the metabolism of labeled pyridoxine in man. Am. J. Clin. Nutr. *18*:185–196.

Johansson, S., S. Lindstedt, and H. G. Tiselium. 1974. Metabolic interconversions of different forms of vitamin B_6. J. Biol. Chem. *249*:6040–6046.

Khera, K. S. 1975. Teratogenicity study in rats given high doses of pyridoxine (vitamin B_6) during organogenesis. Experientia *31*:469–470.

Klosterman, H. J. 1974. Vitamin B_6 antagonists of natural origin. J. Agric. Food Chem. *22*:13–16.

Krishnaswamy, K. 1974. Isonicotinic acid hydrazide and pyridoxine deficiency. Int. J. Vitam. Nutr. Res. *44*:457–465.

Lieck, H., and H. Sondergaard. 1958. The content of vitamin B_6 in Danish foods. Int. J. Vitam. Res. *29*:68–77.

Linkswiler, H., and M. S. Reynolds. 1950. Urinary and fecal elimination of B_6 and 4-pyridoxic acid on three levels of intake. J. Nutr. *41*:523–532.

Matthews, D. M. 1974. Pyridoxine and related compounds. *In* D. H. Smyth (ed.), Intestinal Absorption, Biomembranes, Vol. 4B, Plenum Press, London/New York, pp. 894–896.

Mayes, R. W., R. M. Mason, and D. C. Griffin. 1974. Nomenclature for vitamins B_6 and related compounds. Biochem. J. *137*:417–421.

McCoy, E. E., and C. Colombini. 1972. Interconversions of vitamin B_6 in mammalian tissue. J. Agric. Food Chem. *20*:494–498.

McDawson, R., ed. 1962. Data for Biochemical Research. Oxford Univ. Press, New York, pp. 126–127.

Mueller, J. F., and R. W. Vilter. 1950. Pyridoxine deficiency in human beings induced by desoxypyridoxine. J. Clin. Invest. *29*:193–201.

Neary, J. T., R. L. Meneely, M. R. Grever, and W. F. Diven. 1972. The interactions between biogenic amines and pyridoxal, pyridoxal phosphate, and pyridoxal kinase. Arch. Biochem. Biophys. *151*:42–47.

Okuda, K., J. M. Hsu, and B. F. Chow. 1960. Effect of feeding D-sorbitol on the intestinal absorption of vitamin B_6 and vitamin B_{12} in rats. J. Nutr. *72*:99–104.

Orr, M. L. 1969. Pantothenic acid, vitamin B_6, and vitamin B_{12} in foods. U.S. Dep. Agric. Home Econ. Res. Rep. No. 36:53 pp.

Pelletier, O., and R. Madere. 1974. Automated and manual determination of pyridoxine in multivitamin preparations. Can. J. Pharm. Sci. *9*:99–103.

Rabinowitz, J. C., and E. E. Snell. 1947. The vitamin B_6 group. XI. An improved method for assay of vitamin B_6 with *Streptococcus faecalis*. J. Biol. Chem. *169*:631–642.

Rabinowitz, J. C., and E. E. Snell. 1949. Vitamin B_6 group. XV. Urinary excretion of pyridoxal, pyridoxamine, pyridoxine, and 4-pyridoxic acid in human subjects. Proc. Soc. Exp. Biol. Med. *70*:235–240.

Reddy, S. K., M. S. Reynolds, and J. M. Price. 1958. The determination of 4-pyridoxic acid in human urine. J. Biol. Chem. *233*:691–696.

Rosenberg, H. R. 1945. Vitamin B_6-pyridoxine. Chemistry and Physiology of the Vitamins. Interscience Publ., New York, pp. 197–216.

Schroeder, H. A. 1971. Losses of vitamins and trace minerals resulting from processing and preservation of foods. Am. J. Clin. Nutr. *24*:562–573.

Schwartz, R., and N. O. Kjeldgaard. 1951. The enzymatic oxidation of pyridoxal by liver aldehyde oxidase. Biochem. J. *48*:333–337.

Scudi, J. V., K. Unna, and W. Antopol. 1940. A study of the urinary excretion of vitamin B_6 by a colorimetric method. J. Biol. Chem. *135*:371–376.

Serebro, H. A., H. M. Solomon, J. H. Johnson, and T. R. Hendrix. 1966. The intestinal absorption of vitamin B_6 compounds by the rat and hamster. Bull. Johns Hopkins Hosp. *119*:166–171.

Sharma, P. S., E. E. Snell, and C. A. Elvehjem. 1946. The vitamin B_6 group. VIII. Biological assay of pyridoxal, pyridoxamine, and pyridoxine. J. Biol. Chem. *165*:55–63.

Smith, M. A., and L. S. Dietrich. 1971. Preparative thin-layer chromatography for the separation of the various forms of vitamin B_6 in tissues. Vitamin B_6 contents of chick embryo liver during the midperiod of development. Biochim. Biophys. Acta *230*:262–270.

Snell, E. E. 1950. Microbiological methods. G. Vitamin B_6. 1. Extraction from natural materials. *In* P. Gyorgy (ed.), Vitamin Methods, Vol. 1, Academic Press, New York, pp. 406–408.

Snell, E. E. 1963a. Non-enzymatic reactions of pyridoxal and their significance. *In* E. E. Snell, P. M. Fasella, A. Braunstein, and A. R. Fanelli (eds.), International Symposium on Biological and Chemical Aspects of Pyridoxal Catalysis, Macmillan Co., New York, pp. 1–12.

Snell, E. E. 1963b. Vitamin B_6. Compr. Biochem. *2*:48–58.

Snell, E. E., and B. E. Haskell. 1971. Metabolism of water-soluble vitamins. Compr. Biochem. *21*:47–71.

Snell, E. E., and A. N. Rannefeld. 1945. The vitamin B₆ group. III. The vitamin activity of pyridoxal and pyridoxamine for various organisms. J. Biol. Chem. *157*:475–489.

Spencer, R. P., and T. M. Bow. 1964. *In vitro* transport of radiolabeled vitamins by the small intestine. J. Nucl. Med. *5*:251–258.

Stokes, J. L., A. Larsen, C. R. Woodward, Jr., and J. W. Foster. 1963. A neurospora assay for pyridoxine. J. Biol. Chem. *150*:17–24.

Storvick, C. A., and J. M. Peters. 1964. Methods for the determination of vitamin B₆ in biological materials. Vitam. Horm. *22*:833–854.

Swaminathan, M. 1940. Chemical estimation of vitamin B₆ in foods by means of the diazo reaction and the phenol reagent. Nature *145*:780–781.

Tani, Y., and K. Ogata. 1970. Acid phosphatase having pyridoxine-phosphorylating activity. Methods Enzymol. *18A*:626–630.

Thier, S. O., and S. Segal. 1972. Cystinuria. *In* J. B. Stanbury, J. B. Wyngaarden, and D. S. Fredrickson (eds.), The Metabolic Basis of Inherited Disease, 3rd ed., McGraw-Hill, New York, pp. 1504–1517.

Unna, K. 1940. Studies on the toxicity and pharmacology of vitamin B₆ (2-methyl-3-hydroxy-4,5-bis(hydroxymethyl)-pyridine). J. Pharmacol. Exp. Ther. *70*:400–407.

Vilter, R. W., J. P. Biehl, J. F. Mueller, and B. I. Friedman. 1954. Some abnormalities of vitamin B₆ metabolism in human beings. Fed. Proc. *13*:776–779.

Wada, H. 1970. Pyridoxine phosphate oxidase. *In* D. B. McCormick and L. D. Wright (eds.), Methods in Enzymology, Vitamins and Coenzymes, Vol. 18, Part A, Academic Press, New York/London, pp. 626–630.

Windholz, M., ed. 1976. Pyridoxal 5-phosphate. The Merck Index, 9th ed., Merck & Co., Inc., Rahway, N.J., p. 1035.

Zbinden, G. 1973. Progress in Toxicology, Vol. 1, Springer-Verlag, New York/Heidelberg/Berlin, pp. 60–65.

Ziegler, E., L. Reinken, and H. Berger. 1969. Die ausscheidung von pyridoxinsaeure beim neugeborenen und ihre beeinflussung durch pyridoxinbelastung. Int. J. Vitam. Res. *39*:192–202.

2

Vitamin B$_6$ Relationship in Tryptophan Metabolism

L. M. HENDERSON *and* J. D. HULSE

The metabolism of amino acids in general and tryptophan in particular involves pyridoxal phosphate-dependent enzymes. In addition to the usual aminotransferase, other classes of pyridoxal phosphate enzymes function in tryptophan degradation. The initial attack on L-tryptophan does not involve transamination. However an aminotransferase catalyzes the conversion of indole pyruvate to L-tryptophan providing a mechanism for utilizing D-tryptophan by some mammalian species that possess sufficient D-amino acid oxidase activity (Langner and Berg, 1955; Loh and Berg, 1971; Triebwasser *et al.*, 1976). The other reactions include kynurenine aminotransferase (at least two), kynureninase, and aromatic L-amino acid decarboxylase, which acts on tryptophan or its 5-hydroxy derivative to give tryptamine or serotonin. In addition the *E. coli* enzyme, tryptophanase, participates in disposal of approximately 3 percent of the dietary tryptophan intake. The indole, so formed, is apparently absorbed from the intestine, hydroxylated by a liver microsome system, conjugated with sulfate in the liver, and excreted as the salt, indican.

The recognition of xanthurenic acid as an excretory product of ab-

21

normal tryptophan metabolism was the result of feeding tryptophan to vitamin B_6-deficient rats (Lepkovsky *et al.*, 1943). This became a classical indicator of vitamin B_6 deficiency. It is the controversy regarding the validity of this indicator for human studies that will be a major concern here. Because species vary so much with regard to the quantities of urinary excretory products, this discussion will be confined largely to excretion patterns in human subjects.

Figure 2-1 shows the complex interplay between the metabolism of

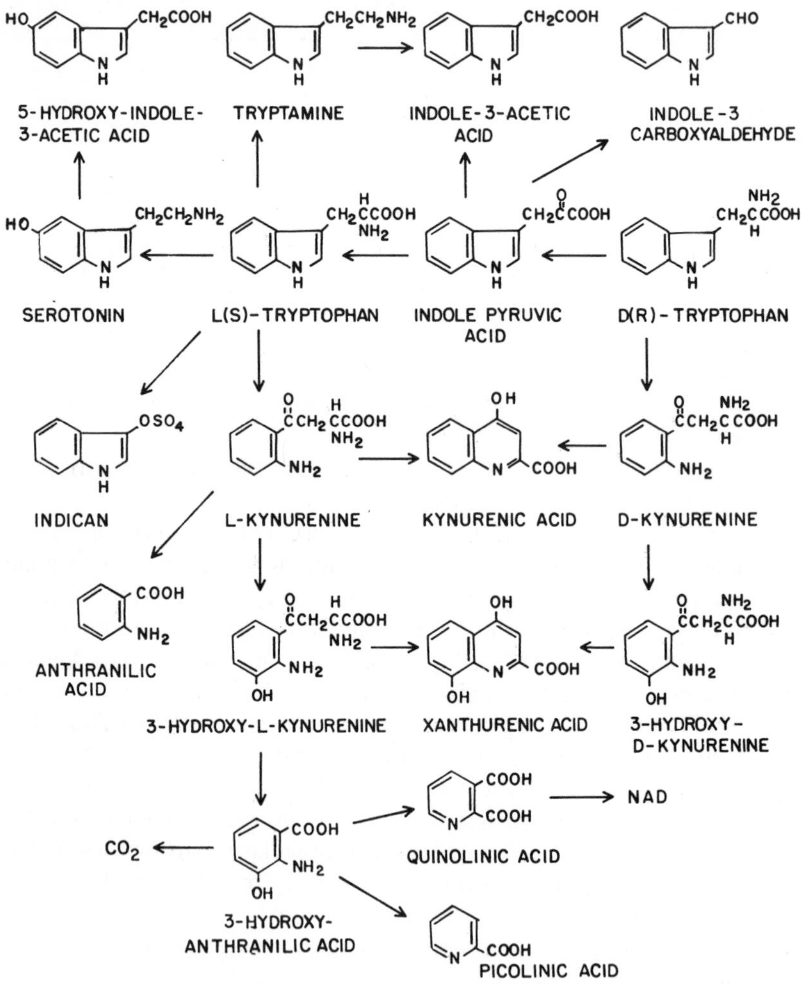

FIGURE 2-1   The metabolic fate of D- and L-tryptophan in mammals.

D- and L-tryptophan (Triebwasser *et al.*, 1976). In addition to the interconversion of the enantiomers, both form their corresponding stereoisomer of kynurenine, the D-isomer by the action of indoleamine-2,3-dioxygenase of intestine and liver as described in the rabbit (Hirata and Hayaishi, 1972) and the rat (Rodden and Berg, 1974). The D-kynurenine so formed is converted to 3-hydroxy-D-kynurenine. Action of D-amino acid oxidase on these two unusual D-amino acids leads to the same kynurenic acid and xanthurenic acid as are formed from L-tryptophan metabolites by transamination. This added complication (i.e., excretion of D-kynurenine and hydroxy-D-kynurenine) underlines the wisdom of using only L-tryptophan for metabolic studies, especially when dealing with a species such as the human, in which the utilization of the D-isomer is poor and a large part of a test dose is excreted in the urine chiefly as D-tryptophan, D-kynurenine, and D-hydroxy-kynurenine (Hankes *et al.*, 1972).

Let us now focus on the kynurenine pathway for L-tryptophan, where dietary and hormonal perturbations have been studied. The involvement of vitamin B₆ in the major pathway to pyridine nucleotides and CO_2 occurs where kynureninase catalyzes the removal of alanine from hydroxykynurenine forming 3-hydroxyanthranilate. That vitamin B₆ is involved in later reactions leading to pyridine nucleotides and CO_2 in man has not been clearly established, but in vitamin B₆ deficiency, increased excretion of hydroxyanthranilate (Price *et al.*, 1972), even without a tryptophan load, and of quinolinate after tryptophan loading (Brown *et al.*, 1965) have been reported. The much investigated indirect effect of vitamin B₆ deficiency on the kynurenine pathway results from requirement for pyridoxal phosphate for the transaminase, which forms the α-keto acids corresponding to kynurenine and 3-hydroxykynurenine, which in turn undergo Schiff's base cyclization to yield the end products, kynurenate and xanthurenate. A somewhat less confounding issue is the action of kynureninase on kynurenine, a substrate which competes with the regular substrate, hydroxy-kynurenine, to give a minor metabolite, anthranilate. The continued attention to the involvement of vitamin B₆ in tryptophan metabolism has resulted from the fact that the pattern of urinary products has been so readily influenced not only by a mild deficiency of vitamin B₆ but also by hormonal changes that result from pregnancy and exposure to the estrogens in oral contraceptives. These observations suggested either that functional deficiency was resulting from estrogens or that estrogens and their metabolic products were exerting a specific effect on kynureninase, which was reversed by vitamin B₆ in amounts in excess of those generally considered adequate by other criteria (Price *et al.*, 1967). The failure of other functions requiring vitamin B_6 to be affected by the hormonal stimuli raises the question of whether the altered tryptophan metabolite excretion pattern is of pathological significance (Leklem *et al.*, 1975a; Lumeng *et al.*, 1974).

The design and interpretation of experiments dealing with hormonal effects on tryptophan metabolism has been influenced by the well-documented effect of steroids on the initial enzyme of this pathway, i.e., tryptophan 2,3-dioxygenase. Much effort has been expended in attempts to show that elevation of the activity of this enzyme is responsible for the increased excretion of kynurenine and the products it forms when it accumulates. Milholland and Rosen (1971) examined this question in rats, where the vitamin B_6 deficiency was hastened and accentuated by feeding deoxypyridoxine. The lack of correlation between the dioxygenase of the liver and the xanthurenate excretion following a tryptophan load was very pronounced. Cortisol induced the enzyme but had no effect on xanthurenate excretion either with or without a tryptophan load. Tryptophan elevated the xanthurenate excretion almost as well in the untreated as in the cortisol-treated rats. These observations support the conclusions of Kim and Miller (1969) that the increase in metabolic products of the oxygenase is due to elevated substrate levels and not to increase in enzyme activity as observed *in vitro*. Other data suggest that the elevation of the level of the initial enzyme in tryptophan degradation by hormones is not responsible for the increased excretion of metabolites caused by hormones. With this in mind let us look at the pattern of excretory products observed in humans as affected by vitamin B_6 deficiency, pregnancy, and oral contraceptives to see if a cause and effect relationship exists.

We have chosen to present the summary data assembled by Wolf (1974) representing the results of his experiments as well as those from many other laboratories. Figure 2-2 shows the excretion of indican and the kynurenine and niacin metabolites expressed as μM per 24 h before and after a 2-g load of L-tryptophan. The metabolites shown are two conjugates of anthranilic acid, its glucuronide and its glycine conjugate, 2-amino hippurate, plus the kynurenine metabolites, arranged so that the abscissa labels represent the metabolic pathway and the ordinate the 24-h excretion, a style of presentation popularized by the Wisconsin group. Note that the units on the ordinates change, but otherwise the ensuing figures are the same to facilitate comparison. The 2-g tryptophan load has relatively little effect on the excretion of metabolites in the normal subject. Figure 2-3 shows a very similar pattern for experiments, where during both preloading and loading periods, large doses

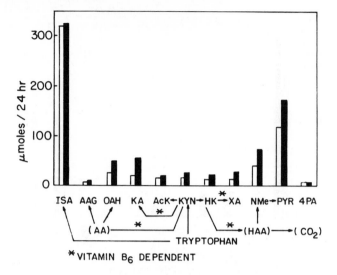

FIGURE 2-2 Average urinary excretion of indican, kynurenine pathway metabolites, and 4-pyridoxic acid with (■) and without (□) a loading dose of 2-g L-tryptophan by normal male subjects. The following abbreviations are used: ISA, indoxyl sulfate; AAG, anthranilic acid glucuronide; OAH, o-aminohippuric acid; KA, kynurenic acid; ACK, acetyl kynurenine; KYN, kynurenine; HK, 3-hydroxykynurenine; XA, xanthurenic acid; NMe, N-methylnicotinamide; PYR, N-methyl-2-pyridone-5-carboxamide; 4-PA, 4-pyridoxic acid; AA, anthranilic acid (not measured); HAA, 3-hydroxyanthranilic acid (not measured). Adapted from Wolf (1974).

of vitamin B₆ were given. Aside from the expected increase in 4-pyridoxic acid, resulting from the vitamin B₆ supplement, no changes were seen in excretion pattern as compared to Figure 2-2.

Figure 2-4 shows the effect of 5–7 weeks of vitamin B₆ depletion followed by 2 days of supplementation with 100 mg/day of vitamin B₆. Indican was not measured in this experiment. The striking elevations of kynurenine, acetylkynurenine, hydroxykynurenine, and xanthurenic acid and the return to normal when vitamin B₆ is given clearly isolate the biochemical lesion at hydroxykynureninase. In Figure 2-5 are shown the effects of pregnancy on the excretion of metabolic products compared to normal nonpregnant women and to the excretion observed after giving 6 mg/day of vitamin B₆ for 11 days. This dosage, well above the requirement, was not sufficient to reduce the values to those of the control subjects. The key metabolites remained at about twice the normal values.

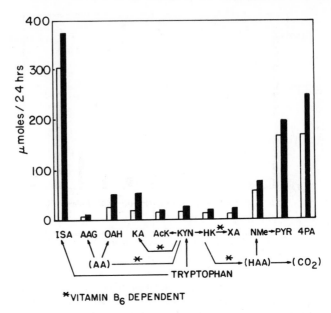

FIGURE 2-3 Average urinary excretion of indican, kynurenine pathway metabolites, and 4-pyridoxic acid during vitamin B_6 supplementation (100 mg/day of pyridoxine ·HCl for 2 days) with (■) and without (□) a loading dose of 2-g L-tryptophan by 15 normal male subjects. Adapted from Wolf (1974).

Figure 2-6 presents a comparison of the excretory patterns of control subjects with those of oral contraceptive users both before and after they received massive doses of vitamin B_6 (100 mg/day for 2 days). Obviously vitamin B_6 corrected the altered pattern completely. The disproportionate elevation of xanthurenate compared to kynurenine and hydroxykynurenine is the result of unusually high xanthurenate excretion.

Figure 2-7 illustrates the effect of estrogens (5 mg of diethyl stilbesterol or 12 mg of chlorotrianisene) on the excretion by male subjects. Again xanthurenate was especially high with kynurenine and hydroxykynurenine severalfold increased, kynurenate elevated twofold, and acetylkynurenine fourfold. Supplemental vitamin B_6 (100 mg/day for 2 days) restored all except the niacin metabolites to pretreatment levels. The effect of estrogens and vitamin B_6 on male excretion patterns are summarized in Figure 2-8. For convenience of comparison, controls, controls plus vitamin B_6 subjects, and estrogen-treated plus

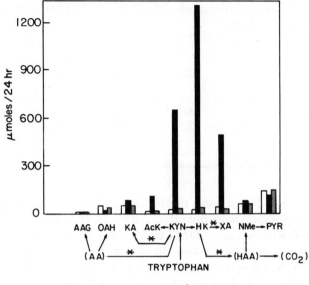

FIGURE 2-4 Average urinary excretion of kynurenine pathway metabolites following a 2-g L-tryptophan load by six male subjects before vitamin B₆ depletion (□), after 32–45 days of vitamin B₆ depletion (■), and after vitamin B₆ supplementation (▨) of 100 mg/day of pyridoxine ·HCl for 2 days. Adapted from Yess *et al.* (1964) and Brown *et al.* (1965).

vitamin B₆ subjects are shown in one bar graph. It is evident that vitamin B₆ had no effect on normal males and that it lowered excretion values to normal in estrogen-treated males.

Finally the mean values for all three groups in Figure 2-8 are compared to vitamin B₆-depleted and estrogen-treated males in Figure 2-9. Vitamin B₆-depleted subjects excreted massive amounts (>13 percent) of the tryptophan as hydroxykynurenine plus the usual high levels of kynurenine and xanthurenate. This unusual elevation of hydroxykynurenine in the vitamin B₆-depleted males compared to the estrogen-treated males and females is interesting and may reflect a block in the transamination of hydroxykynurenine to form xanthurenate.

Tables 2-1 and 2-2 illustrate the distribution of a 2-g load of tryptophan in the urinary products (as shown in Figure 2-9). The values are corrected for control subjects who received no tryptophan load (from

TABLE 2-1   Disposition of a Loading Dose of 2 g of L-Tryptophan in Male Subjects,[a] $\mu M/24$ h

Subjects	ISA	AAG	OAH	KA	ACK	K	HK	XA	NMe	PYR
Nonloaded controls	318	7	27	18	15	15	13	12	41	113
Controls	349	12	43	47	19	29	26	30	67	196
B₆-depleted		5	31	68	110	643	1294	484	76	109
Estrogen-treated	289	14	32	93	79	247	486	557	43	138

[a]Abbreviations used are those identified in Figure 2-2.

Figure 2-2). It will be evident that indican, anthranilate conjugates, and pyridinium products were not increased by the tryptophan load. On the other hand, intermediates of the kynurenine pathway accounted for 0.7 percent of the load in control subjects compared to values of 26.2 percent for the vitamin B_6-depleted and 14.7 percent for the estrogen-treated males. The data on excretion patterns suggest that vitamin B_6-depleted or estrogen-treated subjects would produce substantially less CO_2 from tryptophan. There appear to be no data on the effect of vitamin B_6 depletion on the degradation of tryptophan to CO_2.

The accumulation of compounds derived from tryptophan in a vitamin B_6 deficiency and their ultimate appearance in the urine is most simply explained by the assumption that kynureninase is the enzyme most impaired by this deficiency. The explanation for the leakage past the pyridoxal phosphate-dependent aminotransferase that forms xanthurenate has never been obvious. The matter is complicated by the fact that kynurenine arises in the cytosol while hydroxykynurenine is formed in the mitochondria (Figure 2-10). The latter must be transported back to the cytosol for hydrolytic cleavage by the key enzyme. The aminotransferases have recently been studied intensively by Kido

TABLE 2-2   Response to a 2-g Load of Tryptophan in Male Subjects,[a] %

Subjects	ISA	AAG	OAH	KA	ACK	K	HK	XA	NMe	PYR	Total Kynurenine Products
Control	0	0	0	0.3	0	0.1	0.1	0.2	0.3	0.9	0.7
−B₆	—	0	0	0.7	1.0	6.4	13.1	5.0	0.4	0	26.2
+Estrogen	0	0	0	0.8	0.7	2.5	5.0	5.7	0	0.2	14.7

[a]Abbreviations used are those identified in Figure 2-2.

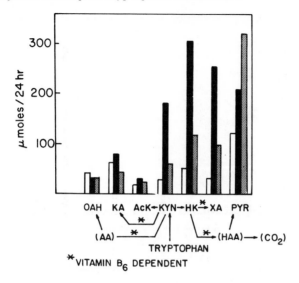

FIGURE 2-5 Average urinary excretion of kynurenine pathway metabolites after a 2-g L-tryptophan loading dose by 14 pregnant women before (■) and after (▨) vitamin B₆ supplementation (6 mg/day of pyridoxine •HCl for 11 days) and by 10 nonpregnant normal women (□). Adapted from Brown *et al.* (1961). *The pyridone value is elevated because of 15 mg of niacinamide present in the multivitamin supplement ingested.

and associates (Nakatani *et al.*, 1974; Noguchi *et al.*, 1975a; Noguchi *et al.*, 1975b). They have presented evidence that two distinct aminotransferases are found in liver, brain, intestine, and kidney, the usual α-ketoglutarate-coupled enzyme and a pyruvate aminotransferase. These are in addition to the usual nonspecific aminotransferases, some of which act on kynurenine. The kidney and liver contain both enzymes in both the supernatant and the mitochondrial fractions (Figure 2-10). In the liver the K_m values for kynurenine are about the same for the pyruvate and α-ketoglutarate enzymes from both fractions. In the kidney the K_m for the pyruvate enzyme is about 15 times lower both in the supernatant and the mitochondria. However, the enzymes present in the two fractions of a given organ appear to be identical, with 50–80 percent of the activity in the supernatant fraction. The pyruvate enzyme has a pH optimum of 8.0-8.5, while that of the α-ketoglutarate enzyme has a pH of 6-6.5.

The distribution of the enzymes of tryptophan degradation in the

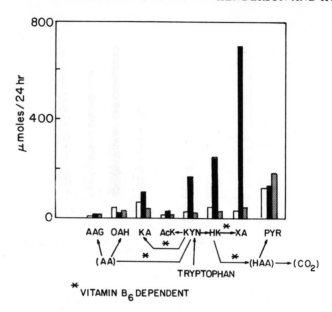

FIGURE 2-6   Average urinary excretion of kynurenine pathway metabolites after a loading dose of 2-g L-tryptophan by normal female subjects treated with an oral contraceptive (Enovid-E[R]) before (■) and after (▨) vitamin B_6 supplementation (100 mg/day of pyridoxine •HCl for 2 days) and excretion by young females not receiving oral contraceptives (□). Adapted from Price et al. (1967).

liver cell suggests that the kynurenine formed in the cytosol has one of three possible fates (Figure 2-10). In normal animals most of it would pass into the mitochondria. In the case of kynurenine accumulation in the cytosol, as occurs in vitamin B_6 deficiency, the lower K_m and higher V_{max} of kynureninase compared to kynurenine aminotransferase should favor formation of anthranilate over kynurenate. The fact that neither is excreted in large amounts by vitamin B_6 deficient humans in response to a tryptophan load suggests that kynureninase and possibly kynurenine aminotransferase are impaired by low pyridoxal phosphate concentrations. Thus, most of the kynurenine formed enters the mitochondria.

Since kynureninase is not present in the mitochondria there are two possible fates for the kynurenine which enters, hydroxylation or transamination. The K_m for the hydroxylase (0.023 mM) is much lower than that for kynurenine-α-ketoglutarate aminotransferase (2.2mM) and kynurenine-pyruvate aminotransferase (2.5 mM), so the kynurenine is

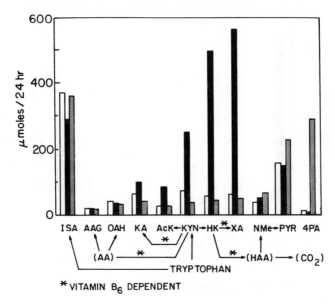

FIGURE 2-7 Average urinary excretion of indican, kynurenine pathway metabolites, and 4-pyridoxic acid after a loading dose of 2-g L-tryptophan before (■) and during (▨) supplementation with pyridoxine ·HCl (100 mg/day for 2 days) by male subjects treated with an estrogen (5 mg of diethylstilbestrol or 12 mg of chloro-trianisene) for 19–56 weeks and by male control subjects (□). Adapted from Wolf (1974).

rapidly hydroxylated. The hydroxykynurenine so formed can be trans-aminated in the mitochondria or diffuse into the cytosol. In the cytosol, two fates are possible, transamination yielding xanthurenate or hy-drolysis via kynureninase to 3-hydroxyanthranilate. In vitamin B₆ defi-ciency these avenues are blocked as they were for kynurenine, since the same supernatant enzymes act on both substrates. Therefore, since xanthurenate is elevated much more than kynurenate in this defi-ciency, it must be arising by transamination where kynurenine is not accumulating, i.e., in the mitochondria. If the mitochondrial kynurenine aminotransferase can be kept saturated with pyridoxal phosphate, it might transaminate hydroxykynurenine in spite of its low affinity for this substrate.

The comparisons of the affinity of involved enzymes for pyridoxal phosphate, then, must include kynurenine aminotransferases of the mitochondria and kynureninase of the cytosol. The lack of pyridoxal

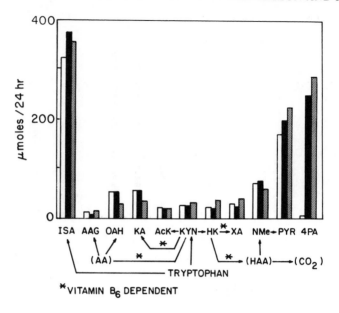

FIGURE 2-8   Average urinary excretion of indican, kynurenine pathway metabolites, and 4-pyridoxic acid after a loading dose of 2-g L-tryptophan by normal male subjects with (■) and without (□) pyridoxine ·HCl (100 mg/day for 2 days) supplementation and normal males ingesting estrogen (5 mg diethylstilbestrol or 12 mg chlorotrianisene) for 19–56 weeks, supplemented with pyridoxine · HCl (100 mg/day for 2 days) (▨). Adapted from Wolf (1974).

phosphate binding by the latter erects the barrier which results in the accumulation of all kynurenine products observed, while the failure of vitamin B_6 deficiency to keep xanthurenate low reflects the tight binding of pyridoxal phosphate by kynurenine aminotransferase in the mitochondria. Few experiments in this area have been done. Ogasawara et al. (1962) reported binding constants for pyridoxal phosphate for partially purified kynureninase and kynurenine aminotransferase from rat liver of 8.8×10^{-7} and 7.0×10^{-6}, respectively. Ueno et al. (1963) reported a K_m for PLP with the aminotransferase of 1.4×10^{-6} and Musajo et al. (1974) reported 8.5×10^{-7}. Thus, tighter binding by the kynurenine aminotransferase is not the explanation for the retention of its activity in the face of the loss of kynureninase. One must invoke some type of protection of mitochondrial kynurenine aminotransferase from the loss of pyridoxal phosphate. While the mitochondrial and cytosol aminotransferases (both pyruvate and α-ketoglutarate

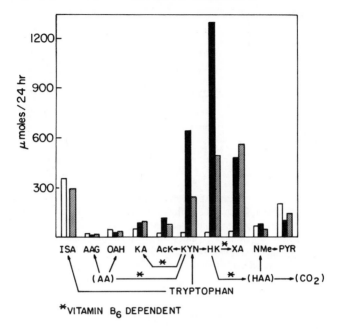

FIGURE 2-9   Average urinary excretion of indican and kynurenine pathway metabolites following a 2-g L-tryptophan load by control males (□), vitamin B₆-depleted males (■), and estrogen-treated males (▨). [The control consists of an average of values for normal males and males with pyridoxine ·HCl (100 mg/day for 2 days) both with and without estrogen treatment (2 mg diethylstilbestrol or 12 mg chlorotrianisene).] Adapted from Brown *et al.* (1965), Yess *et al.* (1964), and Wolf (1974).

coupled) are seemingly identical, this apparent anomaly could be explained if a mitochondrial enzyme had a high affinity for pyridoxal phosphate. There is a precedent for this, in reverse, in the affinity of glutamate-oxalacetate aminotransferase for pyridoxal phosphate as observed by Wada and Morino (1964). In this case the supernatant enzyme had a 600-fold higher affinity than the mitochondrial enzyme.

Another explanation is the possible greater retention of pyridoxal phosphate in the mitochondria during depletion. Ogasawara *et al.* (1962) reported such selective retention as reflected in the minor loss of aminotransferase of the mitochondria compared to 85 percent loss in the supernatant. Leklem *et al.* (1975b) reported that in subjects receiving oral contraceptives and low vitamin B₆ diets the excretion of hydroxykynurenine was very elevated, suggesting that even the

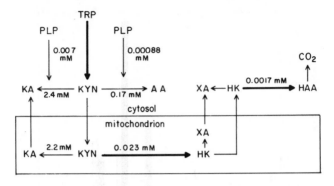

FIGURE 2-10 Subcellular distribution and kinetic constants for the tryptophan-kynurenine pathway in liver. K_m values for the substrate of the reaction in the direction written appear above or below the arrow. Apparent K_m values for pyridoxal phosphate (PLP) are shown beneath the PLP for the corresponding enzymes. K_m values for pyruvate and α-ketoglutarate = 0.3 mM.

mitochondrial kynurenine aminotransferase was stripped of its pyridoxal phosphate in the presence of estrogens.

There appears to be rather general agreement (Lumeng *et al.*, 1974; Leklem *et al.*, 1975b) that pregnancy and oral contraceptive use do not produce a vitamin B_6 deficiency of any practical consequence, even though the altered tryptophan metabolism observed under these conditions is corrected by additional vitamin B_6. The effect of steroid hormones on tryptophan metabolism as affected by vitamin B_6 nutriture has been the subject of extensive investigations. This subject has been reviewed by Mason and Manning (1971) and is discussed elsewhere in this publication (see Chapter 11).

LITERATURE CITED

Brown, R. R., M. J. Thornton, and J. M. Price. 1961. The effect of vitamin supplementation on the urinary excretion of tryptophan metabolites by pregnant women. J. Clin. Invest. *40*:617–623.

Brown, R. R., N. Yess, J. M. Price, H. M. Linkswiler, P. B. Swan, and L. V. Hankes. 1965. Vitamin B_6 depletion in man: Urinary excretion of quinolinic acid and niacin metabolites. J. Nutr. *87*:419–423.

Hankes, L. V., R. R. Brown, J. E. Leklem, M. Schmaeler, and J. Jesseph. 1972. Metabolism of C^{14} enantiomers of tryptophan, kynurenine and hydroxykynurenine in humans with scleroderma. J. Invest. Dermatol. *58*:85–95.

Hirata, F., and O. Hayaishi. 1972. The degradation of 5-hydroxytryptophan and serotonin by intestinal tryptophan 2,3-dioxygenase. Biochem. Biophys. Res. Commun. *47*:1112–1119.

Kim, J. H., and L. L. Miller. 1969. The functional significance of changes in activity of the enzymes, tryptophan pyrrolase and tyrosine transaminase, after induction in intact rats and in the isolated, perfused rat liver. J. Biol. Chem. *244*:1410–1416.

Langner, R. R., and C. P. Berg. 1955. Metabolism of D-tryptophan in the normal human subject. J. Biol. Chem. *214*:699–707.

Leklem, J. E., R. R. Brown, D. P. Rose, and H. M. Linkswiler. 1975a. Vitamin B₆ requirements of women using oral contraceptives. Amer. J. Clin. Nutr. *28*:535–541.

Leklem, J. E., R. R. Brown, D. P. Rose, H. M. Linkswiler, and R. A. Arend. 1975b. Metabolism of tryptophan and niacin in oral contraceptive users receiving controlled intakes of vitamin B₆. Amer. J. Clin. Nutr. *28*:146–156.

Lepkovsky, S., E. Roboz, and A. J. Haagen-Smit. 1943. Vitamin B₆ and its role in the tryptophane metabolism of pyridoxine deficient rats. J. Biol. Chem. *149*:195–201.

Loh, H., and C. P. Berg. 1971. Inversion in the metabolism of D-tryptophan in the rabbit and the rat. J. Nutr. *101*:1351–1358.

Lumeng, L., R. E. Cleary, and T.-K. Li. 1974. Effect of oral contraceptives on the plasma concentration of pyridoxal phosphate. Amer. J. Clin. Nutr. *27*:326–333.

Mason, M., and B. Manning. 1971. Effects of steroid conjugates on availability of pyridoxal phosphate for kynureninase and kynurenine aminotransferase activity. Amer. J. Clin. Nutr. *24*:786–791.

Milholland, R., and F. Rosen. 1971. The role of tryptophan pyrrolase adaptation in the excretions of xanthurenic acid by rats deficient in vitamin B₆. Amer. J. Clin. Nutr. *24*:740–747.

Musajo, L., G. Allegri, A. DeAnton, and C. Costa. 1974. Unpublished data from International Study Group for Tryptophan Research, Padova, Italy.

Nakatani, M., M. Morimoto, T. Noguchi, and R. Kido. 1974. Subcellular distribution and properties of kynurenine transaminase in rat liver. Biochem. J. *143*:303–310.

Noguchi, T., Y. Minatogawa, E. Okuno, M. Nakatani, M. Morimoto, and R. Kido. 1975a. Purification and characterization of kynurenine-2-oxogluterate aminotransferase from the liver, brain and small intestine of rats. Biochem. J. *151*:399–406.

Noguchi, T., M. Nakatani, Y. Minatogawa, M. Morimoto, and R. Kido. 1975b. Subcellular distribution and properties of kynurenine pyruvate transaminase in rat kidney. Z. Physiol. Chem. *356*:1245–1250.

Ogasawara, N., Y. Hagino, and Y. Kotake. 1962. Kynurenine transaminase, kynureninase and the increase of xanthurenic acid excretion. J. Biochem. (Tokyo) *52*:162–166.

Price, J. M., M. J. Thornton, and L. M. Mueller. 1967. Tryptophan metabolism in women using steroid hormones for ovulation control. Amer. J. Clin. Nutr. *20*:452–456.

Price, S. A., D. P. Rose, and P. H. Toseland. 1972. Effect of dietary vitamin B₆ deficiency and oral contraceptives on the spontaneous urinary excretion of 3-hydroxyanthranilic acid. Amer. J. Clin. Nutr. *25*:494–498.

Rodden, F. A., and C. P. Berg. 1974. Enzymatic conversion of L- and D-tryptophan to kynurenine by rat liver. J. Nutr. *104*:227–238.

Triebwasser, K. C., P. B. Swan, L. M. Henderson, and J. A. Budny. 1976. Metabolism of D- and L-tryptophan in dogs. J. Nutr. *106*:642–652.

Ueno, Y., K. Hayaishi, and R. Shukuya. 1963. Kynurenine transaminase from horse kidney. J. Biochem. (Tokyo) 54:75–80.

Wada, H., and Y. Morino. 1964. Comparative studies on glutamic-oxalacetic trans aminases from the mitochondrial and soluble fractions of mammalian tissues. Vitam. Horm. 22:411.

Wolf, H. 1974. Tryptophan metabolism in man. Effect of hormones and vitamin B_6 on urinary excretion of metabolites of the kynurenine pathway. Scand. J. Clin. Lab. Invest. 33, Suppl. 136, 186 pp.

Yess, N., J. M. Price, R. R. Brown, P. B. Swan, and H. Linkswiler. 1964. Vitamin B_6 depletion in man: urinary excretion of tryptophan metabolites. J. Nutr. 84:229–236.

3

Vitamin B$_6$ and the Metabolism of Sulfur Amino Acids

JOHN A. STURMAN

INTRODUCTION

The metabolism of sulfur-containing amino acids is dependent upon the presence of vitamin B$_6$. The pathway of methionine metabolism is illustrated in Figure 3-1. Methionine is first activated in the presence of ATP by methionine adenosyltransferase to s-adenosylmethionine. This compound is the major methyl group donor of the body; it is converted to s-adenosylhomocysteine by various methyltransferases and subsequently to homocysteine by s-adenosylhomocysteine hydrolase. The sulfur atom is then transferred from the three-carbon skeleton of homocysteine to the two-carbon skeleton of serine by the following reaction sequence: Serine is added to homocysteine by cystathionine synthase to form the sulfur-ether cystathionine. This is then cleaved on the other side of the sulfur atom to form cysteine. Cysteine is subsequently oxidized to inorganic sulfate, or to cysteinesulfinic acid, which is then decarboxylated to form taurine. An additional reaction of unknown quantitative significance is the decarboxylation of s-adenosylmethionine, followed by the addition of putrescine to form the polyamine, spermidine (Figure 3-2). Methionine and cysteine are also incorporated into proteins.

37

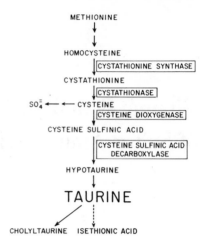

FIGURE 3-1 Pathway of methionine metabolism in mammals.

Vitamin B_6, in the form of pyridoxal 5'-phosphate, is involved as coenzyme with cystathionine synthase, cystathionase, cysteinesulfinic acid decarboxylase, and probably also s-adenosylmethionine decarboxylase.

Each of these enzymatic reactions is discussed in turn, along with its role in normal and abnormal human conditions where applicable.

CYSTATHIONINE SYNTHASE (EC 4.2.1.22)

In mammals, cystathionine is normally formed from serine and homocysteine, as shown in Figure 3-3. This reaction proceeds by the β-activation of serine and the addition of homocysteine. Cystathionine synthase is also capable of carrying out the β-activation of cysteine and synthesizing cystathionine in this fashion (Braunstein et al., 1969, 1971). It should be noted that the sulfur atom is derived from homocysteine in both reactions. The sulfur atom of cysteine can be incorporated into cystathionine, but this requires γ-activation of homocysteine, a reaction mediated by cystathionase, not cystathionine synthase. Cystathionine synthase obtained from human liver has somewhat different properties from that obtained from rat liver, but the enzyme from both sources has been demonstrated to require pyridoxal phosphate as coenzyme (Brown et al., 1966; Nakagawa and Kimura, 1968; Kashiwamata and Greenberg, 1970; Kashiwamata et al., 1970; Brown and Gordon, 1971; Kimura and Nakagawa, 1971; Porter et al., 1974;

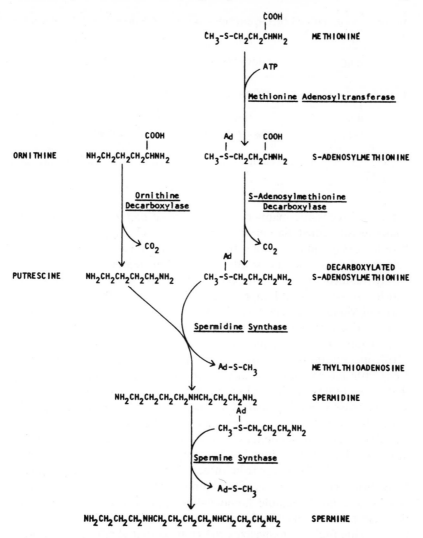

FIGURE 3-2 Pathway for biosynthesis of putrescine and the polyamines spermidine and spermine Ad = adenosyl (Sturman and Gaull, 1975).

Tudball and Reed, 1975; Packman *et al.,* 1976). The coenzyme appears to be tightly bound to the apoenzyme *in vivo,* for a nutritional deficiency of vitamin B$_6$ causes little or no reduction in holocystathionine synthase (Sturman *et al.,* 1969; Pan and Pai, 1970; Finkelstein and Chalmers, 1970; Kashiwamata, 1971).

In the human, cystathionine synthase deficiency is inherited in an

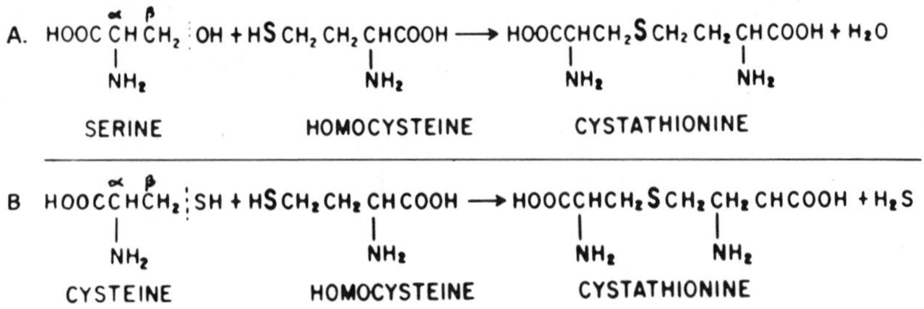

A. HOOC $\overset{\alpha}{C}H\overset{\beta}{C}H_2$ OH + HS CH$_2$ CH$_2$ CHCOOH $\longrightarrow$ HOOCCHCH$_2$S CH$_2$ CH$_2$ CHCOOH + H$_2$O

  | | | |

 NH$_2$ NH$_2$ NH$_2$ NH$_2$

 SERINE   HOMOCYSTEINE   CYSTATHIONINE

B HOOC$\overset{\alpha}{C}$H$\overset{\beta}{C}$H$_2$ SH + HS CH$_2$ CH$_2$ CH COOH $\longrightarrow$ HOOCCHCH$_2$S CH$_2$ CH$_2$ CHCOOH + H$_2$S

  | | | |

 NH$_2$ NH$_2$ NH$_2$ NH$_2$

 CYSTEINE   HOMOCYSTEINE   CYSTATHIONINE

FIGURE 3-3   Some reactions mediated by cystathionine synthase (β-activation) (Tallan et al., 1974).

autosomal recessive manner and is the most common etiology of the characteristic constellation of clinical signs and symptoms associated with the excretion of homocystine in the urine (Gaull et al., 1975). The activity of cystathionine synthase has been demonstrated to be severely reduced, or absent, in liver, in brain, in cultured skin fibroblasts, and in PHA-stimulated lymphocytes (Mudd et al., 1964, 1967; Uhlendorf and Mudd, 1968; Gaull et al., 1969; Goldstein et al., 1972; Fleisher et al., 1973; Uhlendorf et al., 1973). Other biochemical abnormalities include high concentrations of methionine and homocystine and low or zero concentrations of cystine in plasma and urine (Gaull et al., 1975). Very little information is available for organs, but it has been shown that in the brains of affected individuals, cystathionine is virtually absent (Gerritsen and Waisman, 1964; Brenton et al., 1965), whereas it is normally present in high concentrations in the human brain (Tallan et al., 1958). The consequences of this deficiency of cystathionine are unknown, but cystathionine has been implicated as a neurotransmitter (Gaull et al., 1975). Liver from affected individuals does have higher than normal concentrations of methionine but normal concentrations of cystine and no detectable homocystine; thus it does not mirror the biochemical abnormalities found in plasma and urine (Rassin et al., in press). This finding emphasizes the caution that should be exerted in extrapolating blood and urine data to body tissues. The clinical abnormalities may include dislocation of the optic lenses; a malar flush; fair, fine, rather sparse hair; progressive skeletal deformities, including long thin limbs, which are presumably responsible for a peculiar shuffling gait; variable degrees of mental retardation; and severe thromboembolic disease, one of the most devastating features of this condition, which is frequently the cause of death (Gaull et al., 1975).

In some patients, treatment with massive doses of vitamin B$_6$, in the form of pyridoxine hydrochloride, ameliorates the biochemical abnormalities in plasma, urine, and liver, but in other patients, vitamin B$_6$ has no effect on these abnormalities (Gaull *et al.*, 1975). Figure 3-4 illustrates the changes that occur in the plasma of a typical vitamin B$_6$-responsive patient upon the administration of vitamin B$_6$. It is not known if the concentration of cystathionine in the brains of such individuals is altered by vitamin B$_6$ therapy. The mechanism of action of vitamin B$_6$ in those affected individuals who respond to treatment has been the subject of study and speculation for many years. Much of the speculation invoked an abnormal apoenzyme that had a higher requirement of pyridoxal phosphate coenzyme. An increased specific activity of hepatic cystathionine synthase *in vivo* has been demonstrated after treatment with vitamin B$_6$ in some, but not all, responsive cases, but never in nonresponsive cases. Figure 3-5 illustrates such a change for two vitamin B$_6$-responsive siblings and the lack of change for two vitamin B$_6$-unresponsive siblings (Gaull *et al.*, 1974). In general, nonresponsive patients have lower activity of cystathionine synthase than responsive patients, frequently none being detectable.

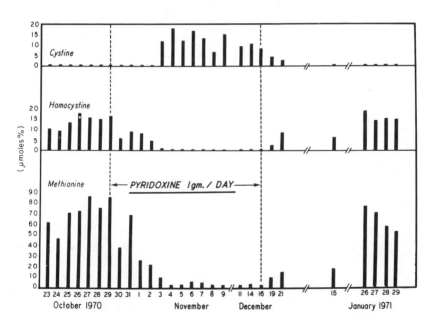

FIGURE 3-4   Effect of pyridoxine treatment on the concentrations of methionine, homocystine, and cystine in plasma of a vitamin B$_6$-responsive, cystathionine synthase-deficient individual.

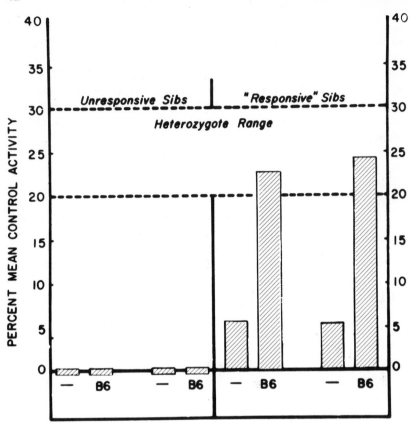

FIGURE 3-5   Response of hepatic cystathionine synthase activity to vitamin B_6 treatment.

There are exceptions, however. There have been some reports of increased activity in extracts of liver and cultured skin fibroblasts from synthase-deficient patients *in vitro* in the presence of high concentrations of pyridoxal phosphate (Gaull *et al.*, 1974; Seashore *et al.*, 1972; Kim and Rosenberg, 1974). There is evidence for a direct effect of pyridoxal phosphate on the enzyme cystathionine synthase in extracts of liver and of cultured skin fibroblasts. When extracts of normal human liver are preincubated at 55° before measuring the activity of cystathionine synthase (Figure 3-6), there is a more than doubling of activity after 3 minutes preincubation followed by a sharp decline in activity after longer preincubation (Longhi *et al.*, 1977). In the presence of 1.3 mM pyridoxal phosphate, the thermal activation of the

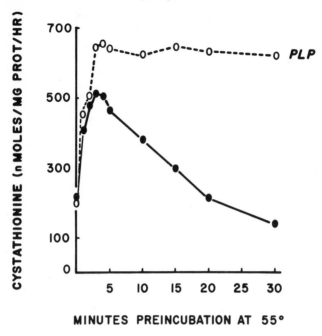

FIGURE 3-6   Effect of preincubation at 55° on specific activity of cystathionine synthase in an extract of normal human liver (Longhi *et al.*, 1977).

enzyme at 3 minutes is followed by no loss of activity during 30 minutes preincubation. Protection against thermal inactivation by pyridoxal phosphate had previously been demonstrated (Mudd *et al.*, 1970). Thus pyridoxal phosphate apparently exerts a direct protective effect against thermal inactivation of normal human cystathionine synthase.

Similar experiments with extracts of liver from vitamin B_6-responsive homocystinuric patients showed some significant differences (Table 3-1). Prior to treatment with vitamin B_6, there was no heat activation of cystathionine synthase, in contrast to the enzyme in normal human liver. After vitamin B_6 therapy, the cystathionine synthase in extracts of liver from the same patients did show thermal activation. Pyridoxal phosphate afforded protection against thermal inactivation both before and after vitamin B_6 therapy (Longhi *et al.*, 1977; Mudd *et al.*, 1970). Irrespective of the mechanism of activation, the demonstration of a qualitative difference, in the response to heat, of cystathionine synthase from homocystinuric patients, which is corrected by vitamin B_6 therapy, is evidence that the vitamin has a direct

TABLE 3-1   Heat-Induced Activation and Inactivation of Human
Hepatic Cystathionine Synthase from Normal and Synthase-Deficient
Individuals

	Relative Specific Activity after Preincubation at 55° for Time (min) Indicated, % of zero-time value		
	0	3	10
Controls (5)	100	263 ± 42	179 ± 14
Synthase-deficient			
1	100	38	60
2	100	88	89
After B$_6$ therapy			
1	100	210	151
2	100	174	126

SOURCE: Longhi et al. (1977).

effect *in vivo* that is not simply the presence of more coenzyme. One
exciting possibility is that the presence of large amounts of vitamin B$_6$
allows responsive-synthase-deficient individuals to synthesize small
amounts of normal enzyme. Then one would postulate that this mechanism did not exist for nonresponsive-synthase-deficient individuals.
These possibilities cannot be properly explored with the tiny fragments
of liver available from occasional biopsies, but they are currently being
investigated in our laboratory with the use of cultured skin fibroblasts.
The heat activation phenomenon is present in normal lines (Figure 3-7),
but not in lines from synthase-deficient patients (Figure 3-8). Pyridoxal
phosphate did afford some protection against thermal inactivation of
extracts of normal lines (Figure 3-7) and some synthase-deficient lines
(Figure 3-8a) but actually enhanced thermal inactivation of extracts of
one synthase-deficient line (Figure 3-8b). This may be a further indication of genetic heterogeneity in this disease. The *in situ* effect of vitamin B$_6$ has not yet been investigated.

An intriguing question of great theoretical genetic interest and of
potential practical importance if enzyme replacement is considered is
whether the total lack of cystathionine synthase activity in extracts of
liver and cultured skin fibroblasts of some affected individuals is due to
the complete failure to synthesize any enzyme protein or is due to the
enzyme protein being so abnormal that it has no enzymatic capability.
One approach is to purify cystathionine synthase from normal tissue,
prepare antiserum against it in an animal such as the rabbit, and test
this against an extract from the affected individual by double im-

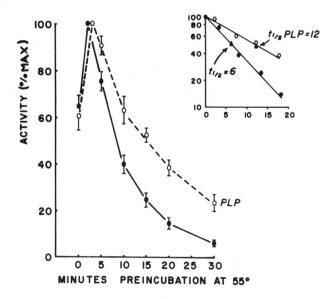

FIGURE 3-7 Effect of preincubation at 55° on specific activity of cystathionine synthase in extracts of cultured human skin fibroblasts from normal individuals.

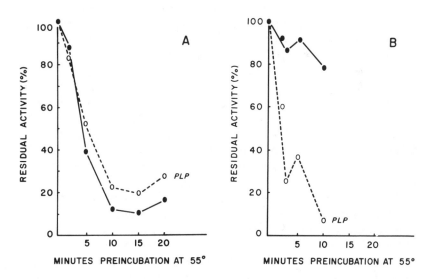

FIGURE 3-8 Effect of preincubation at 55° on specific activity of cystathionine synthase in extracts of cultured human skin fibroblasts from two vitamin B_6-responsive, cystathionine synthase-deficient individuals, illustrating different effects of pyridoxal phosphate.

munodiffusion. Cystathionine synthase from normal human liver has proved to be a very difficult enzyme to purify, and such preparations have only recently been reported (Tudball and Reed, 1975; Packman *et al.*, 1976). One group also reported preparation of antibody to the purified enzyme but did not test it against any extract from a cystathionine synthase-deficient individual (Tudball and Reed, 1975).

It should be noted here that cystathionine synthase activity is present in second-trimester fetal human liver and brain, although the activity is somewhat lower than is present in the adult tissues (Sturman *et al.*, 1970b; Gaull *et al.*, 1972). Thus, this disease is amenable to prenatal detection by culturing cells in amniotic fluid and measuring their cystathionine synthase activity. Such prenatal detection allows termination of the pregnancy if desired and also *in utero* treatment with vitamin B_6 if the fetus is affected with the responsive form, thus minimizing the time it would be exposed to the abnormal metabolic environment (Fleisher *et al.*, 1974).

CYSTATHIONASE (EC 4.4.1.1)

The normal function of cystathionase in mammals is the cleavage of cystathionine in the γ-position to form cysteine (Figure 3-9). It can also catalyze the synthesis of cystathionine from cysteine and homoserine (but not α-oxobutyrate) or homocysteine and the formation of homolanthionine (a symmetrical homologue of cystathionine) from homoserine and homocysteine. In addition, it mediates the degradation of homoserine to α-oxobutyrate and ammonia (homoserine dehydratase); of homocysteine to α-oxobutyrate, ammonia, and H_2S (homocysteine desulfhydrase); and of cysteine to pyruvate, ammonia, and H_2S (cysteine disulfurase) (Tallan *et al.*, 1974). The latter reaction involves activation at the β-carbon of the substrate, whereas all of the other activities involve activation of the γ-carbon. The active site involved in cysteine degradation appears to be different from that involved in the other reactions (Pascal *et al.*, 1972b).

Cystathionase obtained from human liver has somewhat different properties from that obtained from rat liver, although the enzyme from both sources requires pyridoxal phosphate as coenzyme (Pascal *et al.*, 1972b; Frimpter *et al.*, 1969; Tallan *et al.*, 1971). Pyridoxal phosphate does not appear to be very tightly bound to apocystathionase *in vivo*, for a nutritional deficiency of vitamin B_6 causes a dramatic reduction of holocystathionase, with all of the metabolic sequelae expected from such a block in the transsulfuration pathway (Sturman *et al.*, 1969; Pan and Pai, 1970).

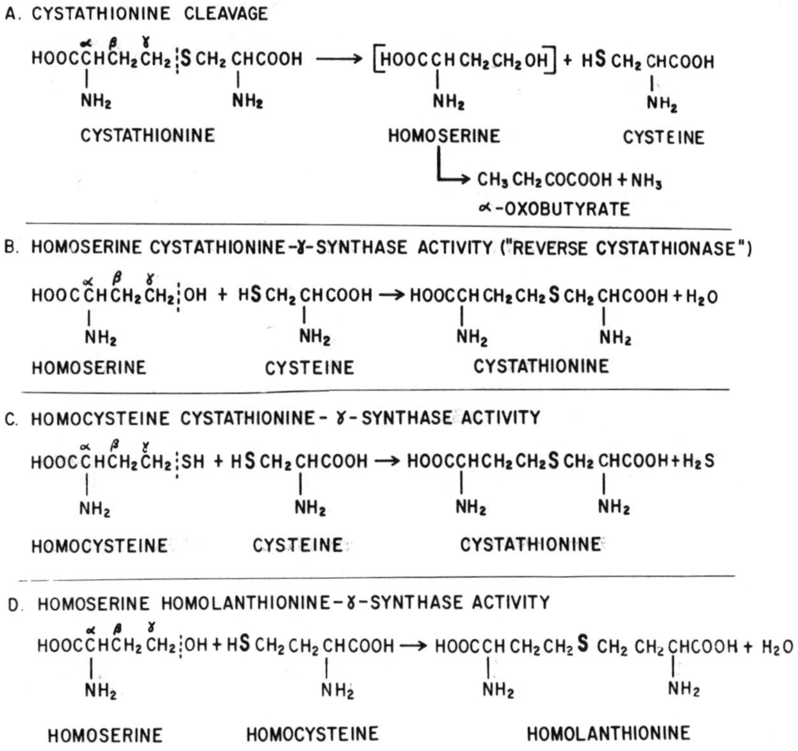

A. CYSTATHIONINE CLEAVAGE

$$\underset{\text{CYSTATHIONINE}}{\text{HOOCCHCH}_2\text{CH}_2\text{SCH}_2\text{CHCOOH}} \longrightarrow \left[\underset{\text{HOMOSERINE}}{\text{HOOCCHCH}_2\text{CH}_2\text{OH}}\right] + \underset{\text{CYSTEINE}}{\text{HSCH}_2\text{CHCOOH}}$$

(with $\overset{\alpha}{C}\overset{\beta}{H}\overset{\gamma}{CH}_2CH_2$ labels, and NH₂ groups)

$$\longrightarrow \underset{\alpha\text{-OXOBUTYRATE}}{\text{CH}_3\text{CH}_2\text{COCOOH} + \text{NH}_3}$$

B. HOMOSERINE CYSTATHIONINE-γ-SYNTHASE ACTIVITY ("REVERSE CYSTATHIONASE")

$$\underset{\text{HOMOSERINE}}{\text{HOOCCHCH}_2\text{CH}_2\text{OH}} + \underset{\text{CYSTEINE}}{\text{HSCH}_2\text{CHCOOH}} \rightarrow \underset{\text{CYSTATHIONINE}}{\text{HOOCCHCH}_2\text{CH}_2\text{SCH}_2\text{CHCOOH}} + \text{H}_2\text{O}$$

C. HOMOCYSTEINE CYSTATHIONINE- γ - SYNTHASE ACTIVITY

$$\underset{\text{HOMOCYSTEINE}}{\text{HOOCCHCH}_2\text{CH}_2\text{SH}} + \underset{\text{CYSTEINE}}{\text{HSCH}_2\text{CHCOOH}} \rightarrow \underset{\text{CYSTATHIONINE}}{\text{HOOCCHCH}_2\text{CH}_2\text{SCH}_2\text{CHCOOH}} + \text{H}_2\text{S}$$

D. HOMOSERINE HOMOLANTHIONINE-γ-SYNTHASE ACTIVITY

$$\underset{\text{HOMOSERINE}}{\text{HOOCCHCH}_2\text{CH}_2\text{OH}} + \underset{\text{HOMOCYSTEINE}}{\text{HSCH}_2\text{CH}_2\text{CHCOOH}} \rightarrow \underset{\text{HOMOLANTHIONINE}}{\text{HOOCCHCH}_2\text{CH}_2\text{SCH}_2\text{CH}_2\text{CHCOOH}} + \text{H}_2\text{O}$$

FIGURE 3-9 Some reactions mediated by cystathionase (γ-activation) (Tallan *et al.*, 1974).

In the human, primary cystathioninuria is the result of an inherited deficiency of cystathionase. The activity of cystathionase has been demonstrated to be deficient, or absent, in liver, in long-term lymphoid cell lines, and in cultured skin fibroblasts (Frimpter, 1965; Finkelstein *et al.*, 1966; Bittles and Carson, 1974; Pascal *et al.*, 1975). The other biochemical abnormalities associated with this defect include the excretion of large quantities of cystathionine in the urine, the presence of detectable cystathionine in plasma (although the renal threshold for this compound is zero) (Pascal *et al.*, 1975), and high concentrations of cystathionine in liver and kidney tissues, where it is normally barely detectable (Brenton *et al.*, 1965). It is possible that the concentration of cystathionine in the brains of affected individuals may be even higher than normal (Brenton *et al.*, 1965), but this is unclear at present because of the lack of available analyses coupled with the fact that the normal brain has a high concentration of cystathionine, possibly a result of the low activity of cystathionase in the normal brain.

Cystathionase deficiency is not reliably associated with a particular constellation of clinical signs and symptoms, and the prevalent view currently held by the investigators of the disease seems to be that it is a "nondisease" or "benign disease."

As found with cystathionine synthase deficiency, treatment with massive doses of vitamin B_6, in the form of pyridoxine hydrochloride, ameliorates or eliminates the cystathioninuria in a large proportion of the affected individuals. As for abnormal cystathionine synthase, the speculation about the mechanism of action of vitamin B_6 in responsive cases of primary cystathioninuria invoked an abnormal apoenzyme that had a higher requirement of pyridoxal phosphate coenzyme. There are reports of increased activity of cystathionase in extracts of liver and of long-term lymphoid cells of affected individuals *in vitro* in the presence of high concentrations of pyridoxal phosphate. (Frimpter, 1965; Pascal *et al.*, 1975). Figure 3-10 illustrates the results obtained for the effects of pyridoxal phosphate on the activity of cystathionase in extracts of long-term lymphoid cells from a normal individual, from a patient with vitamin B_6-responsive cystathioninuria, and from a patient with vitamin B_6-unresponsive cystathioninuria (Pascal *et al.*, 1975). There is no report to date of any direct effect of vitamin B_6 *in vivo* on cystathionase activity in affected individuals.

Cystathionase is virtually absent from second-trimester fetal human liver and brain as demonstrated by activity measurement, radiochemical perfusion studies, and immunochemical investigations (Sturman *et al.*, 1970b; Gaull *et al.*, 1972; Pascal *et al.*, 1972a). No activity could be demonstrated when the concentration of pyridoxal phosphate *in vitro* was greatly increased (Sturman *et al.*, 1970b; Gaull *et al.*, 1972). Measurements on a limited number of liver samples from fetal humans during the third-trimester, from preterm infants and from normal-term infants, suggest that significant cystathionase activity is present only after birth (Table 3-2). This finding suggests that prenatal detection of cystathionase deficiency may not be possible. However, because no ill effects can reliably be associated with a deficiency of cystathionase, the amniocentesis procedure is not justifiable for this purpose. It also raises the possibility that absence of cystathionase activity might be the result of failure to initiate synthesis of the enzyme protein. In this context, it is worth noting that cystathionase can be induced in fetal human liver explants by dexamethasone, glucagon, or dibutyryl cyclic AMP plus theophylline (Heinonen and Räihä, 1974). However, daily treatment of three mothers with 200 mg pyridoxine hydrochloride prior

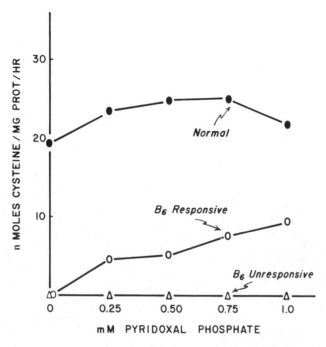

FIGURE 3-10 Effect of increasing concentrations of pyridoxal phosphate on cystathionase activity in extracts of lymphoid cell lines from a normal individual, one with vitamin B_6-responsive cystathioninuria and one with vitamin B_6-nonresponsive cystathioninuria (Pascal *et al.*, 1975).

TABLE 3-2 Activity of Cystathionase in Developing Human Liver

Gestation	Birth Weight, g	Age at Death, h	Cystathionase Activity, nM/mg protein/h
Adult (9)	—	—	126 ± 12
Fetus (24)	—	—	0
Premature	830	11	0
Premature	1000	8	0
Premature	1060	14	0
Premature	1260	3	0
Small-for-date	1500	96	49
Full term	3450	7	9
Full term	4250	72	85
Full term	2730	96	66

SOURCE: Gaull *et al.* (1972).

to abortion failed to elicit any activity of cystathionase in fetal liver or brain (Gaull *et al.*, 1972).

The elegant study illustrated in Figure 3-11 demonstrates that on double immunodiffusion using antiserum to purified human liver cystathionase, a single immunoprecipitin band of identity is present between the extract of normal human liver and that of the normal long-term lymphoid cell line (Pascal *et al.*, 1975). This band joined a precipitin band from the extract of long-term lymphoid cells from a vitamin B_6-responsive patient, indicating the presence of cross-reacting protein. No precipitin band formed, however, with the extract of long-

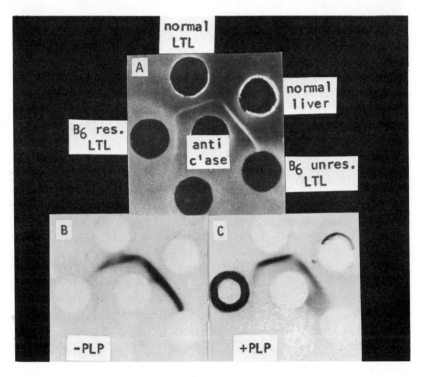

FIGURE 3-11   Agarose double-immunodiffusion plate after 24 h at 23°. Monospecific rabbit antiserum to human liver cystathionase was placed in the center well. Outer wells contained extracts from normal human liver, from normal lymphoid cell line, and from vitamin B_6-unresponsive cystathioninuric lymphoid cell line. (A) Unstained immune precipitate. (B) Same as (A) and stained for cystathionase activity. (C) Result obtained when 1 mM pyridoxal phosphate was added to all extracts before immunodiffusion and then plate was stained as in (B).

term lymphoid cells from a vitamin B_6-unresponsive patient. The gel was then washed to remove unreactive components, and the antigen-antibody complexes were tested for activity of cystathionase by use of a stain employing cystathionine as substrate and reduction of nitro blue tetrazolium. Enzymatic activity in the immune complexes formed with the extracts of normal liver and of normal long-term lymphoid cells was demonstrated, but no cystathionase activity was demonstrated with the extracts of either the vitamin B_6-responsive or the vitamin B_6-unresponsive long-term lymphoid cells. When 1 mM pyridoxal phosphate was added to the long-term lymphoid cell extracts before immunodiffusion, cystathionase activity was demonstrated in the antigen-antibody complex from the vitamin B_6-responsive cells but not from the vitamin B_6-unresponsive cells. These studies provide evidence of a direct effect of pyridoxal phosphate on the enzyme and of two forms of primary cystathioninuria that arise from different mutations. The vitamin B_6-responsive form results from the synthesis of an aberrant enzyme protein exhibiting altered interaction with the coenzyme, thereby resulting in an inherited increase in the requirement for vitamin B_6. The vitamin B_6-unresponsive form results from the complete absence of cystathionase or the synthesis of a protein so greatly altered that it has lost both catalytic activity and immunochemical identity.

CYSTEINESULFINIC ACID DECARBOXYLASE (EC 4.1.1.12)

This enzyme is responsible for the formation of taurine in mammals. It has been demonstrated that the enzyme in rat liver and in rat brain requires pyridoxal phosphate as coenzyme (Bergeret *et al.*, 1955; Hope, 1955; Davison, 1956; Sörbo and Heyman, 1957; Jacobsen *et al.*, 1964; Pasantes-Morales *et al.*, 1976). The pyridoxal phosphate coenzyme appears to be only loosely bound to the apoenzyme in the rat, for a nutritional deficiency of vitamin B_6 soon reduces the holocysteinesulfinic acid decarboxylase to zero, more rapidly in the liver than in the brain (Hope, 1955; Rassin and Sturman, 1975). A further difference is that in liver the apoenzyme is then reduced, eventually to zero, whereas there is no apparent reduction in the apoenzyme in brain.

There are no reports of purification or characterization of this enzyme from human tissue, but this is hardly surprising when one considers the extremely low activity present (Table 3-3). The activity in adult human brain is of the same order of magnitude as human liver, and that in second-trimester fetal human liver and brain is lower still (Gaull *et al.*, 1977). In view of these very low activities, it is doubtful whether

TABLE 3-3   Activity of Cysteinesulfinic Acid
Decarboxylase in Liver

Species	Activity, nM/mg protein/h
Rat	467
Cat	4.5
Human	0.3

SOURCE: Gaull *et al.* (in preparation) and Knopf *et al.* (in press).

cysteinesulfinic acid decarboxylase deficiency could have any meaning
in the human. Our present studies suggest that the human infant, and
probably the adult also, is dependent upon a dietary source of taurine.
Again this is not surprising, because the kitten and cat are clearly
dependent upon a dietary source of taurine, and activity of cysteinesulfinic acid decarboxylase in the organs of the cat is considerably greater
than in those of the human (Hayes *et al.*, 1975; Schmidt *et al.*, 1976;
Berson *et al.*, 1976; Knopf *et al.*, in press). There are some human
conditions in which a deficiency of taurine is implicated: It appears to
be decreased at epileptic foci, and anticonvulsant activity has been
demonstrated during clinical trials with taurine (Barbeau *et al.*, 1975);
an inherited disorder has been recently reported in which neuro-
psychiatric abnormalities occur in association with decreased concentrations of taurine in plasma, cerebrospinal fluid, and brain (Perry *et
al.*, 1975). No measurement of cysteinesulfinic acid decarboxylase activity has been made on tissue from such an individual, however. These
taurine deficiency disorders would appear to be more treatable with
taurine than with vitamin B_6.

S-ADENOSYLMETHIONINE DECARBOXYLASE (EC 4.1.1.50)

This enzyme catalyzes the first step in the synthesis of the polyamines
spermidine (Figure 3-2). Putrescine and the polyamines, spermidine and
spermime, have been implicated in the growth process (Herbst and
Bachrach, 1970; Russell, 1973a; Russell, 1973b; Bachrach, 1973; Raina
and Jänne, 1975) and, more recently, in central nervous system function (Russell *et al.*, 1974; Anderson *et al.*, 1975; Pateman and Shaw,
1975; Russell and Meier, 1975; Sturman and Gaull, 1975; Ingoglia *et al.*,
1976). The enzyme from a number of mammalian tissues, including
human prostate, appears to require pyridoxal phosphate as coenzyme
(Pegg and Williams-Ashman, 1969; Feldman *et al.*, 1972; Zappia *et al.*,
1972; Sturman and Kremzner, 1974). A nutritional deficiency of vita-

TABLE 3-4   Activity of s-Adenosylmethionine
Decarboxylase in Human Liver and Brain

Tissue	Activity, pM CO_2/mg protein/h
Liver	
Adult (5)	12.4 ± 2.0
Fetal (25)	233.8 ± 16.4
Brain	
Adult (6)	351.0 ± 61.2
Fetal (12)	169.4 ± 29.8

SOURCE: Sturman and Gaull (1975).

min B_6 causes a decrease in the holoenzyme in rat liver but no decrease in the apoenzyme (Sturman and Kremzner, 1974).

There are no reported abnormalities in humans involving s-adenosylmethionine decarboxylase, but very little information on this enzyme is available. Activity in normal adult liver is low, although in second-trimester fetal liver it is high (Table 3-4). Activity in both the developing and the mature brain is high. Presumably the high activities present in developing tissues are associated with the higher requirements of polyamines during development, and any deficiency of the enzyme would not be compatible with survival.

EFFECTS OF A NUTRITIONAL DEFICIENCY OF VITAMIN B_6 ON
SULFUR AMINO ACID METABOLISM

As mentioned previously in discussion of the individual enzymes that require pyridoxal phosphate as coenzyme, a nutritional deficiency of vitamin B_6 causes little or no reduction in cystathionine synthase holoenzyme, some reduction in s-adenosylmethionine decarboxylase holoenzyme, and a great reduction of both cystathionase holoenzyme and cysteinesulfinic acid decarboxylase holoenzyme. The metabolic consequences, in the rat, of these reductions are a decreased concentration of spermidine; an increased concentration of cystathionine, accompanied by cystathionine excretion in urine; and, somewhat surprisingly, no change in taurine concentration (Sturman and Rivlin, 1975). Although taurine biosynthesis virtually ceases under these circumstances, taurine is avidly conserved, and excretion of taurine also virtually ceases. The result is a decreased turnover of taurine rather than a decreased concentration (Figure 3-12). Addition of taurine to the diet tends to restore the turnover to normal, suggesting that it may make no

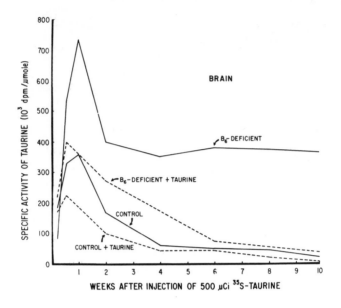

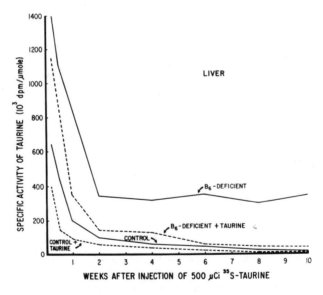

FIGURE 3-12 Specific activity of taurine in brain and liver from rats fed a vitamin B_6-deficient diet, a control diet, a vitamin B_6-deficient diet supplemented with taurine, and a control diet supplemented with taurine after intraperitoneal injection of [35]s-taurine. These results illustrate the reduced turnover of taurine in the vitamin B_6-deficient animals compared to control animals and the correction by taurine supplementation (Sturman and Rivlin, 1975).

difference whether taurine is biosynthesized or provided in the diet (Sturman, 1973). The reason for such avid conservation of taurine is not known. Although it has been implicated as a neurotransmitter or neuromodulater in the central nervous system, it is involved in muscle function, especially in the heart, and it is involved in the structural integrity of the retina, at least.

Methionine and cysteine are both important constituents of proteins, cysteine being especially important because it forms disulfide bridges that maintain the configuration of proteins. Vitamin B_6 deficiency causes little or no change in the incorporation of these amino acids *in vivo* in most tissues, as is illustrated in Figure 3-13 for methionine (Sturman *et al.,* 1970a). There is, however, a dramatic reduction in the incorporation of cystine into hair, a protein which has an extremely high cystine content (Table 3-5) (Sturman and Cohen, 1971). This was of interest because one of the characteristic manifestations of vitamin

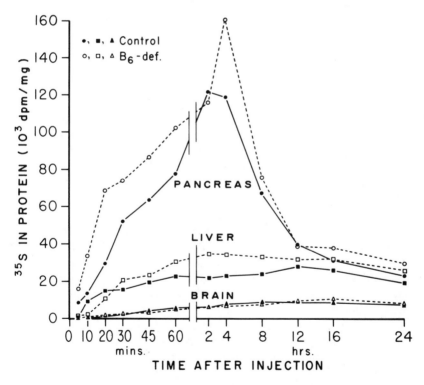

FIGURE 3-13 Specific activity of protein from various organs of rats fed a vitamin B_6-deficient diet or a control diet at different times after injection of ^{35}s-methionine (Sturman *et al.,* 1970a).

TABLE 3-5   Incorporation of [35]s-Cystine into Hair of Control and
Vitamin B$_6$-Deficient Rats

Time after Injection, weeks	Specific Activity of Hair, dpm/mg	
	Control	B$_6$-Deficient
1	917 ± 83	44 ± 13
2	6929 ± 1178	208 ± 55
3	3296 ± 365	351 ± 108

SOURCE: Sturman and Cohen (1971).

B$_6$ deficiency is partial alopecia. This condition is not alleviated by supplementing the diet with cystine, and therefore the vitamin B$_6$ deficiency is affecting some stage of protein synthesis itself rather than causing a deficiency of cysteine.

SUMMARY

The pathways of sulfur amino acid metabolism are very dependent on vitamin B$_6$ in the form of pyridoxal phosphate. These pathways in the mammal, including the human, are considerably affected by a nutritional deficiency of the vitamin. Fortunately, the B$_6$ vitamins occur so widely in nature that there is no pathological syndrome in the human associated with a naturally occurring deficiency of the vitamin. However, there do exist a number of human conditions in which there is a greater *dependency* on vitamin B$_6$, two of which involve sulfur amino acid metabolism, which should be sharply distinguished from true deficiency. The two described in this report involve highly abnormal enzyme proteins with greatly altered requirements for the vitamin B$_6$ coenzyme. The normal daily requirement of vitamin B$_6$ is currently set at approximately 2 mg, whereas daily doses used in the treatment of these dependency conditions have ranged from 10 to 1,500 mg, and the amount necessary has to be determined separately for each affected individual. It is possible, indeed probable, that there exists a range of lesser abnormalities in these enzyme proteins that are not severe enough to result in easily detectable metabolic or clinical changes. Such abnormalities might nevertheless require a greater than normal amount of vitamin B$_6$ for optimal function.

ACKNOWLEDGMENT

Studies performed in the author's laboratory were supported by the New York State Department of Mental Hygiene, National Institutes of Health Clinical Genetics Center Grant GM-19443, and the Lalor Foundation.

LITERATURE CITED

Anderson, D. J., J. Crossland, and G. G. Shaw. 1975. The actions of spermidine and spermine on the central nervous system. Neuropharmacology *14*:571–577.

Bachrach, U. 1973. Function of Naturally Occurring Polyamines, Academic Press, New York.

Barbeau, A., N. Inoue, Y. Tsukada, and R. F. Butterworth. 1975. The neuropharmacology of taurine. Life Sci. *17*:669–678.

Bergeret, B., F. Chatagner, and C. Fromageot. 1955. Quelques relations entre le phosphate de pyridoxal et la décarboxylation de l'acide cystéinesulfinique par divers organs du rat normal an du rat carencé en vitamine B₆. Biochim. Biophys. Acta *17*:128–135.

Berson, E. L., K. C. Hayes, A. R. Rabin, S. Y. Schmidt, and G. Watson. 1976. Retinal degeneration in cats fed casein. II. Supplementation with methionine, cysteine, or taurine. Invest. Ophthalmol. *15*:52–58.

Bittles, A. H., and N. A. J. Carson. 1974. Cystathionase deficiency in fibroblast cultures from a patient with primary cystathioninuria. J. Med. Genet. *11*:121–122.

Braunstein, A. E., E. V. Goryachenkova, and N. D. Lac. 1969. Reactions catalyzed by serine sulfhydrase from chicken liver. Biochim. Biophys. Acta *171*:366–368.

Braunstein, A. E., E. V. Goryachenkova, E. A. Tolosa, I. H. Willhardt, and L. L. Yefremova. 1971. Specificity and some other properties of liver serine sulfhydrase: Evidence for its identity with cystathionine β-synthase. Biochim. Biophys. Acta *242*:247–260.

Brenton, D. P., D. C. Cusworth, and G. E. Gaull. 1965. Homocystinuria: Biochemical studies of tissues including a comparison with cystathioninuria. Pediatrics *35*:50–56.

Brown, F. C., and P. H. Gordon. 1971. Cystathionine synthase from rat liver: Partial purification and properties. Can. J. Biochem. *49*:484–491.

Brown, F. C., J. Mallady, and J. A. Roszell. 1966. The separation of rat liver serine dehydratase and cystathionine synthase. J. Biol. Chem. *241*:5220–5224.

Davison, A. N. 1956. Amino acid decarboxylases in rat brain and liver. Biochim. Biophys. Acta *19*:66–73.

Feldman, M. J., C. C. Levy, and D. H. Russell. 1972. Purification and characterization of s-adenosyl-L-methionine. Biochemistry *11*:671–676.

Finkelstein, J. D., and F. T. Chalmers. 1970. Pyridoxine effects on cystathionine synthase in rat liver. J. Nutr. *100*:467–469.

Finkelstein, J. D., S. H. Mudd, F. Irreverre, and L. Laster. 1966. Deficiencies of cystathionase and homoserine dehydratase activities in cystathioninuria. Proc. Nat. Acad. Sci. U.S.A. *55*:865–872.

Fleisher, L. D., H. H. Tallan, N. G. Beratis, K. Hirschhorn, and G. E. Gaull. 1973. Cystathionine synthase deficiency: Heterozygote detection using cultured skin fibroblasts. Biochem. Biophys. Res. Commun. *55*:38–44.

Fleisher, L. D., R. C. Longhi, H. H. Tallan, N. G. Beratis, K. Hirschhorn, and G. E. Gaull. 1974. Homocystinuria: Investigations of cystathionine synthase in cultured fetal cells and the prenatal determination of genetic status. J. Pediatr. *85*:677–680.

Frimpter, G.W. 1965. Cystathioninuria: Nature of the defect. Science *149*:1095–1096.

Frimpter, G. W., W. F. George, and R. J. Andelman. 1969. Cystathioninuria and B_6 dependency. Ann. N.Y. Acad. Sci. *166*:109–115.

Gaull, G. E., D. K. Rassin, and J. A. Sturman. 1969. Enzymatic and metabolic studies of homocystinuria: Effects of pyridoxine. Neuropädiatrie *1*:199–226.

Gaull, G., J. A. Sturman, and N. C. R. Räihä. 1972. Development of mammalian sulfur metabolism: Absence of cystathionase in human fetal tissues. Pediatr. Res. *6*:538–547.

Gaull, G., J. A. Sturman, and F. Schaffner. 1974. Homocystinuria due to cystathionine synthase deficiency: Enzymatic and ultrastructural studies. J. Pediatr. *84*:381–390.

Gaull, G. E., H. H. Tallan, A. Lajtha, and D. K. Rassin. 1975. Pathogenesis of brain dysfunction in inborn errors of amino acid metabolism. *In* G. E. Gaull (ed.), Biology of Brain Dysfunction, Vol. 3, Plenum Press, New York, pp. 47–143.

Gaull, G. E., D. K. Rassin, N. C. R. Räihä, and K. Heinonen. 1977. Milk protein quantity and quality in low-birth-weight infants. III. Effects on sulfur amino acids in plasma and urine. J. Pediatr. *90*:348.

Gerritsen, T., and H. A. Waisman. 1964. Homocystinuria: Absence of cystathionine in the brain. Science *145*:588.

Goldstein, J. L., B. K. Campbell, and S. M. Gartler. 1972. Cystathionine synthase activity in human lymphocytes: Induction by phytohemagglutinin. J. Clin. Invest. *51*:1034–1037.

Hayes, K. C., R. E. Carey, and S. Y. Schmidt. 1975. Retinal degeneration associated with taurine deficiency in the cat. Science *188*:949–951.

Heinonen, K., and N. C. R. Räihä. 1974. Induction of cystathionase in human fetal liver. Biochem. J. *144*: 607–609.

Herbst, E. J., and U. Bachrach. 1970. Metabolism and function of polyamines. Ann. N.Y. Acad. Sci. *171*: 691–1009.

Hope, D. B. 1955. Pyridoxal phosphate as the coenzyme of the mammalian decarboxylase for L-cysteine sulphinic and L-cysteic acids. Biochem. J. *59*: 497–500.

Ingoglia, N. A., R. Eisner, and J. A. Sturman. 1976. Putrescine is axonally transported in regenerating goldfish optic nerves. Trans. Am. Soc. Neurochem. *7*:246.

Jacobsen, J. G., L. L. Thomas, and L. H. Smith. 1964. Properties and distribution of mammalian L-cysteine sulfinate carboxy-lyases. Biochim. Biophys. Acta *85*:103–116.

Kashiwamata, S. 1971. Brain cystathionine synthase: Vitamin B_6 requirement for its enzymic reaction and changes in enzymic activity during early development of rats. Brain Res. *30*:185–192.

Kashiwamata, S., and D. M. Greenberg. 1970. Studies on cystathionine synthase of rat liver: Properties of the highly purified enzyme. Biochim. Biophys. Acta *212*: 488–500.

Kashiwamata, S., Y. Kotake, and D. M. Greenberg. 1970. Studies of cystathionine synthase of rat liver: Dissociation into two components by sodium dodecyl sulfate disc electrophoresis. Biochim. Biophys. Acta *212*:501–503.

Kim, Y. J., and L. E. Rosenberg. 1974. On the mechanism of pyridoxine responsive homocystinuria. II. Properties of normal and mutant cystathionine β-synthase from cultured fibroblasts. Proc. Nat. Acad. Sci. U.S.A. *71*:4821–4825.

Kimura, H., and H. Nakagawa. 1971. Studies on cystathionine synthetase: Characteristics of purified rat liver enzyme. J. Biochem. *69*:711–723.

Knopf, K., J. A. Sturman, M. Armstrong, and K. C. Hayes. In press. Taurine: An essential nutrient for the cat. J. Nutr.

Longhi, R. C., L. D. Fleisher, H. H. Tallan, and G. E. Gaull. 1977. Cystathionine β-synthase deficiency: A qualitative abnormality of the deficient enzyme modified by vitamin B_6 therapy. Pediatr. Res. *11*:100–103.

Mudd, S. H., J. D. Finkelstein, F. Irreverre, and L. Laster. 1964. Homocystinuria: An enzymatic defect. Science *143*:1443–1445.

Mudd, S. H., L. Laster, J. D. Finkelstein, and F. Irreverre. 1967. Studies on homocystinuria. *In* H. E. Himwich, S. S. Kety, and J. R. Smithies (eds.), Amines and Schizophrenia, Pergamon Press, Oxford, pp. 247–256.

Mudd, S. H., W. A. Edwards, P. M. Loeb, M. S. Brown, and L. Laster. 1970. Homocystinuria due to cystathionine synthase deficiency: The effect of pyridoxine. J. Clin. Invest. *49*:1762–1773.

Nakagawa, H., and H. Kimura. 1968. Purification and properties of cystathionine synthase from rat liver: Separation of cystathionine synthetase from serine dehydratase. Biochem. Biophys. Res. Commun. *32*:208–214.

Packman, S., J. Kraus, and B. Fowler. 1976. Purification and properties of cystathionine synthase from human liver. Fed. Proc. *35*:1660.

Pan, F., and S. Pai. 1970. Dietary vitamin B_6 and enzymes of methionine metabolism in rat liver. J. Chin. Chem. Soc. *17*:46–53.

Pasantes-Morales, H., C. Mapes, R. Tapia, and P. Mandel. 1976. Properties of soluble and particulate cysteine sulfinate decarboxylase of the adult and the developing rat brain. Brain Res. *107*:575–589.

Pascal, T. A., B. M. Gillam, and G. E. Gaull. 1972a. Cystathionase: Immunochemical evidence for absence from human fetal liver. Pediatr. Res. *6*:773–778.

Pascal, T. A., H. H. Tallan, and B. M. Gillam. 1972b. Hepatic cystathionase: Immunochemical and electrophoretic studies of the human and rat forms. Biochim. Biophys. Acta *285*:48–59.

Pascal, T. A., G. E. Gaull, N. G. Beratis, B. M. Gillam, H. H. Tallan, and K. Hirschhorn. 1975. Vitamin B_6 -responsive and -unresponsive cystathioninuria: Two variant molecular forms. Science *190*:1209–1211.

Pateman, A. J., and G. G. Shaw. 1975. The uptake of spermidine and spermine by slices of mouse cerebral hemispheres. J. Neurochem. *25*:341–345.

Pegg, A. E., and H. G. Williams-Ashman. 1969. On the role of s-adenosylmethionine in the biosynthesis of spermidine by rat prostate. J. Biol. Chem. *244*:682–693.

Perry, T. L., P. J. A. Bratty, S. Hansen, J. Kennedy, N. Urquhart, and C. L. Dolman. 1975. Hereditary mental depression and parkinsonism with taurine deficiency. Arch. Neurol. *32*:108–113.

Porter, P. N., M. S. Grishaver, and O. W. Jones. 1974. Characterization of human cystathionine β-synthase: Evidence for the identity of human L-serine dehydratase and cystathionine β-synthase. Biochim. Biophys. Acta *364*:128–139.

Raina, A., and J. Jänne. 1975. Physiology of the natural polyamines putrescine, spermidine and spermine. Med. Biol. *53*:121–147.

Rassin, D. K., and J. A. Sturman. 1975. Cysteine sulfinic acid decarboxylase in rat brain: Effect of vitamin B_6 deficiency on soluble and particulate components. Life Sci. *16*:875–882.

Rassin, D. K., R. C. Longhi, and G. E. Gaull. In press. Free amino acids in liver of patients with homocystinuria due to cystathionine synthase deficiency: Effects of vitamin B_6. Clin. Chim. Acta.

Russell, D. H. 1973a. Polyamines in Normal and Neoplastic Growth. Raven Press, New York.

Russell, D. H. 1973b. The roles of the polyamines, putrescine, spermidine, and spermine in normal and malignant tissues. Life Sci. *13*:1635–1647.

Russell, D. H., and H. Meier. 1975. Alterations in the accumulation patterns of polyamines in brains of myelin-deficient mice. J. Neurobiol. 6:267–275.

Russell, D. H., E. Gfeller, L. F. Marton, and S. M. Legendre. 1974. Distribution of putrescine, spermidine, and spermine in rhesus monkey brain: Decrease in spermidine and spermine concentrations in motor cortex after electrical stimulation. J. Neurobiol. 5:349–354.

Schmidt, S. Y., E. L. Berson, and K. C. Hayes. 1976. Retinal degeneration in cats fed casein. I. Taurine deficiency. Invest. Ophthalmol. 15:47–52.

Seashore, M. R., J. L. Durant, and L. E. Rosenberg. 1972. Studies of the mechanism of pyridoxine-responsive homocystinuria. Pediatr. Res. 6:187–196.

Sörbo, B., and T. Heyman. 1957. On the purification of cysteinesulfinic acid decarboxylase and its substrate specificity. Biochim. Biophys. Acta 23:624–627.

Sturman, J. A. 1973. Taurine pool sizes in the rat. Effects of vitamin B_6 deficiency and high taurine diet. J. Nutr. 103:1566–1580.

Sturman, J. A., and P. A. Cohen. 1971. Cystine metabolism in vitamin B_6 deficiency: Evidence of multiple taurine pools. Biochem. Med. 5:245–268.

Sturman, J. A., and G. E. Gaull. 1975. Polyamine metabolism in the brain and liver of the developing monkey. J. Neurochem. 35:267–272.

Sturman, J. A., and L. T. Kremzner. 1974. Polyamine biosynthesis and vitamin B_6 deficiency: Evidence for pyridoxal phosphate as coenzyme for s-adenosylmethionine decarboxylase. Biochim. Biophys. Acta 372:162–170.

Sturman, J. A., and R. S. Rivlin. 1975. Pathogenesis of brain dysfunction in deficiency of thiamine, riboflavin, pantothenic acid, or vitamin B_6. In G. E. Gaull (ed.), Biology of Brain Dysfunction, Vol. 3, Plenum Press, New York, pp. 425–475.

Sturman, J. A., P. A. Cohen, and G. E. Gaull. 1969. Effects of deficiency of vitamin B_6 on transsulfuration. Biochem. Med. 3:244–251.

Sturman, J. A., P. A. Cohen, and G. E. Gaull. 1970a. Metabolism of L-^{35}s-methionine in vitamin B_6 deficiency: Observation on cystathioninuria. Biochem. Med. 3:510–523.

Sturman, J. A., G. Gaull, and N. C. R. Räihä. 1970b. Absence of cystathionase in human fetal liver: Is cystine essential? Science 169:74–76.

Tallan, H. H., S. Moore and W. H. Stein. 1958. L-Cystathionine in human brain. J. Biol. Chem. 230:707–716.

Tallan, H. H., T. A. Pascal, K. Schneidman, B. Gillam, and G. E. Gaull. 1971. Homolanthionine synthesis by human liver cystathionase. Biochem. Biophys. Res. Commun. 43:303–310.

Tallan, H. H., J. A. Sturman, T. A. Pascal, and G. E. Gaull. 1974. Cystathionine γ-synthesis from homocysteine and cystine by mammalian tissue. Biochem. Med. 9:90–101.

Tudball, N., and M. A. Reed. 1975. Purification and properties of cystathionine synthase from human liver. Biochem. Biophys. Res. Commun. 67:550–555.

Uhlendorf, B. W., and S. H. Mudd. 1968. Cystathionine synthase in tissue culture derived from human skin: Enzyme defect in homocystinuria. Science 160:1007–1009.

Uhlendorf, B. W., E. B. Conerly, and S. H. Mudd. 1973. Homocystinuria: Studies in tissue culture. Pediatr. Res. 7:645–658.

Zappia, V., M. Carteni-Farina, and G. D. Pietra. 1972. s-Adenosylmethionine decarboxylase from human prostate: Activation by putrescine. Biochem. J. 129:703–709.

4

Analysis of Vitamin B$_6$

BETTY E. HASKELL

The analysis of vitamin B$_6$ in biological samples is a continuing challenge to the skill and ingenuity of investigators who are concerned with the metabolism and utilization of this nutrient. The analytical problems are numerous. First, the method must be capable of detecting not a single chemical compound but a group of structurally related substances: pyridoxal, pyridoxine, and pyridoxamine and their corresponding 5′-phosphates. Second, much of the vitamin B$_6$ in biological samples is protein-bound. Different types of biological samples may present unique problems with regard to hydrolysis and extraction. Third, methods suitable for nutritional investigations must permit accurate and reproducible quantitation of a few nanograms of the vitamin in the presence of a wide variety of interfering substances. Finally, satisfactory analysis of vitamin B$_6$ requires that the sample be protected from light. This is particularly true of dilute solutions, which are extremely light sensitive. For example, when a solution of pyridoxal phosphate, 20 ng/ml, pH 7.8, is exposed to ordinary laboratory daylight for 30 minutes, half of it is destroyed (Haskell and Snell, 1972).

This chapter will review methods presently in use for the analysis of vitamin B_6, including microbiological, enzymatic, and fluorometric procedures. In addition, specialized methods developed primarily to follow the metabolism of radioactive vitamin B_6 in biological samples will be discussed briefly.

MICROBIOLOGICAL METHODS

Microbiological assay has been associated with vitamin B_6 since its discovery. It was the discrepancy between the vitamin B_6 content of biological samples as measured by lactobacillus assays as compared to the yeast assay that led to the discovery of pyridoxal and pyridoxamine (Snell, 1944). For many purposes, including the determination of the vitamin B_6 content of foods, microbiological assay still is the method of choice.

The method depends upon the growth response to a standard or sample of a vitamin B_6-requiring microorganism grown in a vitamin B_6-free basal medium. The method is specific, rapid as compared to animal growth assays, and sensitive. Most methods can quantitate 0.1 ng of vitamin B_6 per milliliter of medium. Detailed instructions for assay procedures have been published (Sauberlich, 1967; Storvick *et al.*, 1964; Haskell and Snell, 1970). However, special precautions are necessary to prevent accidental contamination of the basal medium with vitamin B_6. In the author's experience, occasional high blanks invariably have been due to contamination of the basal medium rather than to mutation of the test organism. Usually, the method is satisfactory for quantitation of vitamin B_6 in crude extracts. For certain samples, however, partial purification prior to assay gives superior results (Toepfer and Lehmann, 1961).

Although many different microorganisms may be used for microbiological assay of vitamin B_6 [see Storvick and Peters (1964) for a review], by far the most widely used is *Saccharomyces carlsbergensis* #4228 (ATCC 9080), now renamed *Saccharomyces uvarum* (American Type Culture Collection, 1974). Most cultures of this yeast grow with approximately equal efficiency in response to pyridoxal, pyridoxine, and pyridoxamine. Since these three forms of the vitamin also have equal activity for animals and humans, *S. carlsbergensis* is well suited to the estimation of total vitamin B_6 in foods.

Because this yeast grows only on the free forms of the vitamin, biological samples must be hydrolyzed prior to assay to free the vitamin of phosphate and of protein. The most widely used hydrolysis method is that described by Rabinowitz and Snell (1947), in which a finely divided sample is suspended in 180 ml of 0.055 N HCl and autoclaved for 5 h at 15 lbs pressure. However, a variety of hydrolysis techniques have been developed to improve recoveries from specific biological materials (Saüberlich, 1967; Barton-Wright, 1971).

One objection to *S. carlsbergensis* as an assay organism is that some cultures apparently grow only about 80 percent as well on pyridoxamine as they do on pyridoxal or pyridoxine. To correct for this lower growth response, one can separate pyridoxal, pyridoxine, and pyridoxamine by ion exchange chromatography (Toepfer and Lehmann, 1961; Brin, 1970) and assay the pyridoxamine-containing fraction against pyridoxamine standard. Prior fractionation not only permits one to correct for a possible lower response to pyridoxamine on the part of the test organism but also improves the specificity of the assay, since separation of the three forms of the vitamin results in partial purification of the sample (Toepfer and Lehman, 1961).

Table 4-1 shows that the vitamin B₆ content of four types of food as determined by microbiological assay with *S. carlsbergensis* agrees well with values obtained by rat growth assay (Richardson *et al.*, 1961). This microbiological method is the basis of much of the data on the vitamin B₆ content of foods contained in U.S. Department of Agriculture Home Economics Research Report No. 36 (Orr, 1969).

An advantage of the *S. carlsbergensis* assay is that the yeast is unaffected by the presence of D-alanine and peptides in the sample (Haskell and Wallnofer, 1967; Sauberlich, 1967). By contrast,

TABLE 4-1   A Comparison of the Total Vitamin B₆ Content of Selected Foods as Determined by Rat and Yeast Assay

| Food | Total Vitamin B₆ (μg/g) | |
	Rat Assay	Yeast Assay (fractionated extract)
Beef, lean dried	13.25	15.93
	(10.37–16.91)	(14.55–17.31)
Lima beans, dry	7.13	6.72
	(5.78–8.79)	(6.11–7.33)
Milk solids, nonfat, dry	3.16	4.06
	(2.64–3.80)	(3.73–4.39)
Whole wheat flour	2.94	3.50
	(2.40–3.59)	(3.27–3.73)

SOURCE: Toepfer *et al.*, 1963.
Values in parentheses are low and high values for 95% confidence limits. Rat assays were carried out by the method of Richardson *et al.*, 1961. Yeast assays were carried out with *Saccharomyces carlsbergensis* ATCC 9080 after column separation of pyridoxal, pyridoxine, and pyridoxamine (Toepfer and Lehmann, 1961).

D-alanine and peptides can permit the growth of certain lactic acid bacteria test organisms in media containing no vitamin B_6 by providing preformed an efficiently utilized supply of metabolites whose biosynthesis requires vitamin B_6 (Snell and Guirard, 1943; Snell, 1945; Rabinowitz et al., 1948; Holden and Snell, 1949; Gregory, 1959; Moller, 1950; Kihara and Snell, 1960a; Raines and Haskell, 1968). Interference from these sources received widespread attention when Storvick and Peters (1964) reported that prolonged acid hydrolysis of whole blood produced a startling increase in its apparent vitamin B_6 content for L. casei ATCC #7469 (which grows in response to pyridoxal) and S. faecium $\phi51$ (which grows in response to pyridoxal and pyridoxamine) but did not affect the total vitamin B_6 content of the sample, as measured by S. carlsbergensis. These puzzling data apparently were due to the racemization of L-alanine to D-alanine and to the formation of peptides during prolonged hydrolysis. Figure 4-1 shows that the D-alanine and free amino group content of whole blood increases with hydrolysis time. This increase is reflected in an increase in the apparent vitamin B_6 content of the medium for lactic acid bacteria (Haskell and Wallnofer, 1967).

Some investigators have concluded from the work of Storvick and Peters (1964) that microbiological assay is to be avoided because of the nonspecificity of the test organisms. It should be noted that the experiments described by Storvick and Peters constitute the only known examples of D-alanine and peptide interference in the assay of vitamin B_6. This is not surprising, since D-alanine is rare in nature. It is a highly inefficient substitute for vitamin B_6, 10,000 to 25,000 μg being required to substitute for 1 μg of pyridoxal when L. casei is grown in a peptide-enriched medium (Rabinowitz et al., 1948). Furthermore, the protein content of the sample must be unusually high and the vitamin B_6 content unusually low for D-alanine interference to occur. Moller (1950) has estimated that D-alanine can interfere with the microbiological assay of vitamin B_6 only when the ratio of protein to vitamin is at least 10^4 to 1.

That lactic acid bacteria can be used satisfactorily for assay of pyridoxal in blood is indicated by a recent report of an improved method developed by Anderson et al. (1970) for L. casei. These investigators shortened the hydrolysis time to 1 h to minimize racemization of L-alanine to D-alanine, and they improved the basal medium by supplementation with L-alanine and L-tryptophan. The revised assay permits 200-fold dilution of the blood sample and is 10 times more sensitive than earlier procedures.

Microbiological assay has been used successfully in connection with

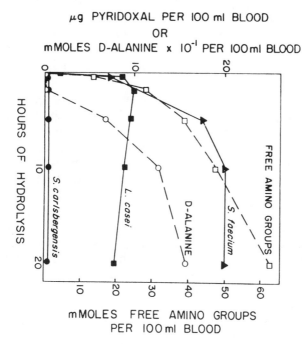

μg PYRIDOXAL PER 100 ml BLOOD
OR
mMOLES D-ALANINE x 10⁻¹ PER 100ml BLOOD

FIGURE 4-1   Effect of hydrolysis time on the apparent vitamin
B_6 content of whole blood. Prolonged hydrolysis in 0.055 N HCl
at 121°C increases the apparent vitamin B_6 content of human
whole blood for *S. faecium* and *L. casei* but not for *S.
carlsbergensis*. Since *L. casei* responds only to pyridoxal and *S.
faecium* only to pyridoxal and pyridoxamine, these microorganisms might be expected to show less growth than *S.
carlsbergensis*, which utilizes all three forms of the vitamin.
Growth of the lactic acid bacteria, *S. faecium* and *L. casei,* but
not of the yeast, reflects the increase in D-alanine and free amino
content of blood samples with hydrolysis time (Haskell and
Wallnofer, 1967).

column chromatography for the quantitative determination of
pyridoxal, pyridoxine, pyridoxamine, and their corresponding phosphates in animal tissue (Bain and Williams, 1960). Although the method
is slow and tedious, it is highly specific and thus, in the author's opin-
ion, more reliable for use with partially purified biological samples than
are fluorometric methods currently in use. The procedure separates
each of the free and phosphorylated forms of vitamin B_6 with citrate
buffers on a two-layered ion exchange column consisting of Dowex 50
(K) on top of Dowex 1 (formate). Separations are clean and reproducible. Each fraction is assayed for vitamin B_6 with *S. carlsbergensis*.

Fractions containing the phosphorylated vitamin are subjected to prior hydrolysis. Overall recovery from the column is 85 percent.

ENZYMATIC METHODS

Sensitive and highly specific enzymatic methods have been developed for the quantitative determination of pyridoxal phosphate, the major coenzyme form of vitamin B_6. These methods depend upon the ability of pyridoxal phosphate to restore activity to a highly purified apoenzyme. Recent methods using either apotryptophanase (Haskell and Snell, 1972) or tyrosine apodecarboxylase (Chabner and Livingston, 1970) are described here.

Tryptophanase needs to be isolated from *E. coli* Blt7A, grown under culture conditions such that tryptophanase comprises 10 percent of the cellular soluble protein (Newton and Snell, 1964). Isolation of an enzyme preparation free of pyridoxal phosphate is facilitated by the ease with which the apoenzyme may be crystallized (Morino and Snell, 1970). Either the crystalline apoenzyme or a highly purified ammonium sulfate preparation is satisfactory for use in assay of pyridoxal phosphate (Haskell and Snell, 1972).

The sequence of reactions in the apotryptophanase assay for pyridoxal phosphate is as follows:

Apotryptophan + pyridoxal phosphate $\longrightarrow$ holoenzyme

L-Tryptophan + water $\xrightarrow[\text{tryptophanase}]{}$ pyruvic acid + indole + ammonia

Indole $\xrightarrow[\text{Ehrlich reagent}]{}$ adsorbance at 570 mu

The apoenzyme is preincubated with pyridoxal phosphate to permit reassociation of apoenzyme with the cofactor. Tryptophan then is added to the reaction flask, and the activity of the holoenzyme measured by indole formation. Indole is estimated colorimetrically with an Ehrlich reagent. The method is similar to that of McCormick *et al.* (1961), but it is simpler and more sensitive. Quantitation is satisfactory, either in the concentration range from 60 to 240 ng or, with minor modifications, in the 3–15 ng range. The final reaction volume is 5 ml.

The method is satisfactory for the quantitation of pyridoxal phosphate in assay mixtures for pyridoxal phosphokinase (McCormick *et al.*, 1961) and pyridoxine ·phosphate oxidase (Wada and Snell, 1961). Recovery of added pyridoxal phosphate standard to either reaction mixture is greater than 90 percent.

Reproducibility is good. The error for duplicates is about 7 percent when the assay is used at the 3- to 15-ng range; 3 percent when the assay is used in the 60- to 240-ng range.

The quantitative determination of pyridoxal phosphate with tyrosine apodecarboxylase has the advantage of using an apoenzyme that may be purchased from a commercial source. The crude commercial product is further purified to obtain a stable apoenzyme preparation suitable for assay of pyridoxal phosphate (Chabner and Livingston, 1970).

The reaction scheme for estimation of pyridoxal phosphate with tyrosine apodecarboxylase is as follows:

Tyrosine apodecarboxylase + pyridoxal phosphate ⟶ holoenzyme

$$\text{L-tyrosine-1-}^{14}\text{C} \xrightarrow{\text{tyrosine decarboxylase}} \text{tyramine} + {}^{14}\text{C-CO}_2$$

Apodecarboxylase is preincubated with standards or samples containing pyridoxal phosphate to allow reconstitution of the holoenzyme. Tyrosine-1-^{14}C is added, and the activity of the holoenzyme measured by ^{14}C-carbon dioxide evolution. The radioactive carbon dioxide is trapped in alkali in the center well of a commercially available reaction flask. The alkali trap and its contents are transferred to a scintillation vial, combined with scintillant, and counted.

The method is reproducible (standard error of the mean for 76 consecutive duplicate determinations, 5.8 percent), sensitive (linear range from 0.5 to 2.0 ng) and specific for pyridoxal phosphate. Recovery of pyridoxal phosphate added to plasma prior to deproteinization averaged 89 percent.

FLUOROMETRIC METHODS

Fluorescent methods for the quantitative determination of vitamin B₆ in biological materials are largely unsatisfactory with the exception of a few that include rigorous purification of the sample to remove interfering materials prior to analysis. One such method that has proved highly satisfactory is that of Reddy *et al.* (1958) for the quantitative determination of 4-pyridoxic acid, an oxidation product of pyridoxal formed in liver and excreted in urine. This compound has neither vitamin B₆ activity nor antivitamin B₆ activity.

The method of Reddy *et al.* (1958) depends upon the increase in fluorescence that occurs when 4-pyridoxic acid is converted to the highly fluorescent lactone. Prior to analysis, the sample is purified on Dowex 1 (Cl) and on Dowex 50 (H). Then it is treated with alkali to convert any lactone formed during column elution to free 4-pyridoxic acid. Finally, the sample is converted to the highly fluorescent lactone and read against its own delactonized blank.

A possible source of error not anticipated at the time this method was developed is the presence in biological samples of 4-pyridoxic acid phosphate. Contrary to earlier reports (Contractor and Shane, 1970), this compound is not a metabolite of vitamin B_6 (Wei *et al.*, 1972). However, traces may occur in biological samples owing to photodecomposition of pyridoxal phosphate. Possible interference from this source can be minimized by protecting the sample from light.

Of more practical importance in connection with the fluorometric analysis of vitamin B_6 is evidence that the so-called "cyanohydrin method" (Bonavita and Scardi, 1959; Bonavita, 1960) for the fluorometric estimation of pyridoxal and pyridoxal phosphate actually results in the cyanide-catalyzed oxidation of these compounds to 4-pyridoxic acid lactone and 4-pyridoxic acid 5'-phosphate, respectively (Ohishi and Fukui, 1968). One might expect that these "cyanohydrin methods" would give unreliable results when applied to crude biological samples containing endogenous 4-pyridoxic acid.

Tamura and Takanishi (1970) have developed a satisfactory method for the fluorometric determination of pyridoxal and pyridoxal phosphate in certain biological samples, including plasma, milk, urine, and tissues. The method is not applicable to whole blood because of low recoveries. Pyridoxal phosphate is determined after quantitative conversion to pyridoxal with potato acid phosphatase (Takanishi and Tamura, 1970). The sample is then purified on Dowex 1 (acetate) and Amberlite CG 120, pH 4. Pyridoxal is oxidized in the presence of cyanide ion to 4-pyridoxic acid lactone and estimated fluorometrically. The column purification removes interfering substances, including NAD, thiamin, riboflavin, and 4-pyridoxic acid.

SPECIALIZED CHROMATOGRAPHIC PROCEDURES

The availability from commercial sources or chemical synthesis of pyridoxine • HCl labeled with carton-14 or tritium has stimulated interest in separation methods developed primarily to follow the metabolism of radioactive vitamin B_6 metabolites in animals. Because of the importance of this research in supplying information fundamental to nutritional investigations, these methods are reviewed briefly here.

A procedure appealing in its simplicity is that of Colombini and McCoy (1970), which separates pyridoxal, pyridoxamine, and pyridoxine and their corresponding phosphates by thin-layer electrophoresis on cellulose in 0.05 M sodium acetate buffer, pH 5.1. The phosphates move toward the cathode; the free forms of the vitamin toward the anode. Distance traveled from the origin at 750 V for 3 h or 600 V for 4 h is as follows: pyridoxamine phosphate, 10.2 cm; pyridoxal phosphate, 7.6 cm; pyridoxine phosphate, 2.5 cm; pyridoxamine, 1.3 cm; pyridoxal, 7.6 cm; and pyridoxine, 15.0 cm.

Extracts containing vitamin B_6 labeled with ^{14}C were cochromatographed with standards, and the spots visualized under uv light. Portions of plate containing radioactive vitamin B_6 compounds were scraped into scintillation vials, combined with scintillant, and counted. Recovery of the radioactive extract from the plate was 95–98 percent.

A limitation of this method is that the electrophoretic mobility of 4-pyridoxic acid was not reported. This compound, as well as the free and phosphorylated forms of the vitamin, may be expected to be present in animal tissue as well as in urine.

An excellent column chromatographic method that gives clean separation of 4-pyridoxic acid, pyridoxal, pyridoxine, pyridoxamine, and their corresponding phosphates has been described by Tiselius (1972). He used a complex gradient elution system with ammonium formate buffers to separate the seven compounds on Dowex AG 50 W, x8. The compounds appear in the following order: pyridoxal phosphate, pyridoxine phosphate, 4-pyridoxic acid, pyridoxamine phosphate, pyridoxal, pyridoxine, and pyridoxamine. Recovery is quantitative. A micro adaptation of the column procedure permitted quantitation of tritium-labeled vitamin B_6 metabolites in 50 μl of rat cerebrospinal fluid (Tiselius, 1972).

A final method deserves mention because it suggests the possibility of developing ion exchange chromatographic methods for separation of vitamin B_6 compounds by high-pressure liquid chromatography. The feasibility of this approach is indicated by the report of Williams *et al.* (1973) that sharp, clean separations of pyridoxal, pyridoxine, and pyridoxamine can be achieved in 10 minutes by liquid chromatography on Zipax SCX (strong cation exchanger), column pressure 1200 psi, with 0.1 M KH_2PO_4 buffer, pH 4.4. The applicability of high-pressure liquid chromatography methods to the analysis of radioactive vitamin B_6 metabolites deserves attention.

LITERATURE CITED

American Type Culture Collection. 1974. Catalog of Strains, 11th ed., Rockville, Maryland. p. 231.

Anderson, B. B., M. B. Peart, and C. E. Fulford-Jones. 1970. The measurement of serum pyridoxal by a microbiological assay using *Lactobacillus casei*. J. Clin. Pathol. *23*:232–242.

Bain, J. A., and H. L. Williams. 1960. Concentrations of B₆ vitamins in tissues and tissue fluids. *In* Inhibition in the Nervous System and Gamma-Aminobutyric Acid, Pergamon Press, New York, pp. 275–293. (Proc. Int. Symp., City of Hope Medical Center, Duarte, Cal., May 22–24, 1959. Sponsor: U.S. Air Force Office of Scientific Research.)

Barton-Wright, E. C. 1971. The microbiological assay of the vitamin B₆ complex (pyridoxine, pyridoxal and pyridoxamine) with *Kloeckera brevis*. Analyst 96:314–318.

Bonavita, V. 1960. The reaction of pyridoxal 5-phosphate with cyanide and its analytical use. Arch. Biochem. Biophys. 88:366–372.

Bonavita, V., and V. Scardi. 1959. Spectrophotometric determination of pyridoxal phosphate. Anal. Chim. Acta 20:47–50.

Brin, M. A. 1970. A simplified Toepfer-Lehmann assay for the three vitamin B₆ vitamers. *In* D. B. McCormick and L. D. Wright (eds.), Methods In Enzymology, Vitamins and Coenzymes, Vol. 18, Part A, Academic Press, New York/London, pp. 519–523.

Chabner, B., and D. Livingston. 1970. A simple enzymatic assay for pyridoxal phosphate. Anal. Biochem. 34:413–423.

Colombini, C. E., and E. E. McCoy. 1970. Rapid thin-layer electrophoretic separation and estimation of all vitamin B₆ compounds and of some 5-hydroxyindoles. Anal. Biochem. 34:451–458.

Contractor, S. F., and B. Shane. 1970. 4-Pyridoxic acid 5'-phosphate: A metabolite of pyridoxal in the rat. Biochem. Biophys. Res. Commun. 39:1175–1181.

Gregory, M. E. 1959. Effect of heat on the vitamin B₆ of milk. I. Microbiological tests. J. Dairy Res. 26:203–214.

Haskell, B. E., and E. E. Snell. 1970. Microbiological determination of the vitamin B₆ group. *In* D. B. McCormick and L. D. Wright (eds.), Methods In Enzymology, Vitamins and Coenzymes, Vol. 18, Part A, Academic Press, New York/London, pp. 512–519.

Haskell, B. E., and E. E. Snell. 1972. An improved apotryptophanase assay for pyridoxal phosphate. Anal. Biochem. 45:567–575.

Haskell, B. E., and U. Wallnofer. 1967. D-alanine interference in microbiological assays of vitamin B₆ in human blood. Anal. Biochem. 19:569–577.

Holden, J. T., and E. E. Snell. 1949. The vitamin B₆ group. XVII. The relation of D-alanine and vitamin B₆ to growth of lactic acid bacteria. J. Biol. Chem. 178:799–809.

Kihara, H., and E. E. Snell. 1960a. Peptide and bacterial growth. VIII. The nature of strepogenin. J. Biol. Chem. 235:1409–1413.

Kihara, H., and E. E. Snell. 1960b. Peptides and bacterial growth. IX. Release of double inhibitions with single peptides. J. Biol. Chem. 235:1415–1418.

McCormick, D. B., M. E. Gregory, and E. E. Snell. 1961. Pyridoxal phosphokinases. I. Assay, distribution, purification, and properties. J. Biol. Chem. 236:2076–2084.

Moller, P. 1950. The interrelationship of alanine and vitamin B₆ with two strains of *Streptococcus Faecalis*. Acta Physiol. Scand. 21:332–335.

Morino, Y., and E. E. Snell. 1970. Tryptophanase *(Escherichia coli B)*. *In* D. B. McCormick and L. D. Wright (eds.), Methods In Enzymology, Vol. 17, Part A, Academic Press, New York/London, pp. 439–447.

Newton, W. A., and E. E. Snell. 1964. Catalytic properties of tryptophanase, a multifunctional pyridoxal phosphate enzyme. Proc. Nat. Acad. Sci. U.S.A. 51:382–389.

Ohishi, N., and S. Fukui. 1968. Further study on the reaction products of pyridoxal and pyridoxal-5'-phosphate with cyanide. Arch. Biochem. Biophys. 128:606–610.

Orr, M. L. 1969. Pantothenic acid, vitamin B$_6$ and vitamin B$_{12}$ in foods. U.S. Dep. Agric. Home Econ. Res. Rep. No. 36:36 pp.

Rabinowitz, J. C., and E. E. Snell. 1947. The vitamin B$_6$ group. X. Extraction procedures for the microbiological determination of vitamin B$_6$. Anal. Chem. *19*:277–280.

Rabinowitz, J. C., N. I. Mondy, and E. E. Snell. 1948. The vitamin B$_6$ group. XIII. An improved procedure for determination of pyridoxal with *Lactobacillus casei*. J. Biol. Chem. *175*:147–153.

Raines, R. C., and B. E. Haskell. 1968. Peptide stimulation of *Streptococcus faecium*, a test organism for pyridoxal and pyridoxamine. Anal. Biochem. *23*:413–421.

Reddy, S. K., M. S. Reynolds, and J. M. Price. 1958. The determination of 4-pyridoxic acid in human urine. J. Biol. Chem. *233*:691–696.

Richardson, L. R., S. Wilkes, and S. J. Ritchey. 1961. Comparative vitamin B$_6$ activity of frozen, irradiated and heat-processed foods. J. Nutr. *73*:363–373.

Sauberlich, H. E. 1967. Vitamin B$_6$. *In* P. Gyorgy and W. N. Pearson (eds.), The Vitamins, 2nd ed., Vol. 7, Academic Press, New York, pp. 169–208.

Snell, E. E. 1944. The vitamin activities of "pyridoxal" and "pyridoxamine." J. Biol. Chem. *154*:313–314.

Snell, E. E. 1945. The vitamin B$_6$ group. VII. Replacement of vitamin B$_6$ for some microorganisms by d(-)alanine and an unidentified factor from casein. J. Biol. Chem. *158*:497–503.

Snell, E. E., and B. M. Guirard. 1943. Some interrelationships of pyridoxine, alanine and glycine in their effect on certain lactic acid bacteria. Proc. Nat. Acad. Sci. U.S.A. *29*:66–73.

Storvick, C. A., and J. M. Peters. 1964. Methods for the determination of vitamin B$_6$ in biological materials. Vitam. Horm. *22*:833–854.

Storvick, C. A., E. M. Benson, M. A. Edwards, and M. J. Woodring. 1964. Chemical and microbiological determination of vitamin B$_6$. *In* D. Glick (ed.), Methods of Biochemical Analysis *XII*, Interscience Publishers, New York, pp. 183–276.

Takanishi, S., and Z. Tamura. 1970. Preliminary studies for fluorometric determination of pyridoxal and of its 5'-phosphate. J. Vitaminol. *16*:129–131.

Tamura, Z., and S. Takanishi. 1970. Fluorometric determination of pyridoxal and pyridoxal 5'-phosphate in biological materials by the reaction with cyanide. *In* D. B. McCormick and L. D. Wright (eds.), Methods In Enzymology, Vitamins and Coenzymes, Vol. 18, Part A, Academic Press, New York/London, pp. 471–475.

Tiselius, H.-G. 1972. A chromatographic separation of the different forms of vitamin B$_6$. Clin. Chim. Acta *40*:319–324.

Toepfer, E. W., and J. Lehmann. 1961. Procedure for chromatographic separation and microbiological assay of pyridoxine, pyridoxal and pyridoxamine in food extracts. J. Assoc. Off. Agric. Chem. *44*:426–430.

Toepfer, E. W., M. M. Polansky, L. R. Richardson, and S. Wilkes. 1963. Comparison of vitamin B$_6$ values of selected food samples by bioassay and microbiological assay. J. Agric. Food Chem. *11*:523–525.

Wada, H., and E. E. Snell. 1961. The enzymatic oxidation of pyridoxine and pyridoxamine phosphates. J. Biol. Chem. *236*:2089–2095.

Wei, K.-T., R. R. Bell, and B. E. Haskell. 1972. Regarding 4-pyridoxic acid 5'-phosphate in animal tissue. Biochem. Biophys. Res. Commun. *48*:1671–1674.

Williams, R. C., D. R. Baker, and J. A. Schmit. 1973. Analysis of water-soluble vitamins by high-speed ion-exchange chromatography. J. Chromatogr. Sci. *11*:618–624.

5

Vitamin B₆ in Foods: Assessment of Stability and Bioavailability

J. F. GREGORY *and* J. R. KIRK

INTRODUCTION

The vitamin B_6 content of American diets has been reported to be 1.1–3.6 mg/day for typical diets and 0.7–1.4 mg/day for "poor" diets (Mangay Chung *et al.*, 1961). These results, when compared to the recommended dietary allowance of 2 mg/day, suggest that the majority of diets contain adequate levels of vitamin B_6. However, the variability observed in addition to the uncertainty of the requirement, raises the question of adequacy of vitamin B_6 nutriture of certain segments of the population.

In this discussion, we will consider some of the factors that affect the content and bioavailability of vitamin B_6 in foods, along with the role of analytical methods in the interpretation of the data.

STABILITY AND BIOAVAILABILITY OF VITAMIN B₆

The various forms of the vitamin in pure solution have been shown to be quite stable to heat, acid, and alkali. Exposure to light, especially in neutral or alkaline media, is highly destructive. Light-induced degradation could therefore be of practical significance in fluid milk and other fluid products exposed to light during their shelf life.

Considering the effects of processing and storage on vitamin B_6 in foods, probably more research has been done with dairy products than with other foods. Milk normally contains about 0.6 mg B_6/l (by microbiological assay), of which 70–95 percent is present as pyridoxal. During milk processing, storage, and even spray drying, only slight losses of vitamin B_6 occur.

Research into losses of bioavailable vitamin B_6 began in the early 1950's when vitamin B_6-responsive convulsions were observed in a few infants fed a commercially sterilized, liquid, milk-based formula (Coursin, 1954). Since the syndrome did not appear in infants receiving the same formula, which had been spray dried rather than sterilized, the loss of available B_6 was assumed to be heat induced. Subsequent research on thermally processed dairy products showed interesting, although as yet not totally explained, results. During the sterilization of canned evaporated milk, rapid losses of vitamin B_6 were observed, followed by a continued progressive loss over about the first 10 days of storage, with little further change up to 1 year (Hassinen *et al.*, 1954). When vitamin B_6 was added in its various forms, pyridoxal and pyridoxamine were found to be destroyed at the same rate as naturally occurring vitamin B_6, whereas added pyridoxine was found to be quite heat stable. Therefore, pyridoxine HCl has been used for fortification purposes. Bioavailability studies on evaporated milk and sterilized infant formulas indicated that the vitamin B_6 activity available to the rat was only about one half of that found by microbiological assay. By contrast, bioassay and microbiological values were equal for unheated milk and products fortified with pyridoxine HCl (Tomarelli *et al.*, 1955; Hodson, 1956; Davies *et al.*, 1959). Therefore, the bioavailability of vitamin B_6 in foods may be significantly affected by thermal processing.

Little research has been directed toward the effects of processing on the bioavailability of vitamin B_6 in foods other than milk and infant formulas. In the early 1950's, studies on the nutritional quality of army field rations showed that the vitamin B_6 availability to support rat growth was less than that predicted by microbiological assay (Register *et al.*, 1950; Tappan *et al.*, 1953). Recent studies concerning the effects of roasting on corn and soybean meal have found thermally induced losses of biologically available vitamin B_6 (Yen *et al.*, 1976). Attempts to correlate losses of the vitamin B_6 available to the rat or chick with microbiological assay results have not been successful. Richardson *et al.* (1961) reported that heat processing by retorting induced variable losses in available vitamin B_6 in a variety of products. Toepfer *et al.* (1963) later showed that significant differences were not observed between bioassay and microbiological values for all foods. Thus, it appears that the chemical composition of the food, in addition to process conditions, affects the net retention of available vitamin B_6; however, further research is needed to identify and quantitate the factors responsible.

MECHANISMS FOR CONTROL OF VITAMIN B_6 LOSSES

In order that processing and storage conditions be designed so that losses are minimized, the mechanisms and kinetics of vitamin B_6 degradation must be elucidated. Relatively little is known to date in this regard.

Fortunately, pyridoxine HCl, when used in food fortification, is quite stable. Recent studies have shown that cereal products fortified with pyridoxine HCl retain essentially all of the added vitamin during processing and storage over a 12-week period (Cort *et al.*, 1976). Thus the fortification of foods with pyridoxine HCl tends to alleviate the problems of processing induced losses of naturally occurring vitamin B_6.

The predominant losses of vitamin B_6 activity in foods occur by reactions involving pyridoxal and pyridoxamine (Hassinen *et al.*, 1954). Relatively little is known regarding the effects of processing on these vitamin B_6 compounds. To explain the losses of bioavailable vitamin B_6 in foods during processing, numerous researchers have proposed various interactions of the vitamin with food proteins and amino acids (Hassinen *et al.*, 1954; Tomarelli *et al.*, 1955; Hodson, 1956; Bernhart *et al.*, 1960; Srncova and Davidek, 1972). The potential mechanisms of interaction of pyridoxal and pyridoxal phosphate with proteins are (1) formation of a Schiff base by interaction of the carbonyl with a free amino group (Matsuo, 1957), (2) formation of a pyridoxylamino acid by reduction of a Schiff base (Heyl *et al.*, 1948), (3) reaction with free sulfhydryl groups to form 4-pyridoxthiol or its disulfide bis-4-pyridoxyl disulfide, by way of the hemimercaptal intermediate (Bernhart *et al.*, 1960).

Whereas the availability of vitamin B_6 in a Schiff base has not been determined, it is presumed to be totally available, since the complex readily dissociates with acid hydrolysis under gastric conditions. The reduction of the Schiff base linkage to form a pyridoxylamino acid has not been demonstrated in food systems.

The biological activity of various pyridoxylamino acids has been found to be quite low (Snell and Rabinowitz, 1948). Preliminary results in our laboratory have shown that the proportion of pyridoxal complexed with protein amino groups, even after heat sterilization at neutral pH, is very small. This study was conducted using mixtures of pyridoxal at 50 μg/ml and heat stable peptides isolated from a peptic hydrolysate of β-lactoglobulin. To investigate the possible effects of carbonyl-amine browning in the presence of a reducing agent, glucose and ascorbic acid were added to the vitamin B_6-peptide system in various combinations, autoclaved for 20 minutes, and then cooled to 4°C. Two mg of sodium borohydride were added to the samples to provide reduction of all Schiff base linkages. The peptide fraction of these samples was isolated by Sephadex G-10 gel filtration, followed by measurement of absorbance at 323 nm. The difference in absorbance at 323 nm between samples that contained pyridoxal and their respective blanks was then used to calculate total bound pyridoxal, the sum of Schiff base and pyridoxylamino B_6 formed during the autoclave sterilization. On the basis of the results of this study, the potential losses of vitamin B_6 activity by such mechanisms would be minimal. Currently, investigations concerning the behavior of pyridoxal phosphate in the same model system are being carried out.

The formation of the vitamin B_6 disulfide compound has been proposed as a possible mechanism for the loss of bioavailability of the vitamin in sterilized condensed milk (Bernhart *et al.,* 1960). Although the compound has been isolated from condensed milk to which a high level of pyridoxal had been added before heat treatments, the reaction has not been confirmed or quantitated.

Further study is obviously required to determine the magnitude of losses of biologically available vitamin B_6 in foods. Assessment of reaction mechanisms, biological activity of reaction products, and factors affecting rates of degradation would then provide a better understanding of processing effects.

ANALYTICAL METHODS AND INTERPRETATION

For the evaluation of the vitamin B_6 content and biological availability in foods the primary requisite should be accuracy and precision of the analytical technique, particularly from one laboratory to another. The literature to date has been based mainly upon several microbiological methods of assay (Stokes *et al.,* 1943; Toepfer and Polansky, 1970). Similarly, the data upon which the recommended dietary allowances for vitamin B_6 are based were derived mainly from studies utilizing the standard microbiological procedures (Food and Nutrition Board,

1974). Despite problems of variability in growth response with various microorganisms and precision between laboratory groups in quantitating the B_6 vitamers, the microbiological methods have been the only methods available.

Considerable effort has been placed on the development of chemical methods for the determination of total vitamin B_6 in foods. The results of several studies utilizing various fluorometric procedures have shown values for most products analyzed to be significantly greater than corresponding microbiological values (Kraut and Imhoff, 1967; Chin, 1975; Gregory and Kirk, in press). Chemically determined values ranged from approximately equal to microbiological values to about a tenfold difference, depending upon the food product analyzed. Recently, an ion exchange chromatography procedure was developed to remove compounds that could potentially interfere with the fluorometric assay for pyridoxine, pyridoxal, and pyridoxamine (Gregory and Kirk, 1977).

These results suggest that the microbiological values may be plagued by inherent artifacts. Microbiologically unavailable complexes of the vitamin may be formed as a result of the acid extraction, or microbial growth may be retarded by substances formed in the food extract, either of which would affect the accuracy of the assay.

Results of these studies, which included pure forms of the vitamin B_6 vitamers, model systems, and food systems, indicate that current microbiological methods for vitamin B_6 may not be totally adequate. Because of this uncertainty, a thorough reevaluation of conclusions based upon microbiological methods is warranted.

LITERATURE CITED

Bernhart, F. W., E. D'Amato, and R. M. Tomarelli. 1960. The vitamin B₆ activity of heat-sterilized milk. Arch. Biochem. Biophys. *88*:267.

Chin, Y. P. 1975. Chromatographic separation and fluorometric determination of pyridoxal, pyridoxamine, and pyridoxine in food system. M.S. Thesis. Michigan State University. 79 pp.

Cort, W. M., B. Borenstein, J. H. Harley, M. Osadca, and J. Scheiner. 1976. Nutrient stability of fortified cereal products. Food Technol. *30*:52–62.

Coursin, D. B. 1954. Convulsive seizures in infants with pyridoxine deficient diet. J. Am. Med. Assoc. *154*:406–408.

Davies, M. K., M. E. Gregory, and K. M. Henry. 1959. The effect of heat on the vitamin B₆ of milk. II. A comparison of biological and microbiological tests of evaporated milk. J. Dairy Res. *26*:215–220.

Food and Nutrition Board. 1974. Recommended Dietary Allowances, 8th ed., National Academy of Sciences, Washington, D.C., 128 pp.

Gregory, J. F., and J. R. Kirk. 1977. Improved chromatographic separation and fluorometric determination of vitamin B₆ in foods. J. Food Sci. *42*:1073–1076.

Hassinen, J. B., G. T. Durbin, and F. W. Bernhart. 1954. The vitamin B₆ content of milk products. J. Nutr. *53*:249–257.

Heyl, D., S. A. Harris, and K. Folkers. 1948. The chemistry of vitamin B₆. VI. Pyridoxylamino acids. J. Am. Chem. Soc. *70*:3429–3431.

Hodson, A. Z. 1956. Vitamin B₆ in sterilized milk and other milk products. J. Agric. Food Chem. *4*:876–881.

Kraut, H., and U. Imhoff. 1967. Forschungsber, Landes, Nordrheim-Westfallen, pp. 1833–1853.

Mangay Chung, A. S., W. N. Pearson, W. J. Darby, O. N. Miller, and G. A. Goldsmith. 1961. Folic acid, vitamin B₆, pantothenic acid, and vitamin B₁₂ in human dietaries. Am. J. Clin. Nutr. *9*:573–582.

Matsuo, Y. 1957. Formation of Schiff base of pyridoxal phosphate. Reaction with metal ions. J. Am. Chem. Soc. *79*:2011–2019.

Register, U. D., U. J. Lewis, W. R. Ruegamer, and C. A. Elvehjem. 1950. Studies on the nutritional adequacy of army combat rations. J. Nutr. *40*:281–294.

Richardson, L. R., S. Wilkes, and R. J. Ritchey. 1961. Comparative vitamin B₆ activity of frozen, irradiated and heat-processed foods. J. Nutr. *73*:363–368.

Snell, E. E., and J. C. Rabinowitz. 1948. The microbiological activity of pyridoxylamino acids. J. Am. Chem. Soc. *70*:3432–3434.

Srncova, V., and J. Davidek. 1972. Reaction of pyridoxal and pyridoxal-5-phosphate with proteins. Reaction of pyridoxal with milk serum proteins. J. Food Sci. *37*:310–312.

Stokes, J. L., L. L. Larson, C. R. Woodward, and J. W. Foster. 1943. A *Neurospora* assay for pyridoxine. J. Biol. Chem. *150*:17–24.

Tappan, D. V., U. J. Lewis, A. H. Methfessel, and C. A. Elvehjem. 1953. Studies concerning the pyridoxine requirements of rats receiving highly processed rations. J. Nutr. *51*:479–490.

Toepfer, E. W., and M. M. Polansky. 1970. Microbiological assay of vitamin B₆ and its components. J. Assoc. Off. Agric. Chem. *53*:546–550.

Toepfer, E. W., M. M. Polansky, L. R. Richardson, and S. Wilkes. 1963. Comparison of vitamin B₆ values of selected food samples by bioassay and microbiological assay. J. Agric. Food Chem. *11*:523–525.

Tomarelli, R. M., E. R. Spence, and F. W. Bernhart. 1955. Biological availability of vitamin B₆ in heated milk. J. Agric. Food. Chem. *3*:338–341.

Yen, J. T., A. H. Jensen, and D. H. Baker. 1976. Assessment of the concentration of biologically available vitamin B₆ in corn and soybean meal. J. Anim. Sci. *42*:866–870.

6

Vitamin B₆: Nutritional and Pharmaceutical Usage, Stability, Bioavailability, Antagonists, and Safety

J. C. BAUERNFEIND *and* O. N. MILLER

INTRODUCTION

Vitamins B₆ was first recognized as a distinct vitamin entity by György (1934; 1935) as the rat acrodynia preventing factor and 2 years later by Lepkovsky *et al.* (1936) as an essential nutrient for chickens. Vitamin B₆ subsequently became known as a complex of active compounds through the research of Snell *et al.* (1942) and Snell and Rannefeld (1945) with microorganisms. Isolation of pyridoxine (pyridoxin or pyridoxol), the principal component, was accomplished in 1938 by five different teams acting independently followed by synthesis by four other teams in 1939. Pyridoxine occurs naturally in plants by biosynthesis, and in animals, as a result of consumption of plant foods. It is a required nutrient (Hawkins and Barsky, 1948; Snyderman *et al.*, 1953; Coursin, 1954; Molony and Parmelee, 1954; Bessey *et al.*, 1957; Coursin, 1964; Canham *et al.*, 1964; Horrigan, 1968) and a necessary component of the daily diet of man. In mammalian tissues, the enzymic conversion compounds, pyridoxal and pyridoxamine (pyridoxamin) are also present, plus the physiologically active forms, pyridoxal phosphate (codecarboxylase) and pyridoxamine phosphate. Vitamin B₆ functions as a coenzyme in the metabolism of protein, carbohydrate, and fat. In protein metabolism it participates in decarboxylation, transamination, dehydration, and transsulphuration of amino acids. It participates in the conversion of tryptophan to niacin or to serotonin. In its functions it interrelates with other vitamins such as riboflavin, cyanocobalamin, ascorbic acid, and vitamin E and minerals such as zinc, potassium, and sodium. It is associated with brain metabolism, the development of immune mechanisms, the formation of endogenous oxalates, the occurrence of dental caries, and anemia.

PYRIDOXINE BY CHEMICAL SYNTHESIS

Pyridoxine as the hydrochloride salt (Table 6-1) has been in commercial production since the early 1940's. Pyridoxine, 2-methyl-3-hydroxy-4,5-bis(hydroxymethyl)pyridine, or 5-hydroxy-6-methyl-3,4-pyridine-dimethanol, has the empirical formula $C_8H_{11}NO_3$, molecular weight 169.28, melting point 160°C; its hydrochloride, molecular weight 205.64, forms platelets or rods that melt with decomposition at 202–206°C. Pyridoxine hydrochloride $C_8H_{11}NO_3 \cdot HCl$ is a white to practically white crystal or crystalline powder. Pyridoxine hydrochloride is soluble in water, ethanol, and propylene glycol, sparingly soluble in acetone, and insoluble in ether or chloroform.

Since the early 1940's to date, production of pyridoxine hydrochloride has constantly increased, and the bulk selling price in terms of dollars per kilo has decreased from several thousand to $50 or less. As currently produced, pyridoxine hydrochloride meets all specifications (Table 6-1) of the U.S. Pharmacopeia XIX (1975) and Food Chemicals Codex II (1972).

TYPE OF USAGE

Pyridoxine hydrochloride is utilized in pharamceutical liquid and dry preparations, in nutritional food supplements, and in the fortification of foods and animal feeds.

In the successful development of acceptable vitamin dosage forms, the compounding pharmacist needs to have (1) knowledge of the fundamental aspects of vitamin chemistry, (2) the application knowledge of the different forms of the vitamin, (3) experience in the different techniques of manufacture, and (4) the judicious employment of adequate overages based on previous trials in the art and science of pharmaceutical manufacturing. Interaction of vitamins among themselves and the general factors in pharmaceutical dosage form preparation such as light, heat, pH, moisture, trace elements, formulation additives, diluents, and excipients influence the successful preparation

TABLE 6-1   Description and Specifications[a] of Pyridoxine
Hydrochloride (Vitamin B_6 Hydrochloride), U.S. Pharmacopoeia and
Food Chemicals Codex

Description
  Pyridoxine hydrochloride is a white, odorless, crystalline powder.

Physical-Chemical Properties
  Empirical formula $C_8H_{11}NO_3 \cdot HCl$
  Molecular weight   205.64
  Structure

  Melting point   202.0–206.0°C
  Solubility at room temperature (23°C)   One g dissolves in 16 ml of
                                          water and about 100 ml of alcohol.
                                          Insoluble in ether.

Specifications
  Pyridoxine hydrochloride meets all the requirements of U.S. Pharmacopoeia XIX and
  the Food Chemicals Codex II when tested according to those methods.
  Identification   Positive
  pH   2.0–4.0 (10% aqueous solution)
  Loss on drying   Maximum 0.1%
  Residue on ignition   Maximum 0.1%
  Chloride content   16.9–17.6% (dry basis)
  Heavy metals   Maximum 20 ppm
  Assay   Minimum 98.0% (dry basis)
  Mesh size   Minimum 95% through
                                          No. 100 U.S. standard sieve

Stability
  Pyridoxine hydrochloride is stable in dry form, but exposure to excessive heat, alkali,
  or light should be avoided. Protect solutions from light.

Uses
  Pyridoxine hydrochloride is used in the manufacture of both dry and liquid pharmaceutical preparations—tablets, capsules, and ampuls. Coated pyridoxine hydrochloride is recommended for chewable tablets.
  Pyridoxine hydrochloride is also widely used in the vitamin nutrification of foods.

FDA Status
  Pyridoxine hydrochloride is generally recognized as safe (GRAS) as a nutrient.

Storage and Handling
  Store at room temperature (15° to 30°C) in a dry place. Protect from light.

Label Suggestion for Product Use
  Label in terms of milligrams of pyridoxine, which is the reference form of vitamin B_6.
  1.21 mg of pyridoxine hydrochloride provide 1.00 mg of pyridoxine and must be listed
  as the ingredient form.

[a]As manufactured by Roche.

TABLE 6-2   Pyridoxine Hydrochloride Injection[a]

Category
  Vitamin B_6 (enzyme cofactor)
Usual dose
  Prophylactic: intramuscular or intravenous, 2 mg once a day
  Therapeutic: intramuscular or intravenous, 10–105 mg 1 to 3 times a day
Usual dose range
  2–600 mg daily
Injections available
  Injection usually available contains the following amounts of pyridoxine hydrochloride: 50 and 100 mg/ml

SOURCE: U.S. Pharmacopoeia, XIX Edition (1975).
[a]Pyridoxine hydrochloride injection is a sterile solution of pyridoxine hydrochloride in water for injection.

of products acceptable to consumers for their intended purpose. In addition to pure crystalline pyridoxine hydrochloride, micronized pyridoxine hydrochloride coated with a mixture of monoglyceride and diglycerides of edible fatty acids is available to industry for incorporation into product dosage forms where odor, flavor, or stability problems are encountered. Pharmaceutical dosage forms containing pyridoxine include pyridoxine hydrochloride injectable (Table 6-2); pyridoxine hydrochloride tablets (Table 6-3); multivitamin parenterals, multivitamin tablets, and multivitamin capsules (Table 6-4).

Pharmaceutical preparations usually contain 1–100 mg of pyridoxine hydrochloride per milliliter or tablet, depending on the product. Par-

TABLE 6-3   Pyridoxine Hydrochloride Tablets[a]

Category
  Vitamin B_6 (enzyme cofactor)
Usual dose
  Prophylactic: 2 mg once a day
  Therapeutic: 10–150 mg 1 to 3 times a day
Usual dose range
  2–600 mg daily
Tablets available
  Tablets usually available contain the following amounts of pyridoxine hydrochloride: 10, 25, 50, and 100 mg

SOURCE: U.S. Pharmacopoeia, XIX Edition (1975).
[a]Pyridoxine hydrochloride tablets contain not less than 95.0 percent and not more than 115.0 percent of the labeled amount of $C_8H_{11}NO_3 \cdot HCl$.

TABLE 6-4   Vitamin Products

Product Type	Range in Pyridoxine Content, mg per dose
Pediatric drops	0.5–1
B-complex supplement	1–3
One-a-day supplement	1–3
High-potency iron supplement with vitamins	1–8
Prenatal nutritional supplement	1–10
High-potency multivitamin supplement	5–20
High-potency B-complex supplement	10–40
Estrogenic steroid supplement	25–50

enteral solutions containing 50–100 mg pyridoxine hydrochloride per milliliter represent the range of most therapeutic vitamin B_6 parenteral formulas. Pharmaceutical preparations (Tables 6-2 to 6-4) of vitamin B_6 alone or multivitamin combinations containing vitamin B_6 may be divided into two major groups: (1) therapeutic and (2) prophylactic. Another division would be vitamin B-complex preparations containing pyridoxine with and without fat-soluble vitamins. There are also parenteral and oral B-complex preparations with and without vitamin C containing pyridoxine hydrochloride in varying amounts. Lastly, there are special purpose dosage forms. Nutritional supplements such as daily vitamin supplements in liquid or dry form entail similar problems in formulation. However, in these prophylactic products the pyridoxine hydrochloride content is lower than that in therapeutic preparations, depending on the age of subjects taking the preparation, their physiological state, and frequency of administration. Vitamin B_6 market forms are available from a number of manufacturers of pharmaceutical and food supplement products.

About 25 years ago the importance of the relationship of vitamin B_6 to infant nutrition and the tragic results that can follow were indicated when physicians observed convulsive seizures in infants fed a commercially prepared modified cow's milk (May, 1954). The likely cause was judged to be vitamin B_6 deficiency. Snyderman et al. (1953) had observed convulsive seizures in a mentally defective infant maintained on a vitamin B_6-free diet. The report of Molony and Parmelee (1954) and several papers by Coursin (Coursin, 1954; 1955a, b; 1956, 1964) quickly established the seizures developed on the milk product to be due to low intake of vitamin B_6. Infants with seizures were treated by intramuscular or oral administration of pyridoxine hydrochloride, and complete recoveries were observed. Furthermore, the offending modified cow's milk product was found to be low in vitamin B$_6$ content. Lastly, Tomarelli *et al.* (1955) reported heat treatment of milk to lower the biological value of vitamin B$_6$ in milk. Coursin's studies showed that a suboptimal intake of 60 μg of vitamin B$_6$ per liter of milk lowers thresholds of central nervous system activity, lowers mineral retention, and increases xanthurenic acid excretion, defects overcome by higher pyridoxine administration. Since the early 1950's many U.S. infant formulas have been fortified with added pyridoxine hydrochloride by manufacturers as a prophylactic measure.

The Panel of the Committee on Food Standards and Fortification Policy of the Food and Nutrition Board, National Research Council/ National Academy of Sciences (1974) proposed that (1) since cereal-grain products constitute 26 percent of the daily caloric intake, (2) since they are suitable carriers for the addition of nutrients to the diet because of their broad usage by almost everyone in the United States, and (3) since there is evidence of potential risk of deficiency of vitamin A, thiamin, riboflavin, niacin, vitamin B$_6$, folacin, iron, calcium, magnesium, and zinc among significant segments of the population, cereal-grain products be nutrified with these 10 nutrients (Table 6-5). A pyridoxine level of 2 mg/lb of cereal-grain product has been proposed. A substantial governmental grant has been made to a university to investigate this proposal and extend available data. Currently, refined

TABLE 6-5   Nutrients and Levels Recommended for Inclusion in Nutrification of Cereal-Grain Products[a]

Nutrient	Levels Recommended	
	mg/lb	mg/100 g
Vitamin A[b]	2.2	0.48
Thiamin	2.9	0.64
Riboflavin	1.8	0.40
Niacin	24.0	5.29
Vitamin B$_6$	2.0	0.44
Folic acid	0.3	0.07
Iron	40	8.81
Calcium	900	198.2
Magnesium	200	44.1
Zinc	10	2.2

SOURCE: Food and Nutrition Board (1974).
[a]Wheat flour, corn grits, cornmeal, rice. Other cereal-grain products in proportion to their cereal-grain content.
[b]Retinol equivalent.

and processed cereal-grain products such as white bread are only nutrified with thiamin, riboflavin, niacin, and iron. Food products to
which pyridoxine hydrochloride has been added include texturized
proteins, instant-type breakfasts, milk replacers, and some breakfast
cereals.

Fuller (1964) concluded 10 years ago that to ensure the well-being of
and to permit maximum expectation of economical production in farm
animals, nutritionists should provide supplemental pyridoxine in feeds
for monogastric animals of all species during the active period of
growth and reproduction. This is essentially what is done today in
many commercial feeds (Bauernfeind, 1974) in the United States (Table
6-6). The amount added varies from 1 to 10 mg/kg of feed, depending on
species, age, activity, stress of performance, formulation of the ration,
and field use experience.

TABLE 6-6 Vitamin Additions to U.S. Commercial Feeds

Added Nutrients	Type of Feed or Ration
Vitamins A, D_3, E, K, thiamin, ribo-flavin, *pyridoxine*, cyanocobalamin, folic acid, niacin, pantothenate, choline	Chicken starter, broiler, breeder; turkey starter, breeder; swine starter, breeder; fish starter, fry, grower, breeder; horse grower, breeder; fur animal grower, breeder; dog and cat dry meals
Vitamins A, D_3, E, K, riboflavin, cyanocobalamin, folic acid, niacin, pantothenate, choline	Chicken grower, developer, layer; turkey grower,[a] finisher[a]; swine grower[a]
Vitamins A, D_3, E	Lamb fattener; sheep breeder; beef cattle fattener, breeder, supplement; dairy cattle, milker, breeder, supplement
Biotin	Chicken breeder; turkey starter, breeder; swine starter, breeder
L-ascorbic acid	Fish starter, fry, grower, breeder; certain stress animal feeds; certain laboratory animal feeds

SOURCE: Bauernfeind (1974).
[a]Pyridoxine is also added.

STABILITY

Fortunately, pyridoxine hydrochloride is a rather stable compound (Table 6-1) and presents less difficulty in incorporating it into products than do many of the other vitamins. Crystalline pyridoxine hydrochloride is stable in air but is slowly affected by sunlight if exposed sufficiently. Acidic solutions of pyridoxine hydrochloride are stable and may be heated 30 minutes at 120°C without decomposition. Likewise, pyridoxine hydrochloride solutions are not easily affected by heating with mild alkali, nitrous acid, and ethyl nitrite. Alkaline or neutral aqueous solutions are sensitive to light with subsequent destruction of the vitamin after sufficient exposure. Discolorations and loss of potency can occur in the presence of trace metal ions such as iron.

Overages above label claim for pharmaceutical preparations are customarily added to vitamin formulations during manufacture as a means of maintaining at least the claimed level of each vitamin for the normal shelf life of the product and to allow for variation in assay performance. The percent overage for each particular vitamin will vary according to the stability pattern of the particular vitamin, the type of product, and the shelf life expectancy of the product. In general, problems of instability of vitamins are much more actue in multivitamin liquids than in single-vitamin liquid formulations or in single-vitamin or multivitamin solid dosage forms. With only a single, active vitamin ingredient, the vehicle and the end product form can be chosen for optimal physical and chemical compatibility with the particular individual vitamin, whereas with multiple formulations, optimal stability must be directed toward an averaged situation or else special formulating techniques must be utilized. The shelf life of pharmaceutical dosage forms should be at least 18 months for a liquid vitamin product and 24 months or more for dry or solid dosage products to be commercially feasible. Storage at normal room temperature for the shelf life and accelerating aging tests are in common practice in the pharmaceutical trade, and manufacturing overages are established on the basis of anticipated stability under such conditions.

Pyridoxine hydrochloride incorporated into an array of pharmaceutical liquid and dry products (Roche Product Development Department data) and stored 1 year at room temperature (23°C) or 6 weeks at high temperature (45°C) usually shows losses of less than 10 percent (Figure 6-1). Hence an overage of 10 to 15 percent is usually quite adequate to maintain claimed vitamin B_6 potency for an extended shelf life period. Attention must be given to ingredients in the formulation, particularly

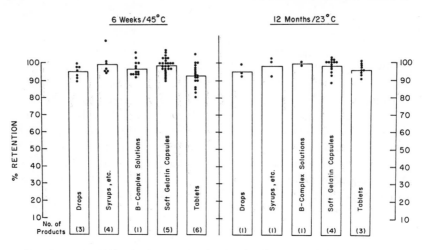

FIGURE 6-1   Stability of added pyridoxine in vitamin preparations (Roche Product Development Department Data).

minerals, as these may influence a stability pattern unfavorably. With experienced research pharmacists developing these products and with long periods of testing prior to marketing, these influences become minimal or nonexistent.

Stability data for foods indicate that pyridoxal and pyridoxamine are significantly less stable than pyridoxine; however, these latter forms of vitamin B_6 are not currently manufactured on a large scale or currently added to pharmaceutical or nutritional products. Vitamin B_6 occurs in natural food products in the three forms—pyridoxine, pyridoxal, and pyridoxamine. Fresh milk contains a high level of pyridoxal in the free and phosphate ester form (Rabinowitz and Snell, 1948). Woodring and Storvick (1960), reviewing natural vitamin B_6 in milk, considered heat treatment such as sterilization to cause lowered vitamin B_6 values because of the greater heat lability of pyridoxal and pyridoxamine present in milk. Hodson (1956) demonstrated the conversion of pyridoxal to pyridoxamine and then to another form during processing and storage of evaporated milk. Bernhart et al. (1960) reported a reaction product of pyridoxal and cysteine to be identical to the form found in evaporated, heat-sterilized milk. Pyridoxal interaction with SH groups during thermal processing is probably responsible for the decrease in natural vitamin B_6 content. Exposure of fluid milk to sunlight has also been reported to destroy vitamin B_6 (Shiroishi and Hayakawa, 1961; Hellström, 1960).

Hassinen et al. (1954) found high losses of natural vitamin B_6 in sterilized liquid infant formula. Added crystalline pyridoxine hydrochloride was much more stable in the infant formulas under the same conditions of heating. Spray drying caused some loss of vitamin B_6 but less than in liquid processing and sterilization. Trials at Roche have also demonstrated good stability of added pyridoxine hydrochloride in heat-processed and stored infant formulas (Table 6-7).

In the milling of hard and soft wheat into flour, 10 to 25 percent of the natural vitamin B_6 content is retained, half or more of which is in the form of pyridoxine (Polansky and Toepfer, 1969). Schroeder (1971) reported extensive data on vitamin and mineral losses in the processing of cereal-grain products. Vitamin B_6 losses were great. Nutrient losses in the processing of food have been reviewed by Nesheim (1974).

In the proposed fortification of cereal-grain products with 10 nutrients including pyridoxine, studies were carried out at Roche to test the stability of the added nutrients in milled white wheat flour, yellow

TABLE 6-7   Stability of Added Pyridoxine in Infant Formula

Product	Condition	Added Pyridoxine, mg/liter	Assayed Pyridoxine Content, mg/liter	Assayed Pyridoxine Content, % retained
Modified cow's milk, heat processed in cans and stored at different conditions	After processing	None	0.46	—
		0.5	0.94	96
	After processing	None	0.52	—
		1.0	1.59	100
	Stored 500 h, 45°C	None	0.47	—
		0.5	0.94	100
		1.0	1.41	94
	Stored 1000 h, 45°C	None	0.43	—
		0.5	0.93	100
		None	0.48	—
		1.0	1.37	89
	Stored 6 months, 23°C	None	0.46	—
		0.5	0.90	88
		None	0.40	—
		1.0	1.33	93
	Stored 12 months, 23°C	None	0.38	—
		0.5	0.84	92
		None	0.43	—
		1.0	1.40	97

SOURCE: Roche Product Development Data.

corn meal, white rice, cooked rice, and baked bread. For the fortification study, special vitamin-mineral premixes were prepared. The stability of added pyridoxine hydrochloride was checked out in the premix,
in the fortified cereal-grain products, and with the heat-treated rice and
bread products (Cort *et al.*, 1976). No stability problems were encountered in any of the products with added pyridoxine hydrochloride (Table 6-8). Hennessy *et al.* (1960) as early as 1960 reported excellent
recoveries of pyridoxine hydrochloride added to flour and then baked
into bread. Bunting (1965) extended these cereal-grain studies. He observed the retention of pyridoxine to be 90 percent or greater in corn
meal and in macaroni following shelf storage for 1 year at 38°C at 50
percent relative humidity. In the making of corn bread, 100 percent of
the pyridoxine present in the meal was retained. In cooking macaroni,
a 50 percent loss was encountered by water drainage. Recently, Anderson *et al.* (1976) reported on the effects of processing and storage on
micronutrients in breakfast cereals. Added pyridoxine hydrochloride
showed excellent stability during storage tests of 3 months at 40°C and
6 months at 22°C. Ample evidence exists now to demonstrate that
fortification of cereal-grain products with added pyridoxine hydrochloride is technically feasible.

TABLE 6-8   Stability of Added Pyridoxine in Cereal-Grain Products

Product	Condition	Assayed Pyridoxine Content, mg/1b	Assayed Pyridoxine Content, % retained
Vitamin-iron premix	Initial	14.8	—
	6 months, 23°C	14.6	99
White wheat flour	Initial	2.35	—
	6 months, 23°C	2.20	94
	12 weeks, 45°C	2.10	90
Baked bread	After baking	9.64	—
	5 days, 23°C	9.82	100
Yellow corn meal	Initial	2.80	—
	6 months, 23°C	2.80	100
	12 weeks, 45°C	2.50	89
Rice premix[a]	Initial	141.0	—
	3 months, 23°C	140.0	99

SOURCE: Cort *et al.* (1976).
[a]No loss in cooking rice at the nutrified level, 2.1 mg/1b.

In the technology involved in the fortification of feed with vitamins, frequently, vitamin-mineral premixes are prepared with variable storage periods before a given premix is introduced into the feed proper. These premixes contain trace mineral salts of copper, iron, manganese, zinc, etc. Partial destruction of pyridoxine in such premixes has been experienced during storage and could occur in similar premixes used for the fortification of foods. To avoid such destructive incidents, low moisture levels are desirable, and coatings are helpful to provide an interphase between reactants. As currently practiced commercially, added pyridoxine hydrochloride to mash and pelleted animal rations is stable (Bauernfeind, 1974).

BIOAVAILABILITY

Bioavailability of pyridoxine from a given product dosage form may be considered as the percentage of vitamin in that product that enters the systemic circulation in an active form after oral administration of the product. Vitamins are nutrients and are natural components of mammalian tissues; hence, it is important to attain maximum absorption of the given dose from a product dosage form. Various biochemical laboratory techniques have been investigated, developed, and employed in assessing bioavailability (Sauberlich *et al.*, 1974). For the water-soluble vitamins (except vitamin B_{12}), urinary excretion of the vitamins or vitamin metabolites (indirect measurements) are most commonly used in assessing bioavailability. The technique for determining bioavailability of water-soluble vitamins for humans was first introduced in 1945 (Melnick *et al.*, 1945; Oser *et al.*, 1945). Normal human subjects consuming average diets without additional supplementation with vitamin products vary widely in the degree of saturation of their tissues with vitamins; hence, relatively uniform excretion patterns can only be achieved by saturating the subjects with the vitamin prior to administering the standard or test doses of the vitamin and measuring appropriate urinary excretions.

Pyridoxine is absorbed readily from the intestinal tract by humans. Only a small fraction of ingested pyridoxine is excreted unchanged in the urine. In man, 4-pyridoxic acid accounts for a large percentage of the urinary excretion products of vitamin B_6 (Rabinowitz and Snell, 1949). In normal human subjects the urinary excretion of 4-pyridoxic acid is directly proportional to the quantity of pyridoxine consumed, provided that at the time of the tests the subjects are subsisting on an adequate diet and that their tissues are saturated with the vitamins under test. The linear dose-response relationship for the test is established by feeding pure pyridoxine in solution (its most completely available form) as a standard and, during another time period, feeding the test product to the same subjects and comparing the test product response to the response of the standard. In our laboratory this technique has been applied to pyridoxine and other water-soluble vitamins.

Data have been obtained on a number of pyridoxine products, and if properly formulated, the pyridoxine contained therein can be demonstrated to be fully biologically available (Table 6-9). Usually, pyridoxine hydrochloride is not chosen as the indicator vitamin in a multivitamin preparation to be tested for biological availability. A less soluble one is selected, on the basis that if it is fully available in the test, those more soluble will be equally available. Emphasis of *in vivo* vitamin absorption has been placed on the excretion of riboflavin, primarily because of its relative insolubility. If a tablet granulation is made with a uniform mixture of the water-soluble vitamins and with water-dispersible beadlets or powders containing the fat-soluble vitamins (a usual procedure), the finding in the urinary excretion test that the riboflavin from the finished tablet is fully available to the body makes it evident that the tablet has disintegrated suitably in the upper portion of the gastrointestinal tract (Table 6-10). After *in vivo* tests such as are described above are correlated with *in vitro* disintegration or dissolution tests for a given product, there is only a need to carry out the *in vitro* tests in routine testing of the manufactured product.

By a perfusion technique of human jejunum, Nelson et al. (1976) have demonstrated that water-soluble vitamins, namely vitamin B_6, may differ in bioavailability from natural food sources, such as orange juice, and synthetic sources and postulated that vitamin-bound forms in natural products may lower absorption performance. Synthetic pyridoxine hydrochloride was judged highly available by this tech-

TABLE 6-9   Bioavailability of Pyridoxine[a] in Formulated Products

Product	No. of Subjects in Test	Dose Adminis- tered, mg	Dose Excreted in 24 h, %	Availability, %
Standard[a]	6	100	38.6	—
Coated pyridox- ine HCl	6	102	38.3	99
Standard[a]	6	5.3	11.7	—
Multivitamin tablet	6	5.3	11.2	95

SOURCE: Roche Product Development Department Data.
[a]Water solution of pyridoxine hydrochloride.

TABLE 6-10 Bioavailability of Water-Soluble Vitamins in a Multivitamin-Mineral Tablet

Vitamin	Product	No. of Subjects on Test	Dose Administered, mg	Dose Excreted in 24 h, %	Availability, %
Thiamin	Standard	5	5.0	18	—
	Test	5	5.9	22	122
Riboflavin	Standard	5	10.0	53	—
	Test	5	10.6	55	104
Niacinamide	Standard	5	50.0	21	—
	Test	5	55.0	20	95
Ascorbic acid	Standard	5	200.0	49	—
	Test	5	173.0	48	98

SOURCE: Oser *et al.* (1945).

nique. Lantz (1939) concluded that the cooking of pinto beans increased the bioavailability of vitamin B_6, suggesting release from a bound form.

DRUG AND CHEMICAL INTERACTIONS; ANTAGONISTS

Drugs can impair vitamin absorption, increase vitamin excretion, or interfere with vitamin utilization, so that a drug-induced vitamin deficiency can occur even when the diet is adequate for normal maintenance. In such instances, administration of larger doses of the vitamin to compensate for that rendered ineffective by the drug is indicated (Roe, 1973).

The antituberculosis drug, isonicotinic acid hydrazide (INH) increases vitamin B_6 excretion in urine, and the higher the drug use, the greater is the loss of the vitamin (Roe et al., 1973; Nutrition Reviews, 1968; Standal et al., 1974). Symptoms of pyridoxine-responsive neuritis (Coyer and Nicholson, 1976; Afifi and Sabra, 1968) or anemia can occur. It is believed that the drug competes with pyridoxal phosphate in the metabolism of tryptophan. Hydrazide drugs form hydrazone complexes with pyridoxal phosphate and inactivate the coenzyme. Penicillamine (Roe, 1973; Kuchinskas and de Vigneaud, 1957; Tomono et al., 1973; Jaffee et al., 1964), a specific antidote in copper poisoning, also forms complexes with pyridoxal. It is used at some centers prophylactically in children with incipient Wilson's disease in the expectation of preventing the onset of overt disease. Prolonged use of penicillamine or high doses can cause vitamin B_6-deficiency symptoms (Smith and Gallagher, 1970; Hollister et al., 1966; Lotz et al., 1966). Penicillamine has chelating properties (Rosen et al., 1964) which raises the question of whether other effective chelating agents, such as ethylenediaminetetraacetic acid (EDTA), a food additive, directly or indirectly interact with the vitamin B_6 function. The antibiotic cycloserine (Roe, 1973; Holtz and Palm, 1964; Cohen, 1969), used in patients resistant to INH, and hydralazine (Roe 1973; Afifi and Sabra, 1968; Raskin and Fishman, 1965; Kirkendall and Page, 1958), an antihypertensive agent, also act as antagonists. The administration of vitamin B_6 along with these drugs helps reduce some of the neurological side effects. Antagonism exists between the anti-Parkinson drug L-dopa (Roe, 1973; Leon et al., 1971; Yahr et al., 1972; Hussar, 1973) and pyridoxine, reflecting the formation of a Schiff base between an amino acid and pyridoxal phosphate. An example of antagonism in which the enzymic potential function of pyridoxine is diminished is the reported block in the conversion of pyridoxine to pyridoxal described in alcoholics (Hines and Cowan, 1970). A high incidence of vitamin B_6 hypovitaminemia has been noted in alcoholics (Leevy *et al.*, 1965; Lunde, 1960).

Various vitamin B_6 antimetabolite structures having unreactive groups at position 4 or 5 on the molecule, such as 5-deoxypyridoxal, 4-deoxypyridoxine, 4-methoxypyridoxine and many others are antagonistic to a greater or lesser degree to vitamin B_6 biologically active structures (Rosen *et al.*, 1964; Umbreit, 1955; McCormick and Snell, 1961; Hoff-Jorgensen, 1966; Sauberlich, 1968; Korytnyk and Lachmann, 1971; Korytnyk *et al.*, 1973). The 4-vinyl analog of pyridoxal is a more potent vitamin B_6 antagonist than 4-deoxypyridoxine according to Korytnyk *et al.* (1973). The pyrimidine moiety (Makino *et al.*, 1954; Shintani, 1956; Scheunert *et al.*, 1956–57; Nishizawa *et al.*, 1975) of thiamin when injected in mice or rats causes convulsions. This effect is eliminated by administration of vitamin B_6. The phosphorylated pyrimidine seems to be a potent antagonist of pyridoxal phosphate. Castrix, 2-chloro-4-dimethylamino-6-methylpyrimidine, a rodenticide, also functions as a vitamin B_6 antagonist (Nishizawa *et al.*, 1975). Other vitamin B_6 antagonists (Table 6-11) are decaborane (Naeger, 1971; Wykes and Laudez, 1967), pentaborane (Mindrum, 1964), procarbazine (Chabner *et al.*, 1969), chloroquine (d'Eshougues *et al.*, 1961), mitomycin C (Fujimoto, 1966; Mastsunaga *et al.*, 1966; Bradner, 1972), bacimethrin (Tanaka *et al.*, 1962), hydrazine (Frierson, 1965; Kirklin *et al.*, 1976; Dubnick *et al.*, 1960), hydrocortisone (Rose and Braidman, 1971), imipramine (Gordon, 1964), phenelzine (Dubnick *et al.*, 1960; Gordon, 1964; Leeson *et al.*, 1959), piperazine (Kulz, 1964), semicarbazide (Banna, 1973), thiosemicarbazide (Eidelberg and Buchwald, 1970; Yamashite, 1974; Davanzo *et al.*, 1961), strophanthin (Eremeev, 1968), and amino carcinogens (Dyer and Morris, 1961; Melicow *et al.*, 1964). Chlorpromazine, promazine, methapyrilene hydrochloride, and methantheline bromide appear also to be antagonists (McLaughlan *et al.*, 1960) in microbial studies. Hydrazine is a component of high-energy rocket fuel, and some people excessively exposed to it exhibit hydrazine poisoning. An excess of choline in the diet of the chick has been shown to be a stress on the metabolic pool of pyridoxal phosphate, which was relieved with supplementary dietary pyridoxine. Rats exposed to carbon disulphide show a distinct decrease in blood plasma level of pyridoxal phosphate. The role of interfering chemicals in the pharmacological aspects of vitamin B_6 has been reviewed by Holtz and Palm (1964) and others (Rosen *et al.*, 1964; Hussar, 1973; Umbreit, 1955; Sauberlich, 1968; Reynolds, 1975; Woodbury, 1969).

TABLE 6-11 Partial List of Chemical Structures Interfering with Vitamin $B_6{}^a$

Compound	Structure	Comment	Reference
Agaritine (β-N-[γ-L(+)-glutamyl]-4-hydroxymethylphenyl-hydrazine)	NHNHCOCH₂CH₂–CHCOO⁻ (with NH₃⁺, CH₂OH)	Constituent of the commercial, edible mushroom, *Agaricus bisporus*; natural compound responsible for vitamin B_6 interference	Klosterman, 1974
l-amino-D-proline		Hydrolyzed compound of linatine present in flax seed and linseed meal; antagonist to vitamin B_6 in animal studies	Klosterman, 1974; Kratzer, 1947; Kratzer and Williams, 1948; Klosterman *et al.*, 1960, 1967
Bacimethrin (4-Amino-2-methoxy-5-pyrimidinemethanol)		Antibiotic substance; produced by *Bacillus megatherium*; interference with antimicrobial action shown by pyridoxine	Tanaka *et al.*, 1962
Canaline	H₂NOCH₂CH₂CHCO₂H (with NH₂)	Hydrolyzed compound of canavanine present in beans; forms oximes with pyridoxal or pyridoxal phosphate; inhibitor of pyridoxal phosphate-dependent enzymes	Klosterman, 1974
Canavanine (2-Amino-4-(guanidinooxy) butyric acid)	NH₂N-CNHCH₂CH₂CHCO₂H (with NH, NH₂)	Present in the jack bean, *Canavalia ensiformis*; natural compound responsible for vitamin B_6 interference	Klosterman, 1974

Compound	Structure	Description	Reference
Carbon bisulfide (dithiocarbonic anhydride)	CS_2	Industrial chemical; inhalation and skin contact causes mental, auditory, visual, and dermal changes; inhalation studies with animals show a distinct plasma pyridoxal phosphase decrease, considered a reflection of binding of B_6 forms with CS_2 metabolites	Gorny, 1971
Chloroquine (7-chloro-4-(4-diethyl-amino-1-methylbutyl-amino) quinoline)	$HN-CH(CH_2)_3N(C_2H_5)_2$, CH_3	Suppressive antimalarial; extraintestinal amebicide; administration of vitamin B_6 suppresses drug intolerance	d'Eshougues et al., 1961
Choline (β-hydroxyethyl) trimethylammonium hydroxide)	OH, $(CH_3)_3\overset{+}{N}CH_2CH_2OH$	Lipotropic agent, nutritional factor; excess choline can stress metabolic pool of pyridoxal phosphate as shown in animal studies	Saville et al., 1967
Cycloserine (D-4-amino-3-isoxazolidinone)		Antibiotic substance; antimicrobial, antimycobacterial; produced naturally by several actinomyces; anti-tubercular drug; inhibitor of pyridoxal phosphate enzymes; pyridoxine reduces cycloserine toxicity in man	Roe, 1973; Holtz and Palm, 1964; Cohen, 1969
β-Cyanoalanine	$N\equiv C-CH_2-CH-COH$, H_2N, O	A neurotoxin from *Vicia* species whose toxic manifestations are partially reversed by pyridoxal in animal studies	Klosterman, 1974

Table 6-11 (Continued)

Compound	Structure	Comment	Reference
Decarborane (DB) (decarboron tetradecahydride)	$B_{10}H_{14}$	Rocket propellant; industrial chemical; nausea, dizziness, tremors result following contact by man; in animal studies, pretreatment with vitamin B_6 lowers antagonism of DB	Naeger, 1971; Wykes and Laudez, 1967
L-Dopa (3-(3,4-dihydroxy-phenyl)-L-alanine)		Drug used in treatment of Parkinson disease; also a natural constituent in the plant tissues of the genus *Mucuna*; antagonizes vitamin B_6; adverse effects alleviated by B_6 forms	Roe, 1973; Leon et al., 1971; Yahr et al., 1972; Hussar, 1973
Ethanol	CH_3-CH_2OH	Toxicant; excessive alcohol inbibing lowers *in vivo* enzymic conversion of pyridoxine to pyridoxal; alcoholics have low vitamin B_6 tissue levels	Hines and Cowan, 1970; Leevy et al., 1965; Lunde, 1960
n-2-fluorenylacetamide (2-acetylamino-fluorene)		Amino carcinogen; enhanced excretion of free and conjugated xanthurenic acid in animals; corrected by supplementary pyridoxine	Dyer and Morris, 1961; Melicow et al., 1964

Compound	Structure	Description	Reference
Gyromitrin	$CH_3CH=NNCHO$ (with CH_3)	Constituent of the desirable wild mushroom. *Gyromitra esculenta*; natural compound responsible for vitamin B_6 interference	Klosterman, 1974
Hydralazine (1-hydrazino-phthalazine)		Antihypertensive agent; dizziness, neuritis develops in man on the drug; pyridoxine supplementation is recommended	Roe, 1973, Afifi and Sabra, 1968; Raskin and Fishman, 1965; Kirkendall and Page, 1958
Hydrazine	H_2NNH_2	Rocket fuel; reducing agent; pyridoxine neuritis develops; useful in treatment of hydrazine poisoning	Frierson, 1965; Kirklin et al., 1976
Hydrocortisone		Adrenocortical steroid: produces an increase in tryptophan metabolites in the urine; prevented by simultaneous administration of vitamin B_6	Rose and Braidman, 1971
4-Hydroxymethyl phenylhydrazine		Hydrolyzed compound of agaritine; present in mushrooms; forms hydrazone derivatives with pyridoxal phosphate	Holtz and Palm, 1964; Klosterman, 1974
Imipramine (5-(3-dimethylamino-propyl)-10,11-dihydro-5H-dibenz[b,f]-azepine)		Antidepressant; tremors, mental confusion occurs in man on the drug; vitamin B_6 administration is recommended	Gordon, 1964

Table 6-11 (Continued)

Compound	Structure	Comment	Reference
Isonicotinic acid hydrazide (isoniazid)		Antitubercular agent; side effects-neuritis CNS stimulation; increases vitamin B_6 excretion in urine; administered pyridoxine prevents neuropathy or drug poisoning in man	Roe, 1973; *Nutrition Reviews*, 1968; Standal *et al.*, 1974; Coyer and Nicholson, 1976; Afifi and Sabra, 1968
Linatine		Constituent of flax seed; natural compound responsible for vitamin B_6 interference	Klosterman, 1974
N-Methyl-N formyl hydrazine	CH_3 H_2NNCHO	Hydrolyzed compound of gyromitrin present in mushrooms; pyridoxine used as an antidote in mushroom poisoning due to hydrazine consumption	Klosterman, 1974
Methylhydrazine	H_2NNHCH_3	Hydrolyzed compound of gyromitrin present in mushrooms; depresses plasma pyridoxal phosphate; a probable inhibitor of pyridoxal kinase reaction; pyridoxine is used to counteract poisoning	Chabner *et al.*, 1969; Klosterman, 1974
Mimosine (3-hydroxy-4-oxo-1(4H)-pyridine; alanine)		Constituent in the seed and foliage of *Mimosa* and *Leucaena*; toxic to animals; effects partially overcome by pyridoxine	Klosterman, 1974

Mitomycin C		Antineoplastic agent; administration of drug lowers pyridoxal tissue levels, especially pyridoxal phosphate in the liver; pyridoxine counteracts some side effects of mitomycin in animal studies; vitamin B_6 administered	Fujimoto, 1966; Mastsunaga et al., 1966; Bradner, 1972
Oral contraceptive steroids			Price et al., 1967; *Nutrition Reviews*, 1973; Luhby et al., 1971; Aly et al., 1971; Lumeng et al., 1974; Baumblatt and Winston, 1970; Winston, 1973; Rose, 1969; Rose et al., 1973; Brown, 1972
Penicillamine (D-3-mercaptovaline)	$\underset{\text{(CH}_3)_2\text{C}-\text{CHCOOH}}{\text{SH}\ \ \ \text{NH}_2}$	Chelating agent in heavy metal poisoning; growth inhibition of L-penicillamine in animals is reversed by pyridoxine; also reduces toxicity of the drug in man	Roe, 1973; Kuchinskas and du Vigneaud, 1957; Tomono et al., 1973; Jafee et al., 1964; Smith and Gallagher, 1970; Hollister et al., 1966; Lotz et al., 1964
Pentaborane (pentaboron nonahydride)	B_5H_9	Pyridoxine counteracts pentaborane intoxication	Mindrum, 1964

Table 6-11 (Continued)

Compound	Structure	Comment	Reference
Phenelzine (β-phenylethyl-hydrazine)	$C_6H_5CH_2CH_2NHNH_2$	Monoamine oxidase inhibitor; antidepressant; side effects—dizziness; pyridoxine protects against toxic doses of phenelzine in animals and man	Dubnick et al., 1960; Gordon, 1964; Leeson et al., 1959
Piperazine (hexahydropyrazine)		Anthelmintic; believed to interfere in vitamin B_6 function	Külz, 1964
Procarbazine (N-isopropyl-α-(2-methylhydrazino)-p-toluamide)	$CONHCH(CH_3)_2$ ... $CH_2NHNHCH_3$	Antineoplastic agent; administration to animals produces rapid and prolonged fall in plasma pyridoxal phosphate	Chabner et al., 1969
Pyridoxine antimetabolites 4-deformyl-4-vinyl-pyridoxal		Analog of pyridoxal: a most potent vitamin B_6 antagonist as shown in animal studies	Rosen et al., 1964; Umbreit, 1955; McCormick and Snell, 1961; Hoff-Jorgensen, 1966; Sauberlich, 1968; Korytnyk and Lachmann, 1971; Korytnyk et al., 1973
5-deoxypyridoxal		Analog of pyridoxal: vitamin B_6 antagonist; converted to phosphorylated form, competes with pyridoxal phosphate	

4-deoxypyridoxine (5-hydroxy-4,6-dimethyl-3-pyridinemethanol)	(structure)	Analog of pyridoxine; vitamin B_6 antagonist commonly used in nutritional studies where an antagonist is desired	Makino et al., 1954; Shintani, 1956; Scheunert et al., 1956-57; Nishizawa et al., 1975
Pyrimidine structures			
2-Chloro-4-dimethyl-amino-6-methyl-pyrimidine (Castrix)	(structure)	Toxicity of the rodenticide in animals is totally inhibited by simultaneous administration of vitamin B_6	
2-Methyl-4-amino-5-oxy-methylpyrimidine (toxopyrimidine)	(structure)	Pyrimidine moiety of thiamin; microbial antagonist to vitamin B_6; causes B_6 deficiency symptoms in animals when added to the diet, corrected by supplementary pyridoxine	
Semicarbazide (aminourea)	$NH_2NHCONH_2$	Pyridoxine interferes with the effects of the compound in animals	Banna, 1973
Strophanthin	Glycoside mixture from *Strophanthus kombe*	Cardiotonic; administration of pyridoxine diminishes toxic effects of the drug	Eremeev, 1968
Thiosemicarbazide	$NH_2CSNHNH_2$	Metal detection agent; pyridoxine administration relieves seizures in animals caused by thiosemi-carbazide administration	Eidelberg and Buchwald, 1970; Yamashita, 1974; Davanzo et al., 1961

[a] As cited in the literature in this incomplete survey.

Oral contraceptive agents (Price *et al.*, 1967; *Nutrition Reviews*, 1973; Luhby *et al.*, 1971; Aly *et al.*, 1971; Lumeng *et al.*, 1974) have been shown to alter the apoenzyme-coenzyme binding of pyridoxal phosphate and lower tissue pyridoxal levels, requiring additional vitamin B_6 intakes for correction. Estrogen as well as estrogen progestogen preparations may cause increased excretion of 3-hydroxykynurenine and xanthurenic acid following a tryptophan load. Administration of pyridoxine causes these abnormalities to return to normal. Depression has been reported in women on the pill, who have responded to supplementary pyridoxine administration (Baumblatt and Winston, 1970; Winston, 1973; Rose, 1969). Impairment of glucose tolerance has been reported to be caused by dietary vitamin B_6 deficiency in oral contraceptive users (Rose *et al.*, 1973). In recent years there has been concern about an increased need for vitamin B_6 in women taking oral contraceptive preparations (*Nutrition Reviews*, 1973; Baumblatt and Winston, 1970; Winston, 1973; Brown, 1972).

Klosterman (1974) recently reviewed vitamin B_6 antagonists of natural origin. Derivatives of carbonyl trapping agents, both hydrazines and hydroxylamines, have been isolated from foods. These agents generally occur in nature in the form of unreactive derivatives; however, enzymes having hydrolase or transferase activity capable of releasing the reactive carbonyl trapping agents are widely distributed in nature, including the digestive tract of mammalians. The presence or release of trapping agents in the digestive process offers the possibility for inactivation of a portion of vitamin B_6 in the metabolic pool.

A factor in linseed meal stable to dry heat but labile to autoclaving was found to have a vitamin B_6-inactivating influence when linseed meal was an ingredient in chick diets regarded as adequate in vitamin B_6 content (Kratzer, 1947). If supplementary pyridoxine is fed with the linseed meal, the toxic effect of linseed ingredient is nullified. About 10 years ago the vitamin B_6 antagonist in linseed meal was isolated and identified (Kratzer and Williams, 1948; Klosterman *et al.*, 1960; 1967) as 1-amino-D-proline, a hydrolyzed compound of linatine. An LD_{50} of 2 mg of linatine per week-old chick can be counteracted by a simultaneous injection of 1 mg of pyridoxine. Linatine is believed to inactivate vitamin B_6 by reacting with the aldehyde, pyridoxal or pyridoxal phosphate, to form stable hydrazones. 1-Amino-D-proline and asymmetrically substituted secondary hydrazines inhibit a variety of pyridoxal phosphate-requiring enzymes isolated from *E. coli*, such as glutamic aminotransferase, tryptophanase, tyrosine decarboxylase, and glutamic decarboxylase.

One of the desirable wild mushrooms *(G. esculenta)* contains

N-methyl-N-formyl hydrazine and methylhydrazine and hydrolyzed compounds of gyromitrin and when partially cooked can cause mild hydrazine poisoning for which pyridoxine is an antidote (Klosterman, 1974). Another mushroom *(A. bysoris)* can release 4-hydroxymethyl phenylhydrazine; a good carbonyl trapping agent from agaritine, the γ-glutamyl derivative of 4-hydroxymethyl phenylhydrazine contained in the mushroom. Canaline, a substituted hydroxylamine, forms oximes with pyridoxal or pyridoxal phosphate and is a potential food vitamin B_6 antagonist (Rahiala *et al.*, 1971). Canaline is formed by enzyme conversion from canavanine, a compound in the *Canavalia* species of Leguminosae, the bean class. Several actinomyces produce D-cyloserine, a substituted hydroxylamine antibiotic previously mentioned as a vitamin B_6 antagonist. L-dopa is found in the seedlings, pod, and beans of *V. faba* (broad bean) and *M. deeringiana* (velvet bean). Other natural antagonists are mimosine, 3-hydroxy-4-keto-1(4H)-pyridinealanine, in the seed and foliage of *Mimosa* and *Leucaena* species and β-cyanoalanine, a neurotoxin from the *Vicia* species (Klosterman, 1974).

Klosterman (1974) comments that known natural vitamin B_6 antagonists occur in relatively low levels, or in foodstuffs that are consumed only occasionally or in small quantities. Under these conditions, the endogenous vitamin B_6 supply is apparently adequate to counteract the harmful effects of small amounts of antagonists in the food. Conceivably, the consumption of larger amounts of ordinary mushrooms over several days could produce a temporary vitamin B_6 deficiency unless offset by supplementary pyridoxine. This effect would probably be aggravated (Klosterman, 1974) if one of the other interfering factors that increases the vitamin B_6 requirement is also present as, for example, L-dopa or an unusually high protein diet. It is accepted that the vitamin B_6 dietary requirement is somewhat directly proportional to the protein content of the diet (Canham *et al.*, 1969).

SAFETY

The toxicity of pyridoxine hydrochloride is regarded as very low. No acute toxicity has been reported in man. Hayes and Hegsted (1973), in a review of the toxicity of the vitamins, state that an intravenous dose of 200 mg of pyridoxine is nontoxic in man and daily oral doses of 100–300 mg have been administered for the alleviation of drug-induced neuritis without side effects. Oral doses up to and exceeding 1,000 mg daily in man without adverse reactions have been reported (Papavasiliou *et al.*, 1972; Pfeiffer *et al.*, 1974; Gibbs and Watts, 1970;

Duvoisin, 1973; Barber and Sapeth, 1969). Some exceptions have been noted. In the Unna and Honig (1968) review, in man, toxic effects were not encountered with daily administration of 50–200 mg pyridoxine over periods of months. In one patient, seizures were aggravated, and in another electroencephalographic pattern changes were observed. Transient electroencephalographic changes have also been reported by Canham *et al.* (1964) at a 200-mg daily intake. Lethargy in one instance and excessive energy and insomnia in another case were reported by Baumblatt and Winston (1970). Lowered folacin tissue levels have been observed from large intakes of pyridoxine as treatment for homocystinuria (Wilcken and Turner, 1973).

Where pyridoxine hydrochloride has been formulated in pharmaceutical products or nutritional supplements, no reports exist to indicate any challenge to human safety by the consumption of these products. It is most likely that even if such consumer products were abused, considering the safety tolerance of the basic vitamin, no untoward effects would be shown.

SUMMARY

Pyridoxine hydrochloride has been in the past and is currently formulated into pharmaceutical and nutritional liquid and dry dosage forms for use by humans. Single-vitamin preparations as well as multivitamin and vitamin-mineral preparations are manufactured in which the pyridoxine content varies, depending on the form and purpose of the preparation. Although conditions contributing to instability of pyridoxine hydrochloride exist, there are no instability problems in properly formulated, packaged, and stored products. When pyridoxine hydrochloride is properly incorporated in pharmaceutical and nutritional products, it is fully available biologically. No indications exist for lack of safety of pyridoxine hydrochloride containing pharmaceutical and nutritional preparations in proper usage.

Insufficient attention has been paid to chemical compounds in the food supply, those taken in drug form and those in which exposure is possible under certain environmental conditions or through certain activities that interfere or may interfere with vitamin B_6 function. This area of research is worthy of further study. In the future determination of allowances for vitamin B_6 by population segments it may be wise to consider the needs of (1) the oral contraceptive user, (2) the alcoholic or the high-alcohol user, and (3) those population segments exposed to vitamin B_6 antagonists for prolonged periods of time.

LITERATURE CITED

Afifi, A. K., and F. A. Sabra. 1968. Treatment of toxic and drug induced neuropathics. Mod. Treat. *5*:1236–1248.

Aly, H. E., E. A. Donald, and M. H. W. Simpson. 1971. Oral contraceptives and vitamin B_6 metabolism. Am. J. Clin. Nutr. *24*:297–303.

Anderson, R. H., D. L. Maxwell, A. E. Mulley, and C. W. Fritsch. 1976. Effect of processing and storage on micronutrients in breakfast cereals. Food Tech. *30*:110–114.

Banna, N. R. 1973. Antagonistic effects of semicarbazide and pyridoxine on cuneate presynaptic inhibition. Brain Res. *56*:249–258.

Barber, G. W., and G. L. Sapeth. 1969. The successful treatment of homocystinuria with pyridoxine. J. Pediatr. *75*:463–478.

Bauernfeind, J. C. 1974. Pyridoxine: A use appraisal in animal feeds. Feedstuffs *46*:30–31.

Baumblatt, M. J., and F. Winston. 1970. Pyridoxine and the pill. Lancet *1*:832–833.

Bernhart, F. W., E. D'Amato, and R. M. Tomarelli. 1960. The vitamin B_6 activity of heat-sterilized milk. Arch. Biochem. Biophys. *88*:267–269.

Bessey, O. A., D. J. Adam, and A. E. Hansen. 1957. Intake of vitamin B_6 and infantile convulsions. Pediatrics *20*:33–44.

Bradner, W. T. 1972. Combination treatment with mitomycin C and pyridoxine hydrochloride. Proc. Am. Assoc. Cancer Res. *13*:22.

Brown, R. R. 1972. Normal and pathological conditions which may alter the human requirement for vitamin B_6. J. Agric. Food Chem. *20*:498–505.

Bunting, W. R. 1965. The stability of pyridoxine added to cereals. Cereal Chem. *42*:569–572.

Canham, J. E., W. T. Nunes, and E. W. Eberlin. 1964. Electroencephalographic and central nervous system manifestations of vitamin B_6 deficiency and induced vitamin B_6 dependency in normal human adults. *In* Proceedings of the Sixth International Congress on Nutrition, E & S Livingstone Ltd., Edinburgh, p. 537.

Canham, J. E., E. M. Baker, R. S. Harding, H. E. Sauberlich, and I. C. Plough. 1969. Dietary protein: Its relationship to vitamin B_6 requirement and function. Ann. N.Y. Acad. Sci. *166*:16–29.

Chabner, B. A., V. T. Devita, N. Considine, and V. T. Oliverio. 1969. Plasma pyridoxal phosphate depletion by the carcinostatic procarbazine. Proc. Soc. Exp. Biol. Med. *132*:1119–1122.

Cohen, A. C. 1969. Pyridoxine in the prevention and treatment of convulsions and neurotoxicity to cycloserine. Ann. N.Y. Acad. Sci. *166*:346–349.

Cort, W. M., B. Borenstein, J. H. Harley, M. Osadca, and J. Scheiner. 1976. Nutrient stability of fortified cereal products. Food Technol. *30*:52–62.

Coursin, D. B. 1954. Convulsive seizures in infants with pyridoxine deficient diet. J. Am. Med. Assoc. *154*:406–408.

Coursin, D. B. 1955a. Symposium on frontiers of human nutrition in relation to milk: Vitamin B_6 in milk. Quart. Rev. Pediatr. *10*:2–9.

Coursin, D. B. 1955b. Vitamin B_6 deficiency in infants. Am. J. Dis. Child. *90*:344–348.

Coursin, D. B. 1956. Effect of vitamin B_6 on the central nervous activity in childhood. Am. J. Clin. Nutr. *4*:354–363.

Coursin, D. B. 1964. Vitamin B_6 metabolism in infants and children. Vitam. Horm. *22*:755–786.

Coyer, J. R., and D. P. Nicholson. 1976. Isoniazid-induced convulsions: Clinical. South. Med. J. *69*:294–297.

Davanzo, J. P., M. E. Greig, and M. A. Cronin. 1961. Anticonvulsant properties of amino-oxyacetic acid. Am. J. Physiol. *201*:833–837.

d'Eshougues, J. R., C. Gille, and A. Smadja. 1961. Intolerance a la chloroquine et deficit en pyridoxine dans 3 cas de maladie lupique. Presse Med. *69*:2524.

Dubnick, B., G. A. Leeson, and C. D. Scott. 1960. Effect of forms of vitamin B_6 on acute toxicity of hydrazines. Toxicol. Appl. Pharmacol. *2*:403–409.

Duvoisin, R. C. 1973. Pyridoxine as an adjunct in the treatment of parkinsonism. Adv. Neurol. *2*:229–248.

Dyer, H. M., and H. P. Morris. 1961. An effect of N-2 fluorenylacetamide on the metabolism of tryptophan in rats. J. Nat. Cancer Inst. *26*:315–329.

Eidelberg, E., and N. A. Buchwald. 1970. Effects of thiosemicarbazide on spinal reflex activity. Neurology *10*:267–270.

Eremeev, V. S. 1968. Effect of vitamin B_6 on the toxic effects of strophanthin. Russ. Pharmacol. Toxicol. *31*:88.

Food Chemicals Codex, Second Edition. 1972. National Academy of Sciences, Washington, D.C., p. 689.

Food and Nutrition Board. 1974. Proposed Fortification Policy for Cereal-Grain Products. National Academy of Sciences, Washington, D.C., 36 pp.

Frierson, W. B. 1965. Use of pyridoxine HCl in acute hydrazine and UDMH intoxication. Ind. Med. Surg. *34*:650–651.

Fujimoto, S. 1966. Effect of pyridoxal phosphate on toxicity and antitumor activity of mitomycin C and 4-deoxypyridoxine hydrochloride in rats: Preliminary observations. Cancer Chemother. Rep. *50*:313–318.

Fuller, H. 1964. Vitamin B_6 in farm animal nutrition and pets. Vitam. Horm. *22*:659–676.

Gibbs, D. A., and R. W. E. Watts. 1970. The action of pyridoxine in primary hyperoxaluria. Clin. Sci. *38*:277–286.

Gordon, E. B. 1964. Vitamin therapy. Br. Med. J. *1*:563.

Gorny, R. 1971. The level of pyridoxal phosphate in the blood plasma of rats exposed to carbon disulfide. Biochem. Pharmacol. *20*:2114–2115.

György, P. 1934. Vitamin B_2 and the pellagra-like dermatitis in rats. Nature *133*:498–499.

György, P. 1935. Investigations on the vitamin B_2 complex: The differentiation of lactoflavin and the "rat antipellagra" factor. Biochem. J. *29*:741–775.

Hassinen, J. B., G. T. Durbin, and F. W. Bernhart. 1954. The vitamin B_6 content of milk products. J. Nutr. *53*:249–257.

Hawkins, W. W., and J. Barsky. 1948. An experiment on human vitamin B_6 deprivation. Science *108*:284–286.

Hayes, K. C., and D. M. Hegsted. 1973. Toxicity of the vitamins. *In* Toxicants Occurring Naturally in Foods, National Academy of Sciences, Washington, D.C., pp. 235–253.

Hellström, V. 1960. The influence of sunlight on vitamin B_6 in milk. Int. Z. Vitaminforsch. *30*:323–327.

Hennessy, D. J., A. M. Steinberg, G. S. Wilson, and W. P. Keaveney. 1960. Fluorometric determination of added pyridoxine in enriched white flour and in bread baked from it. J. Assoc. Off. Agric. Chem. *43*:765–768.

Hines, J. D., and D. H. Cowan. 1970. Studies on the pathogenesis of alcohol-induced sideroblastic bone-marrow abnormalities. N. Engl. J. Med. *283*:441–446.

Hodson, A. Z. 1956. Vitamin B_6 in sterilized milk and other milk products. Food Technol. *10*:221–224.

Hoff-Jorgensen, E. 1966. Antivitamins for vitamin B_6. Nutr. Dieta *8*:160–168.

Hollister, L. E., F. F. Moore, F. Forrest, and J. L. Bennett. 1966. Antipyridoxine effect of D-penicillamine in schizophrenics. Am. J. Clin. Nutr. *19*:307–312.

Holtz, P., and D. Palm. 1964. Pharmacological aspects of vitamin B₆. Pharmacol. Rev. *16*:113–178.

Horrigan, D. L. 1968. Pyridoxine responsive anemias in man. Vitam. Horm. *26*:549–571.

Hussar, D. A. 1973. Drug interactions. Am. J. Pharm. *145*:65–116.

Jaffee, I. A., K. Altman, and P. Merryman. 1964. The antipyridoxine effect of penicillamine in man. J. Clin. Invest. *43*:1869–1873.

Kirkendall, W. M., and E. B. Page. 1958. Polyneuritis occurring during hydralazine therapy. J. Am. Med. Assoc. *167*:427–432.

Kirklin, J. K., K. Watson, C. C. Bardoc, and J. F. Burke. 1976. Treatment of hydrazine induced coma with pyridoxine. N. Engl. J. Med. *294*:938–939.

Klosterman, H. J. 1974. Vitamin B₆ antagonists of natural origin. J. Agric. Food Chem. *22*:13–16.

Klosterman, H. J., R. B. Olsgaard, W. C. Lockhart, and J. W. Magill. 1960. Extraction of the antipyridoxine factor in flax cotyledons. Proc. N.D. Acad. Sci. *14*:81–95.

Klosterman, H. J., G. L. Lamoureux, and J. L. Parsons. 1967. Isolation, characterization and synthesis of linatine: A vitamin B₆ antagonist from flax seed. Biochemistry *6*:170–177.

Korytnyk, W., and B. Lachmann. 1971. Analogs of vitamin B₆ with reactive groups. J. Med. Chem. *14*:641–643.

Korytnyk, W., G. B. Grindey, and B. Lachmann. 1973. 4-Vinyl analog of pyridoxal: A potent antagonist of vitamin B₆. J. Med. Chem. *16*:865–867.

Kratzer, F. H. 1947. Effect of duration of water treatment on the nutritive value of linseed meal. Poultry Sci. *25*:541–542; 1946, *26*:90–91.

Kratzer, F. H., and D. E. Williams. 1948. The relation of pyridoxine to the growth of chicks fed rations containing linseed meal. J. Nutr. *36*:297–305.

Kuchinskas, E. J., and V. du Vigneaud. 1957. An increased vitamin B₆ requirement in the rat on a diet containing L-penicillamine. Arch. Biochem. Biophys. *66*:1–9.

Külz, J. 1964. Die neurotoxischen nebenwirkungen, von piperazinderivaten im EEG von kindern: piperazinadipat, kurzbehandlung, pyridoxin-prophylaxe. Dtsch. Gesundheitswes. *19*:1585–1592.

Lantz, E. 1939. Effect of cooking on the riboflavin and vitamin B₆ content of pinto beans. Bull. Agric. Exp. Sta. N.M. No. 268: pp. 3–16.

Leeson, G. A., B. Dubnick, and C. C. Scott. 1959. Effect of forms of vitamin B₆ on acute toxicity of β-phenylethylhydrazine. Fed. Proc. *18*:414.

Leevy, C. M., H. Baker, W. Tentove, O. Frank, and G. R. Cherrick. 1965. B-complex vitamins in liver disease of the alcoholic. Am. J. Clin. Nutr. *16*:339–346.

Leon, A. S., H. E. Spiegel, G. Thomas, I. Ross, and W. B. Abrams. 1971. Effects of pyridoxine on absorption, metabolism, and clinical activity of levodopa in parkinson's disease. Clin. Pharmacol. Ther. *12*:294–295.

Lepkovsky, S., T. Jukes, and M. Krause. 1936. The multiple nature of the third factor of the vitamin B complex. J. Biol. Chem. *115*:557–566.

Lotz, M., J. T. Potts, Jr., J. M. Holland, W. Kiser, and F. C. Bartter. 1966. D-penicillamine therapy in cystinuria. J. Urol. *95*:257–263.

Luhby, A. L., M. Brin, M. Gordon, P. Davis, M. Murphy, and H. Spiegel. 1971. Vitamin B₆ metabolism in users of oral contraceptive agents. Am. J. Clin. Nutr. *24*:684–693.

Lumeng, L., R. E. Cleary, and T-K. Li. 1974. Effect of oral contraceptives on the plasma concentration of pyridoxal phosphate. Am. J. Clin. Nutr. *27*:326–333.

Lunde, F. 1960. Pyridoxine deficiency in chronic alcoholism. J. Nerv. Ment. Dis. *131*:77–79.

Makino, K., T. Kinoshita, Y. Abramaki, and S. Shintani. 1954. A toxopyrimidine action of vitamins of the vitamin B_6 group. Nature *174*:275–276.

Mastsunaga, F., T. Shimoyama, K. Mikawa, and J. Ishiwata. 1966. A comparative study of administration methods of mitomycin C. Proc. 9th Int. Cancer Congr. Tokyo, Oct. 23–29, p. 439.

May, C. D. 1954. Vitamin B_6 in human nutrition: A critique and an object lesson. Pediatrics *14*:269–279.

McCormick, D. B., and E. E. Snell. 1961. Pyridoxal phosphokinase: Effects of inhibitors. J. Biol. Chem. *236*:2085–2088.

McLaughlan, J. M., K. G. Shenoy, and J. A. Campbell. 1960. Some drug-vitamin interrelationships in microorganisms. Fed. Proc. *19*:415.

Melicow, M. M., A. C. Uson, and T. D. Price. 1964. Bladder tumor induction in rats fed 2-acetamidofluorene and a pyridoxine deficient diet. J. Urol. *91*:520–529.

Melnick, D., H. Hochberg, and B. L. Oser. 1945. Physiological availability of the vitamins: The human assay technique. J. Nutr. *30*:67–79.

Mindrum, G. 1964. Pentaborane intoxication. Arch. Intern. Med. *114*:364–374.

Molony, C. J., A. H. Parmelee. 1954. Convulsions in young infants as a result of pyridoxine deficiency. J. Amer. Med. Assoc. *154:*405–406.

Naeger, L. L. 1971. Mechanisms of decaborane toxicity. Diss. Abstr. Int. B*32:*463–464.

Nelson, E. W., Jr., H. Lane, and J. J. Cerda. 1976. Comparative human intestinal bioavailability of vitamin B_6 from a synthetic and a natural source. J. Nutr. *106*:1433–1437.

Nesheim, R. O. 1974. Nutrient changes in food processing: A current review, Fed. Proc. *33:*2267–2269.

Nishizawa, Y., T. Kodama, and T. Kooka. 1975. Histological investigations on the liver disturbing action of 2-methyl-4-amino-5-hydroxymethyl pyrimidine. J. Vitaminol. *3:*309–321.

Nutrition Reviews. 1973. Oral contraceptive agents and vitamin B_6. *31:*49–50.

Nutrition Reviews. 1968. Vitamin B_6 deficiency following isoniazid therapy. *26:*306–308.

Oser, B. L., D. Melnick, and M. Hochberg. 1945. Physiological availability of the vitamins: Comparison of various techniques for determining vitamin availability in pharmaceutical products. J. Nutr. *30:*67–79.

Papavasiliou, P. S., G. C. Cotzias, and S. E. Düby. 1972. Levodopa in parkinson: Potentiation of central nervous effects with a peripheral inhibitor. N. Engl. J. Med. *286:*8–14.

Pfeiffer, C. C., A. Sohler, C. H. Jenney, and V. Iliev. 1974. Treatment of pyloric schizophrenic (malvaria) with large doses of pyridoxine and a dietary supplement of zinc. J. Orthomolecular Psychiatr. *3:*292–300.

Polansky, M. M., and E. W. Toepfer. 1969. Nutrient composition of selected wheats and wheat products: Vitamin B_6 components. Cereal Chem. *46:*664–674.

Price, J. M., M. J. Thornton, and L. M. Mueller. 1967. Tryptophan metabolism in women using steroid hormones for ovulation control. Am. J. Clin. Nutr. *20:*452–456.

Rabinowitz, J. C., and E. E. Snell. 1948. Distribution of pyridoxal, pyridoxamine and pyridoxine in some natural products. J. Biol. Chem. *176:*1157–1167.

Rabinowitz, J. C., and E. E. Snell. 1949. Vitamin B_6 group: Urinary excretion of pyridoxal, pyridoxamine, pyridoxine and pyridoxic acid in human subjects. Proc. Exp. Biol. Med. *70:*235–240.

Rahiala, E. L., M. Kekomäki, J. Jänne, A. Raina, and N. C. R. Räikä. 1971. Inhibition of pyridoxal enzymes by L-canaline. Biochim. Biophys. Acta 227:337–343.

Raskin, N. H., R. A. Fishman. 1965. Pyridoxine-deficiency neuropathy due to hydralazine. N. Engl. J. Med. 273:1182–1185.

Reynolds, E. H. 1975. Chronic antiepileptic toxicity: A review. Epilepsia 16:319–352.

Roe, D. A. 1973. Drug-induced vitamin deficiencies. Drug Therapy 3:23–32.

Rose, D. P. 1969. Oral contraceptives and depression. Lancet 2:321.

Rose, D. P., and I. P. Braidman. 1971. Excretion of tryptophan metabolites as effected by pregnancy, contraceptive steroids and steroid hormones. Am. J. Clin. Nutr. 24:673–683.

Rose, D. P., J. E. Leklem, R. R. Brown, and H. H. Linkswiler. 1973. Impairment of glucose tolerance by dietary vitamin B₆ deficiency in oral contraceptive users. J. Nutr. 103(7):xviii.

Rosen, F., E. Mihich, and C. A. Nichol. 1964. Selective metabolic and chemotherapeutic effects of vitamin B₆ metabolites. Vitam. Horm. 22:609–653.

Sauberlich, H. E. 1968. Vitamin B₆ group: Active compounds and antagonists. *In* W. H. Sebrell, Jr., and R. S. Harris (eds.) The Vitamins, Academic Press, New York, pp. 33–44.

Sauberlich, H. E., R. P. Dowdy, and J. H. Skala. 1974. Laboratory Tests for the Assessment of Nutritional Status. CRC Press, Cleveland. 136 pp.

Saville, D. G., A. Salvyns, and C. Humphries. 1967. Choline induced pyridoxine deficiency in broiler chickens. Aust. Vet. J. 43:346.

Scheunert, A., H. Haenel, and I. Meyer. 1956–57. Über die Mikrobiologische Antivitamin B₆ wirkung der Thiaminkomponente 2-methyl-4-amino-5-oxymethylpyrimidin. Int. Z. Vitaminforsch. 27:464–476.

Schroeder, H. A. 1971. Losses of vitamins and trace minerals resulting from processing and preservation of foods. Am. J. Clin. Nutr. 24:562–573.

Shintani, S. 1956. Studies on antivitamin B₆ activity of toxopyrimidine. J. Vitaminol. 2:185–192.

Shiroishi, M. and A. Hayakawa. 1961. Effects of sunlight irradiation on vitamin B₆ related compounds. Vitamin (Kyoto) 22:138–141.

Smith, D. B., and B. B. Gallagher. 1970. The effect of penicillamine on seizure threshold: The role of pyridoxine. Arch. Neurol. 23:59–62.

Snell, E. E., and A. N. Rannefeld. 1945. The vitamin B₆ group: The vitamin activity of pyridoxal and pyridoxamine for various organisms. J. Biol. Chem. 157:475–489.

Snell, E., B. Guirard, and R. Williams. 1942. Occurrence in natural products of a physiologically active metabolite of pyridoxine. J. Biol. Chem. 143:519–530.

Snyderman, S. E., L. E. Holt, Jr., R. Carretero, and K. G. Jacobs. 1953. Pyridoxine deficiency in the human infant. Am. J. Clin. Nutr. 1:200–207.

Standal, B. R., S. M. Kao-Chen, G. Y. Young, and D. F. B. Cher. 1974. Early changes in pyridoxine status in patients receiving isoniazid therapy. Am. J. Clin. Nutr. 27:479–484.

Tanaka, F., N. Tanaka, H. Yonehara, and H. Umezawa. 1962. Studies on bacimethrin, a new antibiotic from *B. megatherium*. J. Antibiot. (Tokyo) 15:191–196.

Tomarelli, R. M., E. R. Spence, and F. W. Bernhart. 1955. Biological availability of vitamin B₆ of heated milk. J. Agric. Food Chem. 3:338–341.

Tomono, I., M. Abe, and M. Matsuda. 1973. Effect of penicillamine on pyridoxal enzymes. J. Biochem. (Tokyo) 74:587–592.

Umbreit, W. W. 1955. Vitamin B₆ antagonists. Am. J. Clin. Nutr. 3:291–297.

Unna, K. R., and G. R. Honig. 1968. Vitamin B_6 pharmacology and toxicology. *In* W. A. Sebrell, Jr. and R. S. Harris (ed.), The Vitamins, Academic Press, New York, pp. 104–108.

U.S. Pharmacopeia, XIX Edition. 1975. U.S. Pharmacopeial Convention, Inc., Rockville, Md., p. 429.

Winston, F. 1973. Oral contraceptives, pyridoxine and depression. Am. J. Psychiatr. *130*:1217–1221.

Wilcken, B., and B. Turner. 1973. Homcystinuria: Reduced folate levels during pyridoxine treatment. Arch. Dis. Child. *48*:58–62.

Woodbury, D. M. 1969. Role of pharmacological factors in the evaluation of anticonvulsant drugs. Epilepsia *10*:121–144.

Woodring, M. J., and C. A. Storvick. 1960. Vitamin B_6 in milk: Review of literature. J. Assoc. Off. Agric. Chem. *43*:63–80.

Wykes, A. A., and J. H. Laudez. 1967. Modification of the tissue norepinephrine and serotonin depleting action and toxic effects of decaborane-14 by pyridoxine hydrochloride and pyridoxal phosphate. Fed. Proc. *26*:464.

Yahr, M. D., R. C. Duvoisin, L. Cote, and G. Cohen. 1972. Pyridoxine, dopa and parkinson. Adv. Biochem. Pharmacol. *4*:185–194.

Yamashita, J. 1974. Susceptibility to thiosemicarbazide (an antagonist of vitamin B_6) and phylogenetic and ontogenic development of brain. J. Nutr. Sci. Vitaminol. *20*:113–119.

7

Vitamin B_6 and Blood

BARRY SHANE

METABOLISM OF VITAMIN B_6 IN BLOOD

The red blood cell possesses a full complement of enzymes for the interconversion of vitamin B_6 compounds (Snell and Haskell, 1971). It contains kinase (Hamfelt, 1967b; Lumeng and Li, 1974; Anderson *et al.*, 1971; Anderson and Mollin, 1972; Shane, 1970) for phosphorylation of free vitamin, PNP* oxidase (Lumeng and Li, 1974) for the formation of PLP from PNP or PMP, and a variety of aminotransferases (Raica and Sauberlich, 1964). No mechanism has been detected for the interconversion of nonphosphorylated vitamin in the red cell, and it is unlikely that any such mechanism is present in mammalian tissues (Shane and Snell, 1972, 1975). The level of PLP in the red cell is controlled by the action of a membrane-bound phosphatase (Lumeng and Li, 1974; Anderson *et al.*, 1971). The role of this enzyme in the regulation of tissue PLP levels has only recently become fully appreciated (Lumeng and Li, 1975; Li *et al.*, 1974).

*Vitamin B_6 compounds have been abbreviated, according to published recommendations (IUPAC-IUB Commission on Biochemical Nomenclature, 1970) as follows: PLP, pyridoxal 5'-phosphate; PN, pyridoxine; PL, pyridoxal; PM, pyridoxamine. PIC is 4-pyridoxic acid.

111

Some of these enzymes are also present in leucocytes (Hamfelt, 1967b). They contain higher levels of PL kinase than the erythrocyte, but in terms of total blood enzyme levels, their contribution is minor.

Plasma contains alkaline phosphatases and low levels of some aminotransferases but apparently none of the other vitamin B_6 interconversion enzymes. Although Reinken (1974) reported the presence of PL kinase in plasma, other investigators (Hamfelt, 1967b; Shane, 1970) have not been able to detect this enzyme in plasma.

The levels of PL kinase and PNP oxidase in blood are very low in comparison to levels in other tissues such as kidney and liver (McCormick et al., 1961; Contractor and Shane, 1969), which has led some investigators to conclude that the erythrocytes play only a minor role in the overall metabolism of the dietary vitamin to the active coenzymatic form, PLP (McCormick et al., 1961). Other investigators suggest a possible role for the red cell in the conversion of the plasma vitamin to forms that can be more easily taken up by tissues (Anderson et al., 1971; Anderson and Mollin, 1972).

TRANSPORT OF VITAMIN B_6 BY THE ERYTHROCYTE

Transport of vitamin B_6 by the erythrocyte has been studied extensively by Anderson et al. (1971), Anderson and Mollin (1972), Yamada and Tsuji (1968, 1970), Suzue and Tachibana (1970), Lumeng and Li (1974), and Lumeng et al. (1974a). Some of these data are summarized in Figure 7-1. PLP in plasma and the red cell is tightly bound to protein, mainly albumin (Lumeng et al., 1974a; Anderson et al., 1974) and hemoglobin (Suzue and Tachibana, 1970), which prevents it from crossing the red cell membrane (Anderson et al., 1971; Anderson and Mollin, 1972; Anderson et al., 1974). This binding to protein, which is by means of a Schiff's base complex, also protects PLP to a large

FIGURE 7-1   Transport and metabolism of vitamin B_6 in blood.

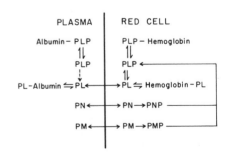

degree from the action of phosphatases. Although albumin-bound PLP is nondialyzable (Lumeng *et al.*, 1974a; Dempsey and Christensen, 1962), alkaline phosphatase will slowly hydrolyze the PLP, even when the phosphatase is enclosed in a dialysis bag (Lumeng *et al.*, 1974a). It appears that a small amount of free PLP is in equilibrium with the protein-bound vitamin. The capacity of plasma proteins to bind PLP greatly exceeds the physiological level of this coenzyme (Lumeng *et al.*, 1974a). In the absence of plasma, however, PLP is slowly transported by the red cell (Suzue and Tachibana, 1970).

PL also binds to protein, but this binding is much looser (Anderson *et al.*, 1974), presumably because this compound exists predominantly in the hemiacetal form, rather than as the free aldehyde, at physiological pH (Metzler and Snell, 1955). PL rapidly crosses the red cell membrane, and its distribution between the red cell and plasma is governed by competing protein binders (Anderson *et al.*, 1974).

PN and PM are also rapidly taken up by the red cell (Yamada and Tsuji, 1968, 1970). They are phosphorylated and oxidized to PLP and after hydrolysis to PL can then be released by the cell (Anderson *et al.*, 1971; Anderson and Mollin, 1972). It has been suggested that PN and PM are actively transported, since their uptake is greatly reduced by decreasing the temperature or by addition of potassium fluoride or the PN analogue, 4'-deoxyPN (Yamada and Tsuji, 1968, 1970). PL uptake is not affected or only slightly affected by these conditions. Also, PN and PM uptake exhibit saturation kinetics, while PL uptake does not. These results, however, are best explained by a diffusion-type uptake of all of these compounds, followed by their intracellular trapping as PLP or PL. Lowering the temperature or the addition of KF or 4'-deoxyPN would decrease the intracellular phosphorylation of these compounds, allowing PN and PM to diffuse out of the cell. This would be similar to the situation in platelets (Gaut and Solomon, 1972), where PN is taken up by diffusion and is trapped by phosphorylation to PNP.

Although PLP binding to protein prevents it from crossing the red cell membrane, it is still available for PLP-requiring apoenzymes. Studies on the activation of apoaminotransferases by albumin-bound PLP (Masugi *et al.*, 1973) have indicated the formation of an intermediate ternary complex between albumin, PLP, and apoenzyme rather than the release of PLP before apoenzyme activation.

One obvious feature of the metabolic routes shown in Figure 7-1 is that red cell metabolism cannot contribute to plasma PLP levels. To investigate the source of plasma PLP, Lumeng *et al.* (1974a) carried out organ ablation studies on dogs. A rapid rise in plasma PLP levels was observed after intravenous injection of PN or PL, and this increase was unaffected by bilateral nephrectomy or by resection of the spleen, stomach, and intestines. After hepatectomy, however, no rise in plasma PLP levels was observed, demonstrating that plasma PLP is derived from the liver. These investigators also suggested that PLP is released by the liver as an albumin-bound complex.

Anderson *et al.* (1971) and Anderson and Mollin (1972) have suggested that PL is the transport form of the vitamin and that red cell metabolism of vitamin B_6 to PL, with its subsequent release into plasma, makes the vitamin available for tissue uptake. Although possible, this role for the red cell is unlikely, since there is evidence from studies with rats and mice that all nonphosphorylated forms of vitamin B_6 can be taken up by mammalian tissues (Johansson *et al.*, 1968; Colombini and McCoy, 1970; Contractor and Shane, 1971; Tiselius, 1973; Johansson *et al.*, 1974) and there is also evidence suggesting that the phosphorylated vitamin is available for tissue uptake. The metabolism of vitamin B_6 by the erythrocyte would seem to be related to the red cell's own needs, and a more general role has not been demonstrated. Apart from the general reactions requiring PLP, erythroblasts and reticulocytes require this cofactor for heme biosynthesis, in particular for the synthesis of δ-aminolevulinic acid (Anderson and Mollin, 1972). Severe vitamin B_6 deficiency leads to an anemia resulting from decreased red cell formation and an even greater decrease in hemoglobin synthesis (Sauberlich, 1968; Keyhani *et al.*, 1974). Severe deficiency also results in changes in red cell membrane lipids (Zehaluk and Walker, 1973), but the mechanism by which these changes occur is not understood.

BLOOD PLP AND AMINOTRANSFERASES AS INDICATORS OF VITAMIN B_6 STATUS

The most commonly used methods for assessing vitamin B_6 status fall into two main categories: (1) the indirect methods, such as the tryptophan load test or the estimation of blood aminotransferase levels, which are based on an enzymatic requirement for PLP, and (2) the more direct approach of assaying blood or urine levels of the vitamin (Cinnamon and Beaton, 1970; Donald *et al.*, 1971; Sauberlich *et al.*, 1972).

Methods for the estimation of blood vitamin levels have not found widespread use, possibly because early methods were more complex than the indirect methods. However, relatively simple enzymatic methods are now available for the assay of PLP (Hamfelt, 1967a; Chabner and Livingston, 1970; Haskell and Snell, 1972).

The levels of various B_6 compounds in whole blood are shown in Table 7-1. These were measured by a fluorimetric technique (Contrac-

TABLE 7-1   Vitamin B_6 Compounds in Blood

Compound	Male, ng/ml	Female, ng/ml
PLP	13.5 ± 2.9 (5)	12.1 ± 2.3 (23)
PNP	0	0
PMP	20.0 ± 5.5	9.3 ± 7.4
PL	1.3 ± 0.9	0.8 ± 0.5
PN	0	0
PM	24.7 ± 19.5	18.0 ± 3.9
PIC	31.9 ± 6.4	31.8 ± 10.1

tor and Shane, 1968, 1970), and the PLP levels agree well with those obtained by enzymatic methods (Lumeng and Li, 1974; Cleary *et al.,* 1975). PLP levels in these control subjects did not vary significantly over several months of study and were unaffected by the menstrual cycle (Contractor and Shane, 1968). A similar stability in individual plasma PLP levels has also been reported (Lumeng and Li, 1974), although with large populations, an age-dependent decrease in plasma PLP levels has been observed (Lumeng and Li, 1974; Hamfelt, 1964). The levels of the other B_6 compounds fluctuated considerably over the period of study (Contractor and Shane, 1968), which suggests that total blood levels of the vitamin are a poorer index of vitamin status than are PLP levels. No PN or PNP was detected in blood. The major advantage in measuring PLP levels, however, is that this is the functional form of the vitamin. It is possible that a vitamin B_6 deficiency caused by impaired formation of PLP, as, for example, by defective phosphorylation or oxidation, may not be detected by measuring total blood levels of the vitamin.

In whole blood, PLP is distributed approximately equally between plasma and erythrocytes (Bhagavan *et al.,* 1975), so that measurement of either would serve equally well as a vitamin status indicator. Leucocytes have a higher PLP content than erythrocytes, but their contribution to total blood levels is negligible (Hamfelt, 1967b). The situation is somewhat different after PN loading. Bhagavan *et al.* (1975) have reported erythrocyte to plasma PLP ratios of up to 50 to 1 after chronic administration of 1 g/day of PN.

Some disagreement exists over whether blood vitamin is mainly phosphorylated or not (Anderson *et al.,* 1971; Sauberlich *et al.,* 1972), and this is probably a consequence of the large variety of assay methods used. The extent of phosphorylation was investigated further by following the metabolism of a tracer dose of [^{14}C]PN in blood (Table 7-2) (Shane, 1970). The labeled vitamin was rapidly removed from

TABLE 7-2   [^{14}C] Vitamin in Blood after Intravenous
Administration of [^{14}C]PN (81 μg) to Nonpregnant
Female

Time, min	Total, % dose	PLP + PIC^a, % dose	PN + PL, % dose
0	100	0	100
2	26	18	7.9
10	17	14	2.7
60	7	6	0.7
240	3	3	—

^{a}[^{14}C] label in this fraction was predominantly [^{14}C]PLP.

blood and, at each time period studied, nonphosphorylated vitamin, represented by the values for PN plus PL, accounted for only a minor share of total blood vitamin.

Large doses of PN are also rapidly cleared from blood (Shane, 1970). Ten minutes after an intravenous (IV) dose of 50 mg PN was administered to healthy female subjects, less than 5 percent of the load could be accounted for in blood. Most of this was in the form of PLP (1.6 percent) with smaller amounts of PN (1.3 percent), PL (0.7 percent), and PIC (0.7 percent).

Experiments with healthy individuals on controlled diets have shown that plasma, erythrocyte, and whole blood vitamin B$_6$ levels fall rapidly during vitamin B$_6$ depletion and rise following supplementation. These changes occur before changes in other biochemical parameters of vitamin status (Donald *et al.*, 1971; Baysal *et al.*, 1966; Kelsay *et al.*, 1968). Blood PLP levels, thus, appear to be a sensitive index of vitamin B$_6$ status in individuals. In pregnancy, an increased requirement for the vitamin is indicated by lowered blood PLP levels in the mother (Table 7-3) (Contractor and Shane, 1970; Cleary *et al.*, 1975; Shane and Contractor, 1975; Wachstein, 1964; Hamfelt and Tuvemo, 1972; Hamfelt and Hahn, 1969; Wachstein *et al.*, 1957). This relative deficiency is a result of fetal sequestration of maternal vitamin (Contractor and Shane, 1970, 1971; Cleary *et al.*, 1975; Wachstein *et al.*, 1960; Karlin *et al.*, 1966; Brin, 1971). Maternal PLP levels decrease throughout pregnancy, however, even after the fetus acquires the ability to phosphorylate the vitamin (Hamfelt and Tuvemo, 1972; Wachstein *et al.*, 1960; Cleary *et al.*, 1975; Contractor and Shane, 1969, 1970).

An increased requirement for the vitamin can also be demonstrated by PLP levels after PN loading. Blood PLP levels peaked about 2 hours after an oral dose of 50 mg PN (Figure 7-2), then fell, but were still

TABLE 7-3   PLP Levels in Blood

Subject	PLP, ng/ml
Male	13.5 ± 2.9 (5)
Female (nonpregnant)	12.1 ± 2.3 (23)
Female (pregnant)	7.7 ± 3.7 (5)
Fetus (cord vein)	27.5 ± 8.1 (5)

considerably higher than preloading levels 48 h after the dose (Shane, 1970; Contractor and Shane, 1970; Wachstein *et al.*, 1960). This pattern was observed in pregnant and nonpregnant groups. Maternal PLP levels, however, were significantly lower than in the control groups at each time period studied. The impaired metabolism of vitamin B_6 to PLP, which has been reported in toxemic patients (Shane, 1970; Kleiger *et al.*, 1966; 1969; Gaynore and Dempsey, 1972), is illustrated by the lower PLP levels in this group (Figure 7-2). A similar pattern was also observed with blood PL and PIC levels. These peaked about 2 hours after the loading dose but by 6 hours had dropped almost to preloading levels. However, in these cases, there were no significant differences in levels between pregnant and nonpregnant subjects (Shane, 1970). No elevation in PM or PMP levels were observed after PN loading, and no PN was detected in blood, although it may have been present before the 2-hour sampling (Shane, 1970).

One of the most commonly used methods for assessing vitamin status has involved the estimation of aspartate or alanine amino-

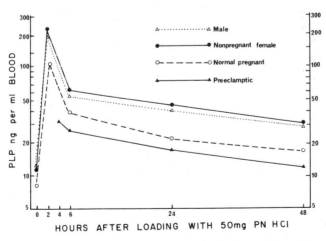

FIGURE 7-2   Levels of PLP in whole blood of various subjects after oral administration of PN.

transferase levels in erythrocytes and their *in vitro* stimulation by PLP (Cinnamon and Beaton, 1970; Donald *et al.*, 1971; Sauberlich *et al.*, 1972). This is usually expressed as an activation factor or the ratio of total enzyme to holoenzyme.

Raica and Sauberlich (1964) investigated the effect of vitamin depletion in control subjects on blood aspartate aminotransferase levels and concluded that the enzyme levels in the erythrocytes, leucocytes, or plasma could not in themselves be used as a measure of vitamin status. However, the *in vitro* stimulation of the erythrocyte enzyme increased during the depletion period and decreased during repletion and appeared to be a useful index of vitamin status. This finding has been confirmed in a number of studies, and the usefulness of this test in assessing vitamin B_6 requirements by controlled depletion-repletion studies appears to be well established (Sauberlich, *et al.*, 1972). These controlled experiments, however, usually involved severe deficiency over a relatively long time period, and measurements were made on individual subjects. The use of this parameter to indicate marginal deficiency has not been adequately demonstrated, nor has its usefulness in pathological conditions, or in physiological states such as pregnancy, in which it may be complicated by hormonal or drug effects, such as have been observed with the tryptophan load test (Rose, 1966; Brin, 1970; Mason *et al.*, 1969; Rose and Cramp, 1970; Altman and Greengard, 1966, Brown *et al.*, 1969).

Erythrocyte alanine aminotransferase levels have also been used as a vitamin B_6 status indicator, but results with this enzyme have been somewhat equivocal. Some investigators have reported that *in vitro* stimulation of this enzyme correlates well with vitamin depletion (Cinnamon and Beaton, 1970), while other investigators have reported no such correlation (Donald *et al.*, 1971).

A comparison of the effectiveness of the two vitamin status tests in assessing vitamin status in pregnancy and oral contraceptive agent users is shown in Table 7-4. In this study, blood samples were analyzed at weekly intervals over a 10-week period, and during the last 4 weeks of the study, the control and oral contraceptive agent users received a daily supplement of 20 mg PN •HCl (Shane and Contractor, 1975). A relative B_6 deficiency or increased requirement for the vitamin was suggested by the significantly lower PLP levels in pregnant women and those receiving oral contraceptives. All the PLP levels in the pregnancy group were lower than the lowest level found in the control group, while PLP levels in the oral contraceptive agent users overlapped those in the control group. This may indicate a mild vitamin deficiency in some, but not all, oral contraceptive agent users (Lumeng *et al.*, 1974b;

TABLE 7-4 Blood PLP Levels and Erythrocyte Aspartate
Aminotransferase Activation Factors in Various Groups

Group	PLP, ng/ml of blood	Range, ng/ml of blood	Aminotransfer-ase Activation Factor
Nonpregnant [12]	9.63 ± 1.67	7.5–12.5	1.69 ± 0.17
+ 20 mg PN per day	47.0 ± 12.8		1.43 ± 0.14
Oral contraceptive users [10]	7.61 ± 1.07	6.3– 8.5	1.64 ± 0.13
+ 20 mg PN per day	42.1 ± 17.1		1.54 ± 0.16
Pregnant (third trimester) [9]	5.06 ± 1.32	2.7– 7.0	1.68 ± 0.12

Brown *et al.*, 1975; Leklem *et al.*, 1975; Miller *et al.*, 1974). The differences in PLP levels were not reflected by the erythrocyte aspartate
aminotransferase activation factors (Table 7-4) nor by total or holoenzyme levels in the erythrocyte (Shane and Contractor, 1975). No correlation was observed between PLP levels and activation factors either on
an individual basis or on a group basis, unless results obtained after PN
loading were included. Hamfelt (1967c) did find a correlation between
these parameters in a large group of individuals, but he was unable to
demonstrate such a relationship in pregnant subjects (Hamfelt and
Tuvemo, 1972).

Conflicting results with the aminotransferase test are not uncommon
in the literature. Some groups have reported an increased activation
factor in pregnancy or in oral contraceptive users, while others have
found no changes in this parameter (Heller *et al.*, 1973; Doberenz *et
al.*, 1971; Salkeld *et al.*, 1973; Aly *et al.*, 1971). There are a number of
possible explanations for these divergent results, not least of which is
the lack of standardization of the experimental procedures used. Data
in Table 7-4 show a 60 percent *in vitro* activation of the enzyme by PLP.
The range reported in the literature for apparently healthy control subjects varies considerably, from about 30 to 80 percent (Cinnamon and
Beaton, 1970; Donald *et al.*, 1971; Sauberlich *et al.*, 1972; Hamfelt,
1967c; Woodring and Storvick, 1970), which means that a large amount
of the enzyme is in the apoenzyme form. Kishi *et al.* (1975) have
recently reported only a 13 percent stimulation of enzyme activity with
student athletes receiving a controlled, nutritionally adequate diet.
These assays were performed on fresh hemolysates. When they were
repeated after storing the hemolysates for 2–3 weeks, the *in vitro*
stimulation increased to over 40 percent, demonstrating that storage
leads to PLP dissociation from the enzyme.

While this may explain some of the discrepancies in the literature, there are a number of other factors that tend to decrease the sensitivity of this test. Vitamin deficiency can lead to loss of apoenzyme (Brin *et al.*, 1960; Pandit and Chakrabarti, 1972), and Kominami *et al.* (1972) have described a protease specific for PLP apoenzymes. Conversely, PN administration may increase enzyme levels (Hamamoto *et al.*, 1970; Greengard and Gordon, 1963), either by enzyme induction or by reducing the rate of degradation. In addition, some aminotransferases are induced by hormones (Rose and Cramp, 1970).

It should be emphasized that deficiencies demonstrated by any of the biochemical tests are relative in that the levels reflecting an absolute deficiency are not known. Although extreme vitamin deficiency is reflected in all of these tests, the converse is not necessarily true. Abnormal results, especially with the indirect methods, may be due to factors unrelated to vitamin B_6. It is often suggested that supplementation with PN brings abnormal test levels back to control levels, which, in the absence of other criteria, are considered to represent the desirable state of vitamin B_6 nutrition. As PLP levels are more sensitive to vitamin depletion and repletion than are the other indices, normalization of the indirect tests usually results in higher than normal blood PLP levels. This effect is compounded in conditions such as pregnancy by the known synergistic effect of hormones on the tryptophan load test and possibly also the aminotransferase activation test.

While PN is considered to be one of the least toxic vitamins, high PLP levels may have an adverse effect under certain circumstances. In pregnancy, a single oral dose of 50 mg of PN leads to high fetal blood levels of PLP (Table 7-5) (Shane, 1970; Contractor and Shane, 1970).

TABLE 7-5   PLP Levels in Maternal and Cord Vein Blood after Oral Administration of 50 mg PN • HCl

Period of Gestation	Time After Loading, hr	Maternal Blood, ng/ml	Cord Blood, ng/ml
Term	3.5	108	167
Term	5.5	38.7	97.7
Term	6.0	31.1	150
Term	6.5	32.1	115
Term	9.0	35.5	109
Term	10.0	16.0	65.7
Term[a]	4.0	34.0	53.0
21 weeks	6.0	6.8	250
25 weeks	6.0	43.0	281

[a]Pre-eclamptic.

This can be compared with the 20 mg/day of PN often recommended in the literature for correcting abnormal tryptophan metabolism or aminotransferase levels in pregnancy. Even higher cord blood levels, up to 300 ng/ml were found in 22- to 25-week-old fetuses. It is possible that high fetal PLP levels may have an adverse effect on the synthesis of fetal PLP enzymes and at worst lead to a high vitamin B_6 requirement at birth. One possible candidate for such an adverse effect is PL kinase. The levels of this enzyme increase in fetal liver and kidney through gestation (Contractor and Shane, 1969), and Ebadi *et al.* (1970) have demonstrated an inverse relationship between the levels of this enzyme and PLP levels in the rabbit brain.

RELATIONSHIP OF BLOOD VITAMIN TO TOTAL VITAMIN STORES

The sensitivity of blood vitamin levels to vitamin deficiency or increased tissue requirements can be anticipated by considering total body stores of the vitamin. Johansson *et al.* (1966) have demonstrated that these can be visualized as a two-compartment system consisting of a rapid-turnover compartment, in which the exogenous vitamin is either excreted into the urine or passed to a second, slow-turnover compartment, which could be compared to tightly bound tissue stores. With three male patients suffering from a variety of disorders, they found total body stores to be equivalent to 40 to 150 mg of PN.

Results from a similar study on healthy subjects (Shane, 1970) are shown in Figures 7-3 and 7-4. Figure 7-3 shows the body retention of

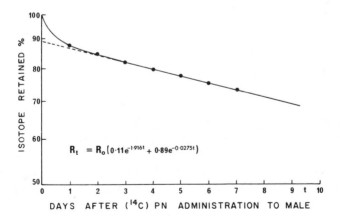

FIGURE 7-3   Whole body retention of [¹⁴C] vitamin after intravenous injection of [¹⁴C]PN (5 μCi).

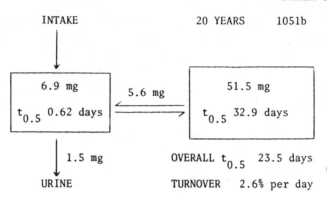

WHOLE BODY VITAMIN B6 COMPARTMENTS IN MALE

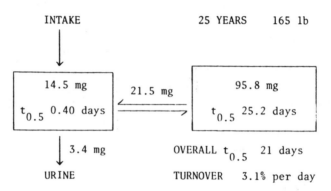

FIGURE 7-4   Total body stores of vitamin B_6 in healthy male and female subjects expressed as PN equivalents. Daily rates for transfer between compartments and for urinary excretion are shown.

the labeled vitamin by a healthy male subject after an IV injection of 5 μCi [^{14}C]PN in a total dose of about 100 μg. About 12 percent of the dose was excreted in the first 24 h and this was followed by a gradual loss of the labeled vitamin. The retention curve can be separated into two first-order components that can be visualized as two body compartments for the vitamin as shown in Figure 7-4.

The total body store in a healthy female subject was about 60 mg PN equivalents (Figure 7-4). About 90 percent was in a slow-turnover compartment with a half-life of 33 days, and the remainder in a fast-turnover compartment with a half-life of about 15 h. The daily excretion of vitamin was equivalent to 1.5 mg PN, 2.6 percent of the total body store. No attempt was made to control the diet in this experiment, and as this model assumes a steady state condition, the average daily absorption of vitamin by this subject can be assessed at 1.5 mg, or slightly less than the RDA.

Equivalent data for a healthy, 25-year-old male are also shown in Figure 7-4. Total body stores in this case were calculated to be approx-about three percent with an overall half-life for the body vitamin of 21 days. Urinary excretion was assessed at 3.4 mg/day, which again one assumes represents the average daily absorption.

The total blood vitamin B_6 content in man is less than 0.5 mg PN equivalents. This is less than one percent of the total body stores, so one would expect an increased tissue requirement for this vitamin to have a pronounced effect on blood levels of the vitamin.

The slow-turnover body compartment probably reflects a protein-bound vitamin, which would be mainly pyridoxal phosphate (Li *et al.*, 1974). This two-compartment model also explains the poor urinary recovery of loading doses of the vitamin (Table 7-6) (Shane, 1970; Snell, 1958). About 30 percent of a 50-mg oral dose of PN was recovered in urine in the first 24 h, predominantly as PIC, and the remainder of the dose was only slowly excreted by the body. Similar results were obtained after a 100-mg loading dose of PN (Shane, 1970; Contractor and Shane, 1968), demonstrating the body's high capacity for vitamin storage. One might expect large doses of the vitamin to disturb the equilibrium of the body compartments, and this was reflected by the 30 percent excretion compared to the 10–15 percent found after administration of a tracer dose of the vitamin.

Oral doses of PL and PLP were less effective in increasing body stores of the vitamin (Table 7-6). In these cases, about 60 percent of the dose was excreted in the first 24 hours. The similarity in results was not surprising, since PLP is probably hydrolyzed during absorption from the gut. The differences in body retention between PN and PL can be

TABLE 7-6   24-Hour Urinary Recovery of PIC after Oral Administration of Equimolar Amounts of PN, PL, and PLP to Nonpregnant Females

Dose		Recovery, %
PN • HCL	(50 mg)	24 ± 2 (3)
PL • HCL	(49.5 mg)	55 ± 7 (3)
PLP	(60.1 mg)	47 ± 4 (3)

explained by the metabolite routes for these compounds. PN can only be metabolized to PIC via PLP, and thus is completely available for tissue storage. PL metabolism can proceed in two directions. It can be phosphorylated to PLP or can be oxidized directly to PIC, which would be excreted.

The importance of phosphorylation in tissue storage has also been demonstrated by the use of the PN analogue, 5′-deoxyPN (Shane and Snell, 1975). In the first 10 minutes after intraperitoneal administration, this compound, which cannot be phosphorylated by PL kinase, was taken up by rat liver and brain to about the same extent as PN. By 2 hours, however, practically all the labeled 5′-deoxyPN had been released by these tissues and was completely recovered in the 24-h urine sample, predominantly as a sulphate ester. Comparable excretion of PN and its metabolites was about 40 percent of the dose.

Although the two body vitamin B_6 compartments should not be considered to have any anatomical meaning, a large proportion of the body PLP is stored in muscle (Krebs and Fischer, 1964; Veitch et al., 1976). Ryan et al. (1976) have shown that increasing the PN intake of the rat leads to a plateau in liver and brain PLP levels while plasma and muscle PLP levels do not saturate. Their data indicate that PLP in plasma and muscle behave as mobilizable storage pools and that plasma PLP is a sensitive indicator of the state of vitamin B_6 nutrition.

SUMMARY

Blood or plasma PLP levels serve as a useful index of vitamin B_6 status. Individual control levels remain relatively constant over long periods of time and they are sensitive to changes in vitamin requirements and body stores. The aminotransferase activation test appears to be a poor index of vitamin status, except in pronounced deficiency or controlled depletion studies, since it is less responsive to vitamin depletion than are blood pyridoxal phosphate levels and suffers from relatively large variations in individual control values. This may be a result of factors unrelated to vitamin B_6.

LITERATURE CITED

Aly, H. E., E. A. Donald, and M. H. W. Simpson. 1971. Oral contraceptives and vitamin B_6 metabolism. Am. J. Clin. Nutr. 24:297–303.

Altman, K., and O. Greengard. 1966. Correlation of kynurenine excretion with liver tryptophan pyrrolase levels in disease and after hydrocortisone induction. J. Clin. Invest. 45:1527–1534.

Anderson, B. B., and D. L. Mollin. 1972. Red-cell metabolism of pyridoxine in sideroblastic anaemias and related anaemias. Br. J. Haematol. 23:159–166.

Anderson, B. B., C. E. Fulford-Jones, J. A. Child, M. E. J. Beard, and C. J. T. Bateman. 1971. Conversion of vitamin B$_6$ compounds to active forms in the red blood cell. J. Clin. Invest. *50*:1901–1909.

Anderson, B. B., P. A. Newmark, M. Rawlins, and R. Green. 1974. Plasma binding of vitamin B$_6$ compounds. Nature *250*:502–504.

Baysal, A., B. A. Johnson, and H. Linkswiler. 1966. Vitamin B$_6$ depletion in man: Blood vitamin B$_6$, plasma pyridoxal phosphate, serum cholesterol, serum transaminases, and urinary vitamin B$_6$ and 4-pyridoxic acid. J. Nutr. *89*:19–23.

Bhagavan, H. N., M. Coleman, and D. B. Coursin. 1975. Distribution of pyridoxal 5'-phosphate in human blood between the cells and the plasma: Effect of oral administration of pyridoxine on the ratio in Down's and hyperactive patients. Biochem. Med. *14*:201–208.

Brin, M. 1970. Pyridoxine, estrogenic contraceptᵃᵉ steroids (ECS) and tryptophan metabolism. Fed. Proc. *29*:824. (abstr.)

Brin, M. 1971. Abnormal tryptophan metabolism in pregnancy and with the oral contraceptive pill. II. Relative levels of vitamin B$_6$-vitamers in cord and maternal blood. Am. J. Clin. Nutr. *24*:704–708.

Brin, M., M. Tai, A. S. Ostashever, and H. Kalinsky. 1960. The relative effects of pyridoxine deficiency on two plasma transaminases in the growing and in the adult rat. J. Nutr. *71*:416–420.

Brown, R. R., D. P. Rose, J. M. Price, and H. Wolf. 1969. Tryptophan metabolism as affected by anovulatory agents. Ann. N.Y. Acad. Sci. *166*:44–56.

Brown, R. R., D. P. Rose, J. E. Leklem, H. Linkswiler, and R. Anand. 1975. Urinary 4-pyridoxic acid, plasma pyridoxal phosphate, and erythrocyte aminotransferase levels in oral contraceptive users receiving controlled intakes of vitamin B$_6$. Am. J. Clin. Nutr. *28*:10–19.

Chabner, B., and D. Livingston. 1970. A simple enzymic assay for pyridoxal phosphate. Anal. Biochem. *34*:413–423.

Cinnamon, A. D., and J. R. Beaton. 1970. Biochemical assessment of vitamin B$_6$ status in man. Am. J. Clin. Nutr. *23*:696–702.

Cleary, R. E., L. Lumeng, and T-K. Li. 1975. Maternal and fetal plasma levels of pyridoxal phosphate at term. Adequacy of vitamin B$_6$ supplementation during pregnancy. Am. J. Obstet. Gynecol. *121*:25–28.

Colombini, C. E., and E. E. McCoy. 1970. Vitamin B$_6$ metabolism. The utilization of [^{14}C]pyridoxine by the normal mouse. Biochemistry *9*:533–538.

Contractor, S. F., and B. Shane. 1968. Estimation of vitamin B$_6$ compounds in human blood and urine. Clin. Chim. Acta *21*:71–77.

Contractor, S. F., and B. Shane. 1969. Pyridoxal kinase in the human placenta and fetus through gestation. Clin. Chim. Acta *25*:465–474.

Contractor, S. F., and B. Shane. 1970. Blood and urine levels of vitamin B$_6$ in the mother and fetus before and after loading of the mother with vitamin B$_6$. Am. J. Obstet. Gynecol. *107*:635–640.

Contractor, S. F., and B. Shane. 1971. Metabolism of [^{14}C]pyridoxol in the pregnant rat. Biochim. Biophys. Acta *230*:127–136.

Dempsey, W. B., and H. N. Christensen. 1962. The specific binding of pyridoxal 5'-phosphate to bovine plasma albumin. J. Biol. Chem. *237*:1113–1120.

Doberenz, A. R., J. P. Van Miller, J. R. Green, and J. R. Beaton. 1971. Vitamin B$_6$ depletion in women using oral contraceptives as determined by erythrocyte glutamic-pyruvic transaminase activities. Proc. Soc. Exp. Biol. Med. *137*:1100–1103.

Donald, E. A., L. D. McBean, M. H. W. Simpson, M. F. Sun, and H. E. Aly. 1971. Vitamin B$_6$ requirements of young adult women. Am. J. Clin. Nutr. *24*:1028–1041.

Ebadi, M. S., E. E. McCoy, and R. B. Kugel. 1970. Interrelationships between pyridoxal phosphate and pyridoxal kinase in rabbit brain. J. Neurochem. *17*:941–948.

Gaut, Z. N., and H. M. Solomon. 1972. Phosphorylation of pyridoxine by human blood platelets: Effects of structure analogs and metabolic inhibitors. Biochem. Pharmacol. *21*:2395–2400.

Gaynor, R., and W. B. Dempsey. 1972. Vitamin B₆ enzymes in normal and pre-eclamptic human placentae. Clin. Chim. Acta *37*:411–416.

Greengard, O., and M. Gordon. 1963. The cofactor-mediated regulation of apoenzyme levels in animal tissues. 1. The pyridoxine-induced rise of rat liver tyrosine transaminase levels *in vivo*. J. Biol. Chem. *238*:3708–3710.

Hamamoto, H., S. Kawashima, and Y. Nose. 1970. Studies on the induction of tyrosine transaminase by large dose administration of vitamin B₆. J. Vitaminol. *16*:268–275.

Hamfelt, A. 1964. Age variation of vitamin B₆ metabolism in man. Clin. Chim. Acta *10*:48–54.

Hamfelt, A. 1967a. Enzymatic determination of pyridoxal phosphate in plasma by decarboxylation of L-tyrosine-¹⁴C(U) and a comparison with the tryptophan load test. Scand. J. Clin. Lab. Invest. *20*:1–10.

Hamfelt, A. 1967b. Pyridoxal kinase activity in blood cells. Clin. Chim. Acta *16*:7–18.

Hamfelt, A. 1967c. Pyridoxal phosphate concentration and aminotransferase activity in human blood cells. Clin. Chim. Acta *16*:19–28.

Hamfelt, A. and L. Hahn. 1969. Pyridoxal phosphate concentration in plasma and tryptophan load testing during pregnancy. Clin. Chim. Acta *25*:91–96.

Hamfelt, A. and T. Tuvemo. 1972. Pyridoxal phosphate and folic acid concentration in blood and erythrocyte aspartate aminotransferase activity during pregnancy. Clin. Chim. Acta *41*:287–298.

Haskell, B. E. and E. E. Snell. 1972. An improved apotryptophanase assay for pyridoxal phosphate. Anal. Biochem. *45*:567–576.

Heller, S., R. M. Salkeld, and W. F. Korner. 1973. Vitamin B₆ status in pregnancy. Am. J. Clin. Nutr. *26*:1339–1348.

IUPAC-IUB Commission on Biochemical Nomenclature. 1970. Nomenclature for vitamins B₆ and related compounds. Biochemistry *9*:4019–4021.

Johansson, S., S. Lindstedt, U. Register, and L. Wadström. 1966. Studies on the metabolism of labeled pyridoxine in man. Am. J. Clin. Nutr. *18*:185–196.

Johansson, S., S. Lindstedt, and H-G. Tiselius. 1968. Metabolism of [³H]pyridoxine in mice. Biochemistry *7*:2327–2332.

Johansson, S., S. Lindstedt, and H-G. Tiselius. 1974. Metabolic interconversions of different forms of vitamin B₆. J. Biol. Chem. *249*:6040–6046.

Karlin, R., R. Bertoye, C. Hours, and N. Berry. 1966. Sur la teneur du sang total en vitamine B₆ chez des femmes gestantes et des femmes temoins, apres l'administration buccale d'une dose test de pyridoxine. C. R. Soc. Biol. *160*:1465–1470.

Kelsay, J., A. Baysal, and H. Linkswiler. 1968. Effect of vitamin B₆ depletion on the pyridoxal, pyridoxamine and pyridoxine content of the blood and urine of men. J. Nutr. *94*:490–494.

Keyhani, M., D. Giuliani, E. R. Giuliani, and B. S. Morse. 1974. Erythropoiesis in pyridoxine deficient mice. Proc. Soc. Exp. Biol. Med. *146*:114–119.

Kishi, H., T. Kishi, R. H. Williams, and K. Folkers. 1975. Human deficiencies of vitamin B₆. I. Studies on parameters of the assay of the glutamic oxaloacetic transaminase by the CAS principle. Res. Commun. Chem. Path. Pharmacol. *12*:557–569.

Kleiger, J. A., J. R. Evard, and R. Pierce. 1966. Abnormal pyridoxine metabolism in toxemia of pregnancy. Am. J. Obstet. Gynecol. *94*:316–321.

Kleiger, J. A., C. H. Altshuler, G. Krakow, and C. Hollister. 1969. Abnormal pyridoxine metabolism in toxemia of pregnancy. Ann. N.Y. Acad. Sci. *166*:288–296.

Kominami, E., K. Kobayashi, S. Kominami, and N. Katunuma. 1972. Properties of a specific protease for pyridoxal enzymes and its biological role. J. Biol. Chem. *247*:6848–6855.

Krebs, E. G., and E. H. Fischer. 1964. Phosphorylase and related enzymes of glycogen metabolism. Vitam. Horm. *22*:399–410.

Leklem, J. E., R. R. Brown, D. P. Rose, and H. M. Linkswiler. 1975. Vitamin B$_6$ requirements of women using oral contraceptives. Am. J. Clin. Nutr. *28*:535–541.

Li, T-K., L. Lumeng, and R. L. Veitch. 1974. Regulation of pyridoxal 5'-phosphate metabolism in liver. Biochem. Biophys. Res. Commun. *61*:677–684.

Lumeng, L., and T-K. Li. 1974. Vitamin B$_6$ metabolism in chronic alcohol abuse. J. Clin. Invest. *53*:693–704.

Lumeng, L., and T-K. Li. 1975. Characterization of the pyridoxal 5'-phosphate and pyridoxamine 5'-phosphate hydrolase activity in rat liver. J. Biol. Chem. *250*:8126–8131.

Lumeng, L., R. E. Brashear, and T-K. Li. 1974a. Pyridoxal 5'-phosphate in plasma: Source, protein-binding, and cellular transport. J. Lab. Clin. Med. *84*:334–343.

Lumeng, L., R. E. Cleary, and T-K. Li. 1974b. Effect of oral contraceptives on the plasma concentration of pyridoxal phosphate. Am. J. Clin. Nutr. *27*:326–333.

Mason, M., J. Ford, and H. L. C. Wu. 1969. Effects of steroid and nonsteroid metabolites on enzyme conformation and pyridoxal phosphate binding. Ann. N.Y. Acad. Sci. *166*:170–183.

Masugi, F., Y. Sumi, S. Shimizu, and S. Fukui. 1973. Transfer of pyridoxal 5'-phosphate from albumin-pyridoxal 5'-phosphate complex to apo-aspartate aminotransferase. J. Nutr. Sci. Vitaminol. *19*:229–236.

McCormick, D. B., M. E. Gregory, and E. E. Snell. 1961. Pyridoxal phosphokinase: I. Assay, distribution, purification, and properties. J. Biol. Chem. *236*:2076–2084.

Metzler, D. E., and E. E. Snell. 1955. Spectra and ionization constants of the vitamin B$_6$ group and related 3-hydroxypyridine derivatives. J. Am. Chem. Soc. *77*:2431–2437.

Miller, L. T., E. M. Benson, M. A. Edwards, and J. Young. 1974. Vitamin B$_6$ metabolism in women using oral contraceptives. Am. J. Clin. Nutr. *27*:797–805.

Pandit, V. I., and C. H. Chakrabarti. 1972. Studies on certain hepatic enzymes and protein biosynthesis in pyridoxine deficient rats. J. Vitaminol. *18*:3–9.

Raica, N., Jr., and H. E. Sauberlich. 1964. Blood cell transaminase activity in human B$_6$ deficiency. Am. J. Clin. Nutr. *15*:67–72.

Reinken, L. 1974. Eine Mikromethode zur Bestimmung der Pyridoxal-Kinase-Activität im Serum. Int. Z. Vitam. Ern. Forsch. *44*:189–194.

Rose, D. P. 1966. Excretion of xanthurenic acid in the urine of women taking progesterone-oestrogen preparations. Nature *210*:196–197.

Rose, D. P., and D. G. Cramp. 1970. Reduction of plasma tyrosine by oral contraceptives and oestrogens: a possible consequence of tyrosine aminotransferase induction. Clin. Chim. Acta *29*:49–53.

Ryan, M. P., L. Lumeng, and T-K. Li. 1976. Validation of plasma pyridoxal 5'-phosphate measurements as an indicator of vitamin B$_6$ nutritional status. Fed. Proc. *35*:660 (Abstract 2508).

Salkeld, R. M., K. Knörr, and W. F. Körner. 1973. The effect of oral contraceptives on vitamin B_6 status. Clin. Chim. Acta 49:195–199.

Sauberlich, H. E. 1968. Biochemical systems and biochemical detection of deficiency. In W. H. Sebrell, Jr., and R. S. Harris (eds.), The Vitamins, Vol. 2, 2nd ed., Academic Press, New York, pp. 67–68.

Sauberlich, H. E., J. E. Canham, E. M. Baker, N. Raica, Jr., and Y. F. Herman. 1972. Biochemical assessment of the nutritional status of vitamin B_6 in the human. Am. J. Clin. Nutr. 25:629–642.

Shane, B. 1970. Metabolism of vitamin B_6 (pyridoxine) in pregnancy. Ph.D. thesis, University of London.

Shane, B., and S. F. Contractor. 1975. Assessment of vitamin B_6 status. Studies on pregnant women and oral contraceptive users. Am. J. Clin. Nutr. 28:739–747.

Shane, B., and E. E. Snell. 1972. The nature of "pyridoxine oxidase" from rabbit liver preparations. Arch. Biochem. Biophys. 153:333–336.

Shane, B., and E. E. Snell. 1975. Metabolism of 5'-deoxypyridoxine in rats: 5'-deoxypyridoxine 4'-sulphate as a major urinary metabolite. Biochem. Biophys. Res. Commun. 66:1294–1300.

Snell, E. E. Some aspects of the metabolism of vitamin B_6. 1958. In Fourth International Congress of Biochemistry-Vitamin Metabolism, Vol. 11, Pergamon Press, New York, pp. 250–265.

Snell, E. E., and B. E. Haskell. 1971. The metabolism of vitamin B_6. In M. Florkin and E. H. Stotz (eds.), Comprehensive Biochemistry, Vol. 21, Elsevier, New York, pp. 47–71.

Suzue, R., and M. Tachibana. 1970. The uptake of pyridoxal phosphate by human red blood cells. J. Vitaminol. 16:164–171.

Tiselius, H-G. 1973. Metabolism of tritium-labelled pyridoxine and pyridoxine 5'-phosphate in the central nervous system. J. Neurochem. 20:937–946.

Veitch, R. L., W. F. Bosron, and T-K. Li. 1976. Distribution of pyridoxal 5'-phosphate binding proteins in rat liver. Fed. Proc. 35:1545 (Abstract 976).

Wachstein, M. 1964. Evidence for a relative vitamin B_6 deficiency in pregnancy and some disease states. Vitam. Horm. 22:705–719.

Wachstein, M., C. Moore, and L. W. Graffeo. 1957. Pyridoxal phosphate levels of circulating leucocytes in maternal and cord blood. Proc. Soc. Exp. Biol. Med. 96:326–328.

Wachstein, M., J. D. Kellner, and J. M. Ortiz. 1960. Pyridoxal phosphate in plasma and leucocytes of normal and pregnant subjects following B_6 load tests. Proc. Soc. Exp. Biol. Med. 103:350–353.

Woodring, M. J., and C. A. Storvick. 1970. Effect of pyridoxine supplementation on glutamic-pyruvic transaminase and in vitro stimulation in erythrocytes of normal women. Am. J. Clin. Nutr. 23:1385–1395.

Yamada, K., and M. Tsuji. 1968. Transport of vitamin B_6 in human erythrocytes. J. Vitaminol. 14:282–294.

Yamada, K., and M. Tsuji. 1970. Transport of vitamin B_6 in human erythrocytes. J. Vitaminol. 16:237–242.

Zehaluk, C. M., and B. L. Walker. 1973. Effect of pyridoxine on red cell fatty acid composition in mature rats fed an essential fatty acid-deficient diet. J. Nutr. 103:1548–155t

8

Vitamin B₆ and Biogenic Amines in Brain Metabolism

MANUCHAIR EBADI

Pyridoxal phosphate and pyridoxamine phosphate, the catalytically active forms of vitamin B₆, influence brain function by participating at stages in metabolism of proteins, lipids, carbohydrates, other coenzymes, and hormones (Tower, 1956; Braunstein, 1960; Harris *et al.* 1964; Snell *et al.,* 1963; Holtz and Palm, 1964; Fasella, 1967; Ebadi and Costa, 1972). The following enumerates the involvement of vitamin B₆ in the metabolism of other vitamins and in hormonal actions (Kutsky, 1973). Vitamin B₆ deficiency results in a lowered concentration of coenzyme A in blood, in reduced absorption and storage of vitamin B₁₂, and in increased excretion of vitamin C. Furthermore, vitamin B₆ acts synergistically with vitamin E to control metabolism of unsaturated fats, with vitamin C in tyrosine metabolism, and with niacin in its action and participates in niacin synthesis. In addition, vitamin B₆ deficiency results in insufficiency of insulin and in alteration of the functions of adrenal and pituitary glands, since it is involved in the synthesis of growth hormone, follicle-stimulating hormone, luteinizing hormone, aldosterone, glucagon, cortisol, estradiol, testosterone, and epinephrine. These above-mentioned hormones, whose metabolism is

129

vitamin B_6-dependent, play decisive roles in maintaining the functional integrity of the peripheral and central nervous systems.

Vitamin B_6 participates in the metabolism of amino acids in the form of decarboxylation, transamination, deamination, racemization, and desulfhydration reactions (Snell, 1953). The crucial roles that these coenzymes play in the maintenance of functional integrity of the brain become evident when one realizes that all compounds implicated as neurotransmitters are synthesized and/or metabolized by the aid of the vitamin B_6-dependent enzymatic reactions. These include dopamine, norepinephrine, and serotonin (Lovenberg *et al.*, 1962), tyramine, tryptamine (Meister, 1965), taurine (Jacobson and Smith, 1968), histamine (Buffoni, 1966; Kahlson and Rosengram, 1965), gamma aminobutyric acid (Roberts and Frankel, 1950; Baxter and Roberts, 1958), and even acetylcholine indirectly (Yamada *et al.*, 1956; Williams and Hata, 1959). In recent years, the above-mentioned biogenic amines have become of considerable interest to neurobiologists who are investigating the etiology and the pathological manifestations of many disorders of the central nervous system (CNS), such as Parkinsonism (cf. Calne, 1973), Huntington's chorea (cf. Barbeau *et al.*, 1973), minimal brain disfunction (cf. Wender, 1971), schizophrenia (cf. Smythies, 1963), depression (cf. Cole and Wittenhorn, 1966), sleep disorders (cf. Kales, 1969), and seizure disorders (cf. Huxtable and Barbeau, 1976). In this report, the recent advances dealing with the interrelations among vitamin B_6, γ-aminobutyric acid (GABA) and CNS excitability and with the interrelations among vitamin B_6, dopamine, and Parkinsonism will be discussed.

VITAMIN B_6 AND GABA IN THE CENTRAL NERVOUS SYSTEM

Many findings support the concept that short chain ω amino acids, namely, taurine and GABA, have inhibitory actions on the central nervous system. Observations that have been reviewed recently (Baxter, 1970; Obata, 1972; Roberts, 1974; Meldrum, 1975) indicate that (1) GABA and its synthesizing enzyme, glutamic acid decarboxylase, are present in synaptosomes; (2) a high affinity and selective uptake mechanism remains operational for GABA; (3) stimulation of inhibitory but not excitatory neurons results in release of GABA; (4) the iontophoretic application of GABA alters membrane conductance to chloride ions similar to that produced by stimulating physiologically functioning inhibitory neurons; and finally (5) GABA receptor site blocking compounds, such as bicuculline, block not only the inhibitory action of

GABA released by neurons, but also that introduced through iontophoretic application.

Metabolism of GABA

In the central nervous system, GABA, which does not penetrate the blood brain barrier, is formed primarily from glutamic acid (Roberts and Frankel, 1950; Baxter and Roberts, 1958) by the aid of a pyridoxal phosphate-dependent L-glutamic acid decarboxylase (L-glutamate-1-carboxyl-lyase; EC 4.1.1.15), a soluble enzyme that is predominantly of synaptosomal origin (Haber *et al.*, 1970). The rate of binding of pyridoxal phosphate to apoglutamate decarboxylase reveals a "two step mechanism involving rapid initial formation of an enzyme pyridoxal phosphate complex followed by slow formation of the catalytically active enzyme pyridoxal phosphate Schiff base" (O'Leary and Malik, 1971). Glutamic acid decarboxylase I, which is inhibited by anions and by amino-oxyacetic acid, is differentiated from glutamic acid decarboxylase II, which is activated by anions and amino-oxyacetic acid and is localized in glial cells, kidney, heart, and adrenal and pituitary glands, through lack of immunological cross reactivity (Saito *et al.*, 1973). Glutamic acid decarboxylase I, which has been purified from mouse brain, has a molecular weight of 85,000 and catalyzes the rapid α-decarboxylation of L-glutamic acid (Wu *et al.*, 1973) at a pH optimum of 7.0. Electrophoretic studies using sodium dodecyl sulphate polyacrylamide gels suggested that glutamic acid decarboxylase I may be a hexamer consisting of 15,000 dalton subunits (Matsuda *et al.*, 1973).

GABA is catabolized by undergoing a reversible transamination with α-ketoglutarate to yield glutamate and succinic semialdehyde. GABA-transaminase (4-aminobutyrate: 2-oxyglutarate amino transaminase, EC 2.6.1.19), a particulate enzyme, requires pyridoxal phosphate, as a coenzyme (Nishizawa, *et al.*, 1959; Baxter and Roberts, 1958). In contrast to glutamic acid decarboxylases, pyridoxal phosphate is bound tightly to GABA-transaminase. Although localized in other tissues (Nakamura and Bernheim, 1962; Caciappo, *et al.*, 1959), in the CNS, GABA-transaminase is found primarily in gray matter. The purified GABA-transaminase (Schousboe *et al.*, 1973) has a molecular weight of 109,000 and can be split into two unequal subunits. In addition to GABA, other ω amino acids such as β-alanine can serve as substrates. However, α-ketoglutarate is the only keto acid that functions as an amino group acceptor.

The product of the transaminase reaction, succinic semialdehyde, is metabolized to succinic acid by the aid of succinic-semialdehyde dehydrogenase (succinic semialdehyde: NAD (p)+ oxidoreductase, EC 1.2.1.16). Succinic acid in turn is oxidized via the reactions of the tricarboxylic acid cycle. GABA-transaminase and succinic semialdehyde dehydrogenase are two closely coupled mitochondrial enzymes (Salganicoff and De Robertis, 1965) that have their pH optima in the alkaline range (Waksman and Roberts, 1965).

In an attempt to reveal the factors regulating its activity, purified glutamic acid decarboxylase from mouse brain has been studied (Wu and Roberts, 1974). The steady state concentrations of GABA in various brain areas are governed by glutamic acid decarboxylase and not by GABA-transaminase. Several facts are known about the purified decarboxylase; these are as follows: The presence of aldehyde, sulfhydryl, and positively charged groups has been suspected at or near the active site of the enzyme. The purified mouse brain glutamic acid decarboxylase is highly sensitive to the inhibitory action of sulfhydryl reagents such as DTNB (5'5'-dithiobis [2-nitrobenzoic acid]) and PCMB (P-chloromercuribenzoate). Iodoacetamide or iodoacetic acid were less inhibitory in nature.

It has been known for some time that other decarboxylases such as s-adenosylmethionine decarboxylase (Wickner *et al.*, 1970), histidine decarboxylase (Chang and Snell, 1968), acetoacetate decarboxylase (Autor and Fridovich, 1970), and L-ornithine decarboxylase (Janne and Williams-Ashman, 1971) were sensitive to sulfhydryl reagents. Among carbonyl trapping agents, amino-oxyacetic acid was the most potent inhibitor, followed by hydroxylamine, hydrazine semicarbazide, and D-penicillamine in descending order (reviewed by Holtz and Palm, 1964). Mercapto acids such as 3-mercapto propionic acid and 2-mercapto propionic acid were competitive inhibitors with Ki of 1.8 μM and 300 μM, respectively. These compounds not only could react with the disulfide moiety at or near the active site of the enzyme but also have been shown previously to form a thiohemiacetal with the aldehyde group of the pyridoxal phosphate (Boyer, 1959; Buell and Hansen, 1960). No other known vitamin B_6-requiring enzyme is so sensitive to the inhibition by mercapto acids as brain L-glutamic acid decarboxylase. Indeed, some vitamin B_6-containing enzymes such as muscle phosphorylase (Buell and Hansen, 1961) and vitamin B_6-requiring enzymes such as L-ornithine decarboxylase (Janne and Williams-Ashman, 1971) are activated or protected by these compounds.

Like bacterial glutamate decarboxylase (Fonda, 1972), carboxylic acids with a net negative charge such as D-glutamate, α-ketoglutarate, fumarate, and L-aspartate were shown to be potent inhibitors of purified mouse brain L-glutamate decarboxylase. The intermediate of glycolysis had no significant effects. Compounds with one carbon less, such as succinic and oxalacetic acids, or with one carbon more, such as adipic or α-ketoadipic acids, were less inhibitory. The monovalent cations Li, Na, NH_4, and CS had no effects on L-glutamic acid decarboxylase in concentrations of up to 10 mM; whereas, the divalent ions were most potent inhibitors. It is interesting that zinc was the most potent inhibitor, inhibiting to the extent of 50 percent at 10 mM. The decreasing order of inhibitory strength was Zn > Cd = Hg = Cu > Ni > Mn > Co > Ba > Ca > Mg > Sr. The anions I, Br, Cl, and F were only weak inhibitors. Consequently, it is believed that Zn might play an important role in regulating the activity of glutamic acid decarboxylase I (Wu and Roberts, 1974). The relationships among the concentration of Zn, the activity of pyridoxal kinase, and L-glutamic acid decarboxylase deserve special attention and perhaps critical analysis. In the brain, the regional distributions of Zn (Lehmann, *et al.*, 1971; Backer, 1967), glutamic acid decarboxylase (Roberts and Kuriyama, 1968), and pyridoxal kinase (McCormick *et al.*, 1961) are identical and highest in gray matter. Unlike glutamic acid decarboxylase, which is inhibited by Zn (Wu and Roberts, 1974), pyridoxal kinase is preferentially activated by it (McCormick and Snell, 1959). The synthesis of GABA is dependent upon glutamic acid decarboxylase, whose activity in turn is dependent on pyridoxal phosphate, which is synthesized by pyridoxal kinase. Zn on one hand activates glutamic acid decarboxylase through coenzyme activation of enzyme but on the other hand inhibits it through other unknown mechanisms. Whether or not this reciprocal antagonism is operational *in vivo* to control the synthesis of GABA remains to be seen.

In continuing with the discussion of factors that might control the synthesis of GABA, Wu and Roberts (1974) have shown that biogenic amines such as norepinephrine and serotonin were potent inhibitors; whereas, acetylcholine, dopamine, and histamine were less effective inhibitors of glutamic acid decarboxylase. Nucleotides such as ATP, ADP, AMP, cyclic AMP, GTP, GDP, GMP, and cyclic GMP were weak inhibitors of this enzyme (Wu and Roberts, 1974).

Regional Distribution of GABA and Its Abnormality in Huntington's Chorea

Like other substances in brain (Duffy *et al.*, 1972), the concentration of GABA increases very rapidly after death (Lovell *et al.*, 1963; Shaw and

Heine, 1965; Minard and Mushawar, 1966; Shank and Aprison, 1971). The unequal postmortem changes in the concentrations of GABA in different regions of the brain (highest in the hypothalamus) may be closely related to the varied activity of glutamic acid decarboxylase (Albers and Brady, 1959). Microwave irradiation techniques and sodium acetate extraction procedures were used to redetermine the regional distribution of GABA in brain (Balcom *et al.*, 1975). The highest levels of GABA (3.50–4.60 μM/g tissue) were found in septal nuclei, hypothalamus, substantia nigra, and nucleus accumbens; the intermediate levels (2.0–3.50 μM/g tissue) were detected in hippocampus, striatum, amygdala-pyriform cortex, thalamus, inferior colliculus, olfactory tubercle, midbrain tegmentum, and superior colliculus; while the lowest levels (1.25–2.0 μM/g tissue) appeared in cortex, cerebellum, and pons medulla. The regional distribution of GABA, determined after microwave irradiation procedure, which inactivates enzymes responsible for altering the levels of various compounds in the brain (Schmidt *et al.*, 1971; Stavinoha *et al.*, 1973), is considerably lower but in good agreement with those concentrations reported previously using the decapitation techniques (Baxter and Roberts, 1959; Okada, *et al.*, 1971).

Huntington's chorea, a degenerative and progressive disease, is characterized by the onset of chorea and dementia. At autopsy, a marked loss of cells is observed in the caudate nucleus and putamen and to a lesser extent in the cerebral cortex (Myrianthopoulos, 1966; Perry *et al.*, 1973; Shoulson and Chase, 1975). Biochemical analyses of the autopsy materials have shown that the concentration of GABA was considerably lower in the substantia nigra and putamen-globus pallidus of patients dying from Huntington's chorea as compared with those obtained from neurologically normal patients (Perry *et al.*, 1973; Bird and Iverson, 1974; Stahl and Swanson, 1974). Similarly, the activity of glutamic acid decarboxylase is considerably lower (Bird and Iverson, 1974; Stahl and Swanson, 1974). In addition, the activity of choline acetyltransferase is subnormal (Bird and Iverson, 1974). No inhibitor of glutamic acid decarboxylase nor the presence of an isoenzyme with decreased affinity for glutamate was detected. The activity of GABA-transaminase is normal (Urquhart *et al.*, 1975). The observation, however, is not specific to chorea, since the activity of glutamic acid decarboxylase is equally low in Parkinson's disease (E. G. McGeer *et al.*, 1971; P. L. McGreer *et al.*, 1971; Lloyd and Hornykiewicz, 1973; Klawans and Rubovits, 1972). Chronic dietary deficiency of vitamin B_6 may not be a likely explanation for the reduced activity of glutamic acid decarboxylase and the reduced concentration of GABA because the concentration of cystathionine, the end product of cystathionase, another vitamin B$_6$-requiring enzyme, is normal (Perry *et al.*, 1973). In addition, the administration of pyridoxine does not ameliorate the symptomatology of patients with Huntington's chorea (Wood *et al.*, 1972).

GABA *Binding Sites in Brain and Its Abnormality in Huntington's Chorea*

Immunochemical localization techniques at the level of the electron microscope were used to study glutamic acid decarboxylase in the cerebellum, a region which is richly endowed with inhibitory synapses (McLaughlin *et al.*, 1975). Glutamic acid decarboxylase is highly localized in certain synaptic vesicles and mitochondria but not within these organelles. Similarly, reaction products for glutamic acid decarboxylase are associated with presynaptic functional membranes (McLaughlin *et al.*, 1975).

The subcellular binding sites of GABA (Zukin *et al.*, 1974; Enna and Snyder, 1975; Enna *et al.*, 1975) and other neurotransmitters (Yamamura and Snyder, 1974; Burgen *et al.*, 1974; Beid and Ariens, 1974; Bennett and Aghaganian, 1974; Snyder, 1975; Bennett and Snyder, 1975; Snyder and Bennett, 1975; Alexander *et al.*, 1975; Zatz *et al.*, 1976) have been studied extensively. In measuring the distribution of specific [3H]-GABA binding in subcellular fractions of whole rat brain, Zukin *et al.* (1974) found that the largest amount of binding was recovered in the crude mitochondrial fraction (P$_2$), which contained both synaptosomes and free mitochondria. Total specific binding in the P$_2$ pellet was as great or greater than that of the whole homogenate. No specific binding could be detected in the crude mitochondrial pellet. The crude synaptic membrane fraction contained about 10 times as much GABA binding as the mitochondria-myelin pellet (Zukin *et al.*, 1974).

Regional distribution of [3H]-GABA binding to synaptic membrane fractions obtained from brain revealed the greatest binding in the cerebellum; intermediate levels in the thalamus, hippocampus, hypothalamus, cerebral cortex, midbrain, and corpus striatum; whereas, the lowest levels were detected in the pons, medulla oblongata, and spinal cord (Zukin *et al.*, 1974). In general, the regional distribution of [3H]-GABA binding sites does not correlate with the content of endogenous transmitter as reported by other workers (Baxter and Roberts, 1959; Okada *et al.*, 1971; Balcom *et al.*, 1975). Zukin *et al.* (1974) feel that "receptor density need not correlate with the content of endogenous transmitter in presynaptic boutons. The relative surface area of postsynaptic membrane may vary throughout the brain independently of the volume or transmitter content of associated nerve terminals." Furthermore, no apparent correlation was shown to exist between the relative density of muscarinic cholinergic receptors and the endogenous levels of acetylcholine (Yamamura *et al.*, 1974; Hiley and Burgen, 1974) and between the lysergic acid diethylamide binding sites and the endogenous levels of serotonin (Bennett and Snyder, 1975).

Although the concentration of GABA is lower in the substantia nigra and putamen-globus pallidus of patients with Huntington's chorea, the GABA receptor binding sites are not (Enna *et al.*, 1976). On the other hand, the muscarinic cholinergic receptor binding substances are reduced (Hiley and Bird, 1974; Enna *et al.*, 1976).

Vitamin B_6 Deficiency, Glutamic Acid Decarboxylase, and GABA

The subcellular distribution of pyridoxal phosphate in brain, which is highest in supernatant and crude mitochondrial fractions (Bain and Williams, 1960; Loo and Mack, 1971; and Pérez de la Mora *et al.*, 1973), corresponds closely with several vitamin B_6-requiring enzymes such as alanine aminotransferase, aspartate aminotransferase, GABA aminotransferase, and glutamic acid decarboxylase (Salganicoff and De Robertis, 1965; Van Kempen *et al.*, 1965; Fonnum, 1968). Consequently, reduction in the concentration of B_6 vitamins, created by dietary deficiency or by administration of vitamin B_6 antimetabolites, should be expected to result not only in reduced activity of soluble enzymes (decarboxylases) and particulate enzymes (aminotransferases), but also in a notable diminution in the concentrations of their end products. For example, Pérez de la Mora *et al.* (1973) have shown that treatment of mice with pyridoxal phosphate-γ-glutamyl hydrazone decreased the concentration of pyridoxal phosphate in several fractions but especially in the soluble fractions. In addition, this treatment inhibited glutamic acid decarboxylase, which in general was greater in those fractions in which pyridoxal phosphate reduction was the highest. The inhibition of glutamic acid decarboxylase is probably secondary to inhibition of pyridoxal kinase, the enzyme that synthesizes the coenzyme pyridoxal phosphate. Consistent with these views is the observation that only those compounds that inhibited pyridoxal kinase, such as 5-phosphate hydrazone of L-glutamyl γ-hydrazone, inhibited glutamic acid decarboxylase; whereas, those compounds that did not inhibit pyridoxal kinase significantly, such as isonicotinylhydrazine or thiosemicarbazide, proved not to be inhibitory to glutamic acid decarboxylase (Tapia and Awapara, 1967, 1969). Furthermore, the degree of inhibition of glutamic acid decarboxylase may be related directly to ability of inhibitors to interact by combining with the aldehyde group of the "loosely bound" versus "firmly bound" pyridoxal phosphate at the active sites of the enzymes. For example, aminooxyacetic acid is a more potent inhibitor of mouse brain glutamic acid decarboxylase than is pyridoxal-5'-phosphate oxime-*o*-acetic acid (Tapia and Sandoval, 1971). This latter compound is thought to combine with the loosely bound and dialyzable pyridoxal phosphate, whereas amino-oxyacetic acid combines with both dialyzable and nondialyzable coenzymes. In short, the influence of pyridoxal phosphate in modulating the action of glutamic acid decarboxylase is demonstrated by the findings of Tapia *et al.* (1970), who measured the concentration of pyridoxal phosphate and the activity of glutamic acid decarboxylase in brains of carp, pigeon, and mouse. Carp had the lowest amount of pyridoxal phosphate and the lowest activity of glutamic acid decarboxylase.

"Mild" and "severe" vitamin B₆ deficiencies result in lower concentration of GABA in whole brain (Tews and Lovell, 1967), in various parts of brain (Bayoumi and Smith, 1973), and in the developing brain (Stephens *et al.*, 1971; Bayoumi and Smith, 1973). This effect appears to be due to inhibition of glutamic acid decarboxylase and not GABA aminotransferase (Stephens *et al.*, 1971). However, the influence of vitamin B₆ on the apoenzyme as compared to the holoenzyme of glutamic acid decarboxylase should be differentiated. For example, Bayoumi and Smith (1973) working with suckling and adult vitamin B₆-deficient rats and measuring glutamic acid decarboxylase in hypothalamus, midbrain, thalamus, corpus striatum, cerebral cortex, hippocampus, medulla, pons, and cerebellum, found that the activity of the holoenzyme (assayed without pyridoxal phosphate) was reduced significantly, whereas the activity of the apoenzyme (assayed with pyridoxal phosphate) showed no change in all regions tested, except in cerebellum where it increased. In contrast to adult animals, the apoenzyme increased substantially in all regions of vitamin B₆-deficient suckling rats.

The Antivitamin B₆ Effects of Compounds of Pharmacological Importance

Isoniazid, the hydrazid of isonicotinic acid, is a highly effective tuberculostatic drug. In tuberculosis patients receiving isoniazid, the urinary excretion of vitamin B_6 (Biehl and Vilter, 1954) and xanthurenic acid after tryptophan load (Biehl and Vilter, 1954; Rajtar and Leontiew, 1970) became increased. The administration of vitamin B_6 rectified both abnormalities (Biehl and Vilter, 1954). In addition, the administration of isoniazid produces peripheral neuropathy (Ross, 1958; Kalinowski et al., 1961), which is initially sensory and may later show signs of motor involvement. The pathological manifestations of neuropathy (reviewed by Aita and Calame, 1972) are characterized by "primary axonal degeneration with subsequent fragmentation of the myelin sheath (Wallerian degeneration) of small- to medium-sized fibers with sparing of large sensory fibers to the muscle spindles plus concomitant remyelination and collateral sprouting of spared motor axons terminally. This degeneration is more severe distally and may later involve the ventral roots and still later, the dorsal roots and possibly the posterior columns. The collateral sprouting represents motor fiber regeneration and is at a sufficient rate to compensate for lost fibers; thus, clinically, the neuropathy is initially and usually sensory."

The incidence of isoniazid-induced peripheral neuritis is increased in malnutrition and in situations where the concentration of hydrazide is increased in the body, such as after chronic administration of large dosages and in patients who are slow metabolizers of this compound (Ross, 1958; Krishnamurthy et al., 1967; Biehl and Vilter, 1954; Ochoa, 1970; Davadatta et al., 1960; Gammon et al., 1953; Money, 1959).

In addition to peripheral neuritis, other manifestations of the neurotoxicity of isoniazid include generalized seizure, optic neuritis followed by atrophy, muscle twitching, dizziness, ataxia, paresthesias, stupor, and toxic encephalopathy. Furthermore, mental abnormalities such as euphoria, transient impairment of memory, separation of ideas and reality, loss of self-control, and psychosis have been reported following the administration of isoniazid (Robson and Sullivan, 1963; Mitchell, 1967; Fox, 1968). Although the mechanisms of tuberculostatic and tuberculocidal actions of isoniazid are not known (Youatt, 1969), the antipyridoxine effects of the compound have been established. For example, the isoniazid-induced neurotoxicities may be prevented, arrested, or reversed by the administration of vitamin B_6 (Carlson et al., 1956; Ross, 1958). Consistent with these views is the observation that the neurotoxicity of isoniazid is increased in malnutrition and in conditions causing secondary vitamin B_6 deficiency, such as pregnancy, hyperthyroidism, infections, and malignancy (Holtz and Palm, 1964). Isoniazid may cause vitamin B_6 deficiency by chelating pyridoxal phosphate to form pyridoxal phosphate hydrazone, which in turn inhibits pyridoxal kinase, the enzyme that synthesizes the catalytically active coenzyme. Therefore, isoniazid reduces the tissue concentration of pyridoxal phosphate directly and indirectly.

Although the antivitamin B_6 effects of isoniazid are well known, there are many other drugs of hydrazine derivation whose chronic effects on the metabolism and functions of vitamin B_6 have not been studied in detail. Among compounds of pharmacological interest, antihypertensive preparations, antianginal agents, cancer chemotherapeutic drugs, immunosuppressive medications, tranquilizers, antidepressants, antiviral substances, antihistamines, antimicrobials, and antiasthmatics (Juchau and Horita, 1972) may be enumerated.

Standal *et al.* (1974), using the criterion of Sauberlich *et al.* (1972) for vitamin B_6 deficiency, determined the vitamin B_6 status of a normal population and compared it with that of patients who were receiving isonicotinic acid hydrazid. The three experimental groups were (1) healthy individuals; (2) persons receiving isoniazid who had shown positive reactions to the tuberculin test but who did not show active tuberculosis; and (3) patients who were hospitalized with active tuberculosis and were receiving in addition to isoniazid, ethambutol and pyridoxine daily. Standal *et al.* (1974) detected vitamin B_6 deficiency in control healthy subjects on "self-selected diets" and patients who were receiving isoniazid without pyridoxine who were on a similar diet to those in the control group. These data indicate that the anti-pyridoxine effects of hydrazine derivatives of pharmacological importance, along with other nonhydrazine compounds such as cycloserine and penicillamine (Holtz and Palm, 1964), probably deserve special attention and careful analytical studies.

Vitamin B₆, GABA, and Convulsion

"The brain, in Lennox's phrase, 'is built to convulse'. Among the built-in defense mechanisms which prevent epilepsy in the majority of mankind, pyridoxine has a definite but uncertain place" (Bower, 1965). In the human, the effects of vitamin B_6 on CNS excitability became dramatically established in 1952 when it was found that pyridoxine-deficient dried milk produced neonatal convulsion (Snyderman *et al.*, 1953). The convulsion due to vitamin B_6 deficiency, which has been reported as early as 3 hours after birth (Hunt *et al.*, 1954) and which has resulted in at least one case of mortality (Scriver, 1960), can be controlled and corrected by administration of vitamin B_6 (Hunt *et al.*, 1954; Scriver, 1960). Autopsy of one infant with persistent convulsions revealed "astrocytic hyperplasia moderate in the cortex and pronounced in the basal ganglia, and nerve loss in the thalamus" (Scriver, 1960). In addition to the human, vitamin B_6 deficiency in experimental animals, such as chicks (Lepkovsky and Kratzer, 1942), swine (Wintrobe et al., 1943), calf (Johnson et al., 1950), and ducks (Hegsted and Rao, 1945), led to neurological disturbances including convulsions. The underlying mechanism(s) is mostly unknown.

The relation among pyridoxine, anticonvulsants, and epilepsy is highly interesting. For example, it has been shown that the plasma concentration of pyridoxal (Davis et al., 1975), but not pyridoxal phosphate (Hagberg et al., 1966), was low in "institutionalized" and "cryptogenic" epileptics, respectively. In addition, not only did the administration of vitamin B_6 produce favorable effects in combating seizures in "vitamin B_6 dependency syndrome" (Waldinger, 1964), but it also was of benefit in certain cases of anticonvulsant-resistant seizure (Hansson and Hagberg, 1968; Ernsting and Ferwerda, 1952). The influence of vitamin B_6 on brain metabolism has been attributed to a "GABA shunt," which permits the decarboxylation of glutamic acid to GABA primarily if not exclusively in the brain. The reason for attaching much significance to the "GABA shunt" in vitamin B_6 deficiency or vitamin B_6 dependency convulsions originates from some interesting but inconclusive circumstantial evidence that has been reviewed previously to a certain extent by Scriver (1960) and Frimpter et al. (1969). The findings may be summarized as follows:

• A reduction in the concentration of pyridoxal phosphate resulting from (1) dietary deficiency of pyridoxine and (2) inhibition of pyridoxal kinase by various means (reviewed by Holtz and Palm, 1964) causes inhibition of glutamic acid decarboxylase.

• A reduction in the activity of glutamic acid decarboxylase decreases GABA formation (Killam and Bain, 1967; Killam, 1967).

• Glutamic acid decarboxylase is more susceptible to vitamin B_6 deficiency in comparison to other vitamin B_6-requiring enzymes such as aromatic L-amino acid decarboxylase (Scriver and Hutchison, 1963).

• Convulsion inhibits oxygen consumption, and GABA is a substrate for cerebral oxidative metabolism (Sokoloff et al., 1959). Vitamin B_6 can reverse the inhibition of brain oxygen consumption brought about during vitamin B_6-dependent convulsion in the human (Frimpter et al., 1969). With the exception of trimethadione, all anticonvulsants share the property of pyridoxine in protecting against hypoxic convulsion (Caillard et al., 1975).

• Barbiturate withdrawal produces seizure (Essig, 1968), which is blocked by the administration of amino-oxyacetic acid, which increases the concentration of GABA in the brain of many experimental animals (Wallach, 1961).

Altogether, these observations suggested that in the brain, pyridoxal phosphate controls the activity of glutamic acid decarboxylase, which in turn influences CNS excitability through the synthesis of an inhibitory transmitter, namely, GABA. Unfortunately, a meaningful correlation among vitamin B_6 deficiency, concentration of GABA, and convulsion has not been established. For example, some studies revealed that certain agents such as hydroxylamine (Baxter and Roberts, 1960), hydrazine (Maynert and Kaji, 1962), or amino-oxyacetic acid (Davanzo *et al.*, 1961) produced seizures in animals whose brains contained either normal or elevated levels of GABA. Other investigators postulated that perhaps inhibition of glutamic acid decarboxylase (Tapia *et al.*, 1967) reduced glutamic acid-GABA- α-ketoglutarate metabolism (Balzer *et al.*, 1960), or the altered binding and retention of GABA (Sze *et al.*, 1971), independent of the total concentration of GABA in brain, played a role in the etiology of vitamin B_6 deficiency-induced convulsion. However, no direct correlation between the onset of seizures and the degree of inhibition of glutamic acid decarboxylase was noted (Balzer *et al.*, 1960; Wood and Abrahams, 1971; Wood and Peesker, 1972). Others (Wood and Peesker, 1975), working with amino-oxyacetic acid, produced convulsions in mice that have been attributed to two different mechanisms. One mechanism "involves GABA metabolism, develops relatively slowly, and is long lasting, becoming progressively more important as the brain GABA level increases with time after administration of the amino-oxyacetic acid. The second mechanism does not involve GABA metabolism, is relatively fast developing, and is of relatively short duration, becoming negligible 6 h after administration of the amino-oxyacetic acid."

It should be recalled that biogenic amines other than GABA may be involved in the genesis of hyperexcitability in the CNS (Schlesinger and Uphouse, 1972; Jobe *et al.*, 1973). For example, in a paper reviewing "pyridoxine dependency and central nervous system excitability," Schlesinger and Uphouse (1972) have shown that in "dilute mice" treatment that lowered the concentration of brain serotonin, such as administration of reserpine, tetrabenazine, or parachlorophenylalanine, increased audiogenic, electroconvulsive, or pentylene-tetrazol, induced seizure; whereas, agents that raised the concentration of serotonin, such as the administration of 5-hydroxytryptophan or monoamine oxidase inhibitors, decreased seizure susceptibility. In this regard, it has been suggested that several anticonvulsants such as phenobarbital and phenytoin elevated serotonin in the brain (Bonnycastle *et al.*, 1957), and this effect may be related to their antiepileptic actions (Anderson *et al.*, 1962; Meyer and Frey, 1973). Furthermore, Chadwick *et al.* (1975) showed that the concentration of

5-hydroxyindoleacetic acid rose in cerebrospinal fluid (CSF) of epileptic patients treated with anticonvulsants. "It was of interest that those of our patients who were well controlled had higher CSF amine metabolite and serum anticonvulsant levels than the poorly controlled group" (Chadwick *et al.*, 1975). The concentration of CSF 5-hydroxyindoleacetic acid rose only when the anticonvulsant concentration in blood reached therapeutic levels (cf. Ebadi, 1975). In addition, the anticonvulsant-induced intoxication such as nystagmus, ataxia, confusion, and drowsiness (cf. Ebadi, 1975), which simulates tryptophan intoxication (Oates and Sjoerdsma, 1960), may be mediated by higher than normal concentration of serotonin brought about by antiepileptic agents.

Besides serotonin, other biogenic amines such as dopamine and norepinephrine may be involved in the genesis of the hyperexcitability state. For example, Schlesinger and Uphouse (1972) reviewed the reports that the treatments that lowered the concentration of norepinephrine, such as administration of reserpine, tetrabenazine, or α-methyl-tyrosine, produced effects similar to those produced by depletion of serotonin. In contrast, the administration of dopa, which increased the concentration of norepinephrine in the brain, decreased seizure susceptibility. Similarly, raising the concentration of GABA by amino-oxyacetic acid decreased seizure susceptibility similar to that produced by raising the concentrations of norepinephrine or serotonin by the agents discussed previously. Pyridoxine deficiency potentiated the drugs that enhanced seizure susceptibility (Schlesinger and Uphouse, 1972). The mechanism through which vitamin B_6 protects against convulsion is not always clear. For example, Castrix (2-chloro-4-dimethylamino-6-methyl pyrimidine) produces convulsions that are prevented and protected by vitamin B_6 (Karlog and Knudsen, 1963). It has been suggested that the "electron donating property of Castrix may be responsible for its convulsant effects" (Murakami and Makino, 1973), since Castrix does not deplete pyridoxal phosphate, does not inhibit the pyridoxal phosphate synthesizing enzymes such as pyridoxal kinase or pyridoxine phosphate oxidase, and does not inhibit glutamic acid decarboxylase (Murakami *et al.*, 1972). The above-mentioned observations speak of the important roles that vitamin B_6 plays in "stabilizing" the hyperexcited neurons. An in-depth and extensive search delineating the involved mechanisms will prove highly revealing scientifically and rewarding clinically.

VITAMIN B6 AND DOPAMINE IN THE CNS

Blaschko (1957) suggested that dopamine, in addition to serving as a precursor in the synthesis of norepinephrine, might possess an independent function, which later was proposed to be that of a neurotransmitter (Carlsson, 1959). The differences between dopamine and norepinephrine as neurotransmitters have been reviewed by Hornykiewicz (1966) and include the following:

• In the periphery, dopamine has a weak sympathomimetic property, whereas norepinephrine has a strong one.

• Dopamine is a vasodilator, whereas norepinephrine is a vasoconstrictor.

• In some organs, such as bronchi, lung, and liver, dopamine is the only available catecholamine.

• The regional distributions of dopamine and norepinephrine in the brain are not identical.

• The norepinephrine receptor site blocking agents do not interact selectively with dopamine receptor sites and vice versa.

• The neuroinhibitory action of dopamine in most instances is not shared by norepinephrine.

The above-enumerated differences paved the way in searching for a role for dopamine in health and in diseases.

Metabolism of Dopamine

The synthesis and degradation of dopamine, which was realized by the discovery of dopa decarboxylase by Holtz *et al.* (1938) and consolidated by the inductive reasoning of Blaschko (1939) proceeds via the following reactions:

Tyrosine → Dopa → Dopamine → Norepinephrine → Epinephrine

Tyrosine is converted to dopa by the aid of tyrosine hydroxylase, which utilizes L-tyrosine as substrate specifically and requires tetrahydropteridine, O_2, and Fe^{++} for cofactors. Tyrosine hydroxylase, which is present in the brain (Iyer *et al.*, 1963; McGeer *et al.*, 1965) and other tissues, is inhibited by many analogues of tyrosine, such as α-methyl-L-tyrosine. The consequence of this inhibition is a reduction in the concentration of norepinephrine (Udenfriend, 1966).

Dopa is converted to dopamine by L-aromatic amino acid decarboxylase (Lovenberg *et al.*, 1962), which utilizes many substrates (e.g., phenylalanine, tyrosine, tryptophan, 5-hydroxytryptophan) and requires pyridoxal phosphate for cofactor. L-aromatic amino acid decarboxylase, which is present in brain and in particularly high concentrations in mammalian liver and kidney (Davis and Awapara, 1960), is inhibited by many compounds including α-methyldopa (Sourkes, 1954), α-methyl-m-tyrosine (Rosengren, 1960), and many hydrazine derivatives (Porter et al., 1962).

Dopamine is converted to norepinephrine by the aid of dopamine β-oxidase, which utilizes nonspecifically many phenylethylamine derivatives and requires ascorbic acid and oxygen for cofactors. Dopamine β-oxidase, located in sympathetic nerve endings in many tissues including brain (Udenfriend and Creveling, 1959), is inhibited by disulfiram, benzylamine, and benzylhydrazine (Goldstein, 1966).

Norepinephrine is converted to epinephrine by the aid of phenylethanolamine N-methyl transferase, which shows specificity for norepinephrine, requires s-adenosylmethionine as a cofactor, and is localized primarily in the adrenal glands (Axelrod, 1966).

The Involvement of Pyridoxal Phosphate in Regulating the Activity of the Dopa Decarboxylase

"A simple way to demonstrate the pyridoxal nature of dopa decarboxylase is to prepare a liver extract from a rat reared on a diet deficient in vitamin B_6. The enzymatic activity of such an extract is normally low but it can be brought up to a normal level by adding pyridoxal phosphate *in vitro*" (Blaschko, 1966). Recent evidence indicates that the pyridoxal phosphate and pyridoxal kinase influence the activity of dopa decarboxylase, which may influence the synthesis of monoamines such as dopamine, norepinephrine, serotonin, and gamma-aminobutyric acid (cf. Ebadi, 1973, for review). The effect of vitamin B_6 deficiency on the activity of glutamic acid decarboxylase and GABA formation has already been discussed.

L-aromatic amino acid decarboxylase of mammalian tissues is unsaturated at physiological conditions. Its activity and the products of its reactions can be increased by incubation with pyridoxal phosphate *in vitro*, by administration of pyridoxine *in vivo*, and by agents that elevate the concentration of pyridoxal phosphate in the body.

Christenson et al. (1970), working with a pure L-aromatic amino acid decarboxylase isolated from hog kidney, reported that the purified enzyme contained 0.7 to 1.1 M of pyridoxal phosphate per 112,000 g of protein. This enzyme "catalyzed significant decarboxylation without exogenous pyridoxal phosphate, but the addition of 1×10^{-7} to 1×10^{-3} M pyridoxal phosphate stimulated the activity twofold to fivefold, with a broad maximum in the range of 5×10^{-6} to 1×10^{-4} M.

Using the brains of patients who died from non-neurological disorders, Lloyd and Hornykiewicz (1970) have shown that the highest dopa decarboxylase activity was found in caudate nucleus, putamen, and hypothalamus, whereas the activity of this enzyme was low in cerebellar cortex and cerebral cortex. The caudate nucleus, putamen, and hypothalamus are known to be heavily endowed with dopamine, norepinephrine, and serotonin, whereas the white matters of cerebellar cortex and cerebral cortex are very poor sources of these biogenic amines (Hornykiewicz, 1966). Lloyd and Hornykiewicz (1970) reported: "It is noteworthy that the decarboxylation of L-dopa as determined with our assay procedure was pyridoxal phosphate dependent; omission of this cofactor reduced the production of $^{14}CO_2$ to blank values."

Similarly, Robins *et al.* (1967) reported an extremely low level of 5-hydroxytryptophan decarboxylase in human brain; it was fourfold to 40-fold less than in any other mammalian species studied.

In addition, the activity of dopa decarboxylase is activated *in vivo* by administration of pyridoxine. In a series of experiments, Pfeiffer and Ebadi (1972) demonstrated that the intraperitoneal administration of a 100-mg/kg dose of L-dopa per day in divided doses for 4 days increased the level of dopamine from 6.66 to 8.61 μg/g in the rat's basal ganglia. Similarly, the administration of a 100-mg/kg dose of pyridoxine given intravenously also increased the level of dopamine in the same region from a baseline of 6.66 to 9.74, 8.09, and 8.73 μg/g at 6, 12, and 30 h respectively. This higher level of dopamine most probably results from its increased synthesis by the accelerated activity of dopa decarboxylase, which is a pyridoxal phosphate-dependent enzyme, through the catalytic action of pyridoxal kinase (EC 2.7.1.35) (McCormick *et al.*, 1961). The administration of pyridoxine increases the concentration of pyridoxal phosphate in the brain (Ebadi *et al.*, 1970), which in turn activates dopa decarboxylase, which is not saturated with coenzyme under physiological conditions (Sourkes, 1966).

Pharmacological agents that alter the concentration of pyridoxal phosphate enhance the activity of dopa decarboxylase. In normothermic animals, chlorpromazine increases the cerebral turnover of dopamine (Burkard *et al.*, 1967) and the level of homovanillic acid (Andén *et al.*, 1964; Roos, 1965; Werdinius, 1966) as well as accelerates the catabolism of catecholamines after inhibition of their synthesis (Neff and Costa, 1966; Corrodi *et al.*, 1967). The acceleration in metabolism of catecholamines is thought to be mediated through alteration in the activity of tyrosine hydroxylase, the rate-limiting enzyme

(Burkard *et al.*, 1967; Gey and Pletscher, 1968; and Nyback *et al.*, 1967). However, the possibility of chlorpromazine-induced activation of dopa decarboxylase has been similarly considered (Gey and Burkard, 1969; Ebadi, 1970).

The intraperitoneal injection of female rats with 10 mg/kg of chlorpromazine significantly increased the activity of brain dopa decarboxylase (Gey and Burkard, 1969). The chlorpromazine-induced enhancement in the activity of dopa decarboxylase, which is noticeable as early as 1 h and has a duration of action of 16 h, is blocked by pretreatment of the rats with cycloheximide or actinomycin D (Gey and Burkard, 1969). Similarly, it is interesting to note that the dopa decarboxylase of untreated brain was activated either by administration of chlorpromazine or by exogenous incubation with pyridoxal phosphate. However, dopa decarboxylase of chlorpromazine-treated brain did not become activated further by incubation with pyridoxal phosphate. In addition, it was shown that the dopa decarboxylase-enhancing dosage of chlorpromazine increased the concentration of pyridoxal phosphate (Gey and Burkard, 1969; Ebadi, 1970). This effect was mediated through increasing the activity of pyridoxine phosphate oxidase, synthesizing more coenzyme, and not by inhibiting the activity of pyridoxine phosphate phosphatase (Ebadi, 1970).

The chlorpromazine-induced increase in the rate of turnover of dopamine in brain (Burkard *et al.*, 1967; Neff and Costa, 1966; Corrodi *et al.*, 1967) might be due to coenzyme-induced activation of dopa decarboxylase. This hypothesis is compatible with the observation of Lin *et al.* (1958) that the activities of tyrosine and tryptophan transaminase are enhanced by increasing the concentration of their coenzyme, pyridoxal phosphate. On the other hand, vitamin B_6 deficiency states reduced the activity of apocysteine sulfinate decarboxylase (Hope, 1955) and threonine dehydrase (Bergeret *et al.*, 1955). In addition, the activity of L-aromatic amino acid decarboxylase was also shown to be inhibited by using 5-hydroxytryptophan (Buxton and Sinclair, 1956; Weissback *et al.*, 1957), dopa (West, 1953; Sourkes *et al.*, 1960), and histidine (Schayer *et al.*, 1959) as substrates. The addition of pyridoxal phosphate restores the activity of the enzyme *in vitro*.

The Relationship between Pyridoxal Kinase and Biogenic Amines in the Brain

It has gradually become apparent that the rate of biogenic amine synthesis is not constant but varies with the degree of sympathetic nerve activity. For example, it is known that exercise and exposure to cold result in increased release of neurotransmitter with a concomitant increase in its synthesis in the brain. Increased catecholamine synthesis has also been demonstrated in heart following electrical stimulation of stellate ganglia and in rat salivary gland. Similar effects have been observed following direct stimulation of the hypogastric nerve using an isolated guinea pig *vas deferens*. With this information at hand, it became desirable to establish the relationship between the concentration of norepinephrine, dopamine, and serotonin and the activity of pyridoxal kinase—the enzyme responsible for the synthesis of the active coenzyme necessary in the metabolism of biogenic amines and/or their precursors. In a series of experiments (Ebadi *et al.*, 1968) an inverse relationship was found to exist between the activity of pyridoxal kinase and the concentrations of brain norepinephrine, dopamine, and serotonin. When the biogenic amine content of the brain was lowered, the activity of pyridoxal kinase rose. Conversely, when the concentration of brain biogenic amines was elevated, depression occurred in the activity of pyridoxal phosphokinase. Neary *et al.* (1972), working with an *in vitro* system and using highly purified enzyme isolated from bovine brain, reported that dopa, dopamine, and norepinephrine inhibited the activity of pyridoxal kinase. Tyrosine demonstrated no similar inhibitory activity. Similarly, serotonin inhibited pyridoxal dinase, whereas tryptophan and 5-hydroxytryptophan were without effect. Similar results were obtained by McCoy *et al.* (1972), using kinase purified from rabbit brain. This relationship, which resembles an *in vivo* allosteric inhibition phenomenon, not only is highly indicative of a relation between the brain vitamin B_6 content and the metabolism of the biogenic amines but also suggests that the concentration of brain biogenic amines might control the production of pyridoxal phosphate (Ebadi *et al.*, 1968; McCoy *et al.*, 1972; Neary *et al.*, 1972).

The results of other experiments carried out in our laboratory indicate that the brain regulates the concentration of pyridoxal phosphate by modifying the activity of pyridoxal kinase. When the concentration of pyridoxal phosphate is below normal, the kinase becomes activated. Conversely, when the level of the coenzyme rises above normal, the activity of kinase becomes depressed (Ebadi *et al.*, 1970). In accordance with the above-mentioned observations are studies which demonstrate an increased requirement for vitamin B_6 in a high-protein diet, in hyperthyroidism, and in fever and neoplasm. It remains to be elucidated whether the above-reported conditions alter the activity of pyridoxal kinase.

Parkinsonism and Striatal Dopamine

A crucial observation by Ehringer and Hornykiewicz (1960) revealed that patients with Parkinsonism had substantially less striatal dopamine in comparison with non-Parkinsonism subjects. For example, Bernheimer *et al.* (1965) provided the following observation:

	Dopamine, μg/g	
Classification of Parkinsonism	Caudate Nucleus	Putamen
Postencephalitic	<0.06	0.05
Idiopathic	0.40	0.03
Arteriosclerotic	0.63	0.20
Control	2.64	3.44

Based on these data, Bernheimer *et al.* (1965) and Hornykiewicz (1973) stated that neurochemically, Parkinsonism is a "striatal dopamine deficiency syndrome." From a clinicopharmacological stand, the normalization of striatal dopamine seems to be at least the best palliative treatment of Parkinsonism. Consequently, the precursor of dopamine, L-dopa, was tried initially in small amounts (Birkmayer and Hornykiewicz, 1961; Barbeau *et al.*, 1962) and subsequently in large and chronic dosage (Cotzias *et al.*, 1967). This later treatment has been successful in combating the "triad of Parkinsonism" in terms of relieving tremor at rest, rigidity, and hypokinesia (for review see Pelton and Chase, 1975). L-tyrosine (Calne and Sandler, 1970) and pteridine cofactor (Kaufman, 1966) are ineffective therapeutically.

Dopa Decarboxylase and Pyridoxine in Parkinsonism

From 1960 to 1970, many investigators including Langemann and Ackermann (1961), Bernheimer and Hornykiewicz (1962), Robins *et al.* (1967), Metzel *et al.* (1969), and Vogel *et al.* (1970) reported either a trace, or no detectable amount, of dopa decarboxylase in human brain, including that of the Parkinsonian. This prompted Robins and his coworkers (1967) to suggest that in the human, L-aromatic amino acid decarboxylase (Lovenberg *et al.*, 1962), rather than tyrosine hydroxylase (Udenfriend, 1966), may control the synthesis of dopamine, norepinephrine, and serotonin. This possibility which has been discussed and reviewed by Costa (1972) and Sandler (1972) awaits scientific documentation.

In 1970, Lloyd and Hornykiewicz reported a detectable but very low activity of dopa decarboxylase in various brain regions of patients with Parkinsonism, which is summarized below (Hornykiewicz, 1973):

L-Dopa Decarboxylase Activity, cpm/mg Protein (Minus Blank)

Brain	Controls	Patients with Parkinson's Disease
Putamen	864 ± 271	38 ± 10
Caudate Nucleus	641 ± 200	55 ± 14
Hypothalamus	238 ± 91	72 ± 21
Cerebellar Cortex	33 ± 9	38 ± 9
Cerebellar White Matter	5	5

Controls were neurologically normal individuals. The addition of pyridoxal phosphate increased the activity of dopa decarboxylase. This observation, along with previously reported beneficial effects of pyridoxine in Parkinsonism (e.g., Duvoisin, 1973, for review), resulted in administration of pyridoxine to patients with Parkinsonism who were receiving L-dopa (Duvoisin *et al.,* 1969).

"Contrary to expectations, pyridoxine not only failed to enhance the 'dopa effect' in Parkinsonism but annulled the benefits of L-dopa treatment altogether. Large doses produced a rapid and complete reversal of the 'dopa effect'; small doses produced a gradual and partial reversal. The adventitious involuntary movements were reduced to tolerable levels in some patients and it seemed at first that perhaps in small doses pyridoxine might be a useful adjunct to L-dopa. However, after extensive experimentation and further observation, we found that we were unable to control the involuntary movements with pyridoxine without losing some of the beneficial effects of L-dopa and that although increasing the dosage of L-dopa could restore the lost therapeutic benefit, doing so also brought back the involuntary movements to their former intensity. It became clear that adding pyridoxine was tantamount to reducing the daily dosage of L-dopa" (Duvoisin, 1973).

Some investigators (e.g., Cotzias and Papavasiliou, 1971; Yahr *et al.,* 1972; Duvoisin *et al.,* 1969, 1973) favor the hypothesis that the nullification of CNS beneficial effects of L-dopa by pyridoxine results from an increase in the decarboxylation of L-dopa to dopamine peripherally, with a consequent decreased availability of L-dopa to the brain. Other investigators (e.g., Calne and Sandler, 1970; Evered, 1971; Johnston, 1971; Pfeiffer and Ebadi, 1972; Sandler, 1973) theorize that the nullification of CNS effects of L-dopa by pyridoxine may also result from the formation of a Schiff base between pyridoxine and L-dopa which results in biochemical and pharmacological inactivation of both compounds. Regardless of the mechanism(s), pyridoxine may be used to overcome some of the side effects of levodopa such as the appearance of involuntary movements (Jameson, 1970). However, pyridoxine seems to be ineffective in reducing drug-induced tardive dyskinesia (Crane et al., 1970).

The chronic administration of L-dopa elevates the plasma and erythrocyte concentrations of pyridoxal phosphate (Mars, 1975). The author feels that "chronic administration of levodopa may result in an adaptive alteration in the decarboxylase system with an increased cellular ability to synthesize pyridoxal phosphate from pyridoxine, possibly through enzyme induction." The effects of levodopa, when given chronically on the activity of pyridoxal kinase and pyridoxine phosphate oxidase, remain to be determined.

SUMMARY AND CONCLUSION

As a coenzyme, vitamin B_6 participates in the biotransformation of many amino acids and the metabolism of proteins, lipids, carbohydrates, purines, pyrimidines, and all compounds implicated as neurotransmitters. Vitamin B_6 deficiency is characterized by anemia, growth retardation, and alteration in neuronal function, including neuropathies, hyperirritability, hyperexcitability, and convulsions. The importance of vitamin B_6 in the study of brain function assumes still greater significance when one considers the effects of nutritional deficiencies on the growth and development of the brain and mental processes and the involvement of vitamin B_6 in some inborn errors of metabolism which result in mental retardation.

Despite the fact that various classes of psychoactive agents alter the level of pyridoxal phosphate, as well as the activities of the vitamin B_6-related enzymes and the vitamin B_6-dependent enzymes of the brain, no theoretical or experimental explanation of the mechanism of these phenomena has been presented. Although various stimulants of the central nervous system reduce the level of pyridoxal phosphate within the CNS and concomitantly cause hyperexcitability and convulsions, the role that vitamin B_6 plays in the maintenance of the integrity of neuronal excitability is obscure. More research on these and similar effects of vitamin B_6 seems indicated. It is hoped that by understanding the factors that regulate the synthesis, binding, storage, and degradation of pyridoxal phosphate in the brain, a better insight into the above mentioned problems may be gained.

LITERATURE CITED

Aita, J. F., and T. R. Calame. 1972. Peripheral neuropathy secondary to isoniazid-induced pyridoxine deficiency. Md. State Med. J., *21*:68–70.

Albers, R. W., and R. O. Brady. 1959. The distribution of glutamic decarboxylase in the nervous system of the rhesus monkey. J. Biol. Chem. *234*:926–928.

Alexander, R. W., J. N. Davis, and R. J. Lefkowitz. 1975. Direct identification and characterization of β-adrenergic receptors in rat brain. Nature *258*:437–440.

Andén, N. E., B. E. Roos, and B. Werdinius. 1964. Effects of chlorpromazine, haloperidol and reserpine on the levels of phenolic acids in rabbit corpus striatum. Life Sci. *3*:149–158.

Anderson, E. G., S. D. Markowitz, and D. D. Bonnycastle. 1962. Brain 5-hydroxytryptamine and anticonvulsant activity. J. Pharmacol. Exp. Ther. *136*:179–182.

Autor, A. P., and I. Fridovich. 1970. The interactions of acetoacetate decarboxylase with carbonyl compounds, hydrogen cyanide, and an organic mercurial. J. Biol. Chem. *245*:5214–5222.

Axelrod, J. 1966. Methylation reactions in the formation and metabolism of catecholamines and other biogenic amines. Pharmacol. Rev. *18*:95–113.

Backer, E. T. 1967. Chloric acid digestion in the determination of trace metals (Fe, Zn, and Cu) in brain and hair by atomic absorption spectrophotometry. Clin. Chem. Acta *24*:233–238.

Bain, J. A., and H. L. Williams. 1960. Concentration of B₆ vitamers in tissues and tissue fluids. *In* E. Roberts (ed.), Inhibition in the Nervous System and Gamma Aminobutyric Acid, Pergamon Press, New York, pp. 275–293.

Balcom, A. J., R. H. Lenox, and J. L. Meyerhoff. 1975. Regional γ-aminobutyric acid levels in rat brain determined after microwave fixation. J. Neurochem. *24*:609–613.

Balzer, H., P. Holtz, and D. Palm. 1960. Untersuchungen über die biochemischen Grundlagen der konvulsiven Wirkung von Hydraziden. Naunyn-Schmiedeberg's Arch. Exp. Pathol. Pharmakol. *239*:520–552.

Barbeau, A., T. L. Sourkes, and G. F. Murphy. 1962. Les catécholamines dans la maladie de parkinson. *In* J. de Ajuriaguerra (ed.), Monoamines et Système Nerveux Centrale, George, Génève, and Masson, Paris, p. 247.

Barbeau, A., T. N. Chase, and G. W. Paulson. 1973. Huntington's chorea. Adv. Neurol. *1*:1–901.

Baxter, C. F. 1970. The nature of γ-aminobutyric acid. Handbook of Neurochem. *3*:289–353.

Baxter, C. F., and E. Roberts. 1958. The γ-aminobutyric acid α-ketoglutaric acid transaminase of beef brain. J. Biol. Chem. *233*:1135–1139.

Baxter, C. F., and E. Roberts. 1959. Elevation of γ-aminobutyric acid in rat brain with hydroxylamine. Proc. Soc. Exp. Biol. Med. *101*:811–815.

Baxter, C. F., and E. Roberts. 1960. Demonstration of thiosemicarbazide-induced convulsions in rats with elevated brain levels of γ-aminobutyric acid. Proc. Soc. Exp. Biol. *104*:426–427.

Bayoumi, R. A., and W. R. D. Smith. 1973. Regional distribution of glutamic acid decarboxylase in the developing brain of the pyridoxine-deficient rat. J. Neurochem. *21*:603–613.

Beid, A. J., and E. J. Ariens. 1974. Stereospecific binding as a tool in attempts to localize and isolate muscarinic receptors. II. Binding of (+)-benzetamide, (−)-benzetamide and atropine to a fraction from bovine tracheal smooth muscle and to bovine caudate nucleus. Eur. J. Pharmacol. *25*:203–209.

Bennett, J. L., and G. K. Aghajanian. 1974. D-LSD binding to brain homogenates: Possible relationship to serotonin receptors. Life Sci. *15*:1935–1944.

Bennett, J. P., Jr., and S. H. Snyder. 1975. Stereospecific binding of D-lysergic acid diethylamide (LSD) to brain membranes: Relationship to serotonin receptors. Brain Res. *94*:523–544.

Bergeret, B., F. Chatagner, and C. Fromageot. 1955. Quelques relations entre le phosphate de pyridoxal et la decarboxylation de l'acide cysteine-sulfinique par divers organes du rat normal ou du rat carence en vitamine B₆. Biochim. Biophys. Acta *17*:128–135.

Bernheimer, H., and O. Hornykiewicz. 1962. Das verhalten einiger Enzyme im Gehirn normaler und Parkinsonkranker menschen. Arch. Exp. Pathol. Pharmakol. *243*:295–296.

Bernheimer, H., W. Birkmayer, O. Hornykiewicz, K. Jellinger, and F. Seitelberger. 1965. Zur differenzierung des Parkinson, Syndrome: Biochemisch-neurohistologische Verglesichsuntersuchungen. *In* Proceedings of the Eighth International Congress of Neurology, Vol. IV, Wiener Medizinische Akademie, Vienna (Abstract).

Biehl, J. P., and R. W. Vilter. 1954. Effect of isoniazid on pyridoxine metabolism: Its possible significance in producing isoniazid neuritis. Proc. Soc. Exp. Biol. Med., *85*:389–392.

Bird, E. D., and L. L. Iversen. 1974. Huntington's chorea: Post-mortem measurement of glutamic acid decarboxylase, choline acetyltransferase, and dopamine in basal ganglia. Brain *97*:457–472.

Birkmayer, W., and O. Hornykiewicz. 1961. Der L-Dioxyphenylalanine (= dopa) Effekt bei der Parkinson-akinese. Wien. Klin. Wochenschr. *73*:787–788.

Blaschko, H. 1939. The specific action of L-dopa decarboxylase. J. Physiol. (London) *96*:50–51.

Blaschko, H. 1957. Metabolism and storage of biogenic amines. Experientia *13*:9–12.

Blaschko, H. 1966. Catecholamines. Pharmacol. Rev. *18*:39–41.

Bonnycastle, D. D., N. J. Giarman, and M. K. Paasonen. 1957. Anticonvulsant compounds and 5-hydroxytryptamine in rat brain. Br. J. Pharmacol. *12*:228–231.

Bower, B. D. 1965. Pyridoxine, tryptophan and epilepsy. Dev. Med. Child. Neurol. *7*:73–83.

Boyer, P. D. 1959. Addition and alkylation reaction of SH groups. *In* P. D. Boyer, H. Lardy and K. Myrbäck (eds.), The Enzymes, Vol. 1, Academic Press, New York, pp. 527–529.

Braunstein, A. 1960. Pyridoxal phosphate. *In* P. D. Boyer, H. Lardy, and K. Myrbäck (eds.), The Enzymes, Vol. 2, Academic Press, New York, pp. 113–184.

Buell, M. V., and R. E. Hansen. 1960. Reaction of pyridoxal-5 phosphate with aminothiols. J. Am. Chem. Soc. *82*:6042–6049.

Buell, M. V., and R. E. Hansen. 1961. On the action of muscle phosphorylase a in vitro. J. Biol. Chem. *236*:1991–1995.

Buffoni, F. 1966. Histaminase related amine oxidases. Pharmacol. Rev. *18*:1163–1199.

Burgen, A. S. V., R. Hiley, and J. M. Young. 1974. The properties of muscarinic receptors in mammalian cerebral cortex. Br. J. Pharmacol. *51*:279–285.

Burkard, W. P., K. F. Gey, and A. Pletscher. 1967. Activation of tyrosine hydroxylation in rat brain in vivo by chlorpromazine. Nature *213*:732–733.

Buxton, J., and H. M. Sinclair. 1956. Pyridoxal phosphate as a coenzyme of 5-hydroxytryptophan decarboxylase. Biochem. J. *62*:1–27.

Caciappo, F., L. Pandolfo, and G. Di Chiara. 1959. Transamination reaction between 4-aminobutyric acid and α-ketoglutaric acid in certain rat tissues. Boll. Soc. Ital. Biol. Sper. *36*:465–467.

Caillard, C., A. Menu, M. Plotkine, and P. Rossignol. 1975. Do anticonvulsant drugs exert protective effect against hypoxia? Life Sci. *16*:1607–1612.

Calne, D. B. 1973. Progress in the treatment of parkinsonism. Adv. Neurol. *3*:1–326.

Calne, D. B., and M. Sandler. 1970. L-dopa and parkinsonism. Nature (London) *226*:21–24.

Carlson, H. B., E. M. Anthony, W. F. Russel, and G. Middlebrook. 1956. Prophylaxis of isoniazid neuropathy with pyridoxine. New Engl. J. Med. *255*:118–122.

Carlsson, A. 1959. The occurrence, distribution and physiological role of catecholamines in the nervous system. Pharmacol. Rev. *11*:490–493.

Chadwick, D., P. Jenner, and E. H. Reynolds. 1975. Amines, anticonvulsants and epilepsy. Lancet *1*:473–483.

Chang, G. W., and E. E. Snell. 1968. Histidine decarboxylase of lactobacillus 30a. III. Composition and subunit structure. Biochemistry *7*:2012–2020.

Christenson, J. G., W. Dairman, and S. Udenfriend. 1970. Preparation and properties of a homogeneous aromatic L-amino acid decarboxylase from hog kidney. Arch. Biochem. Biophys. *141*:356–367.

Cole, J. O., and J. R. Wittenborn. 1966. Pharmacotherapy of Depression. C. C. Thomas, Springfield, Ill., pp. 1–189.

Corrodi, H., K. Fuxe, and T. Hokelt. 1967. The effect of neuroleptics on the activity of central catecholamine neurones. Life Sci. *6*:767–774.

Costa, E. 1972. Appraisal of current methods to estimate the turnover rate of serotonin and catecholamines in human brain. *In* M. Ebadi and E. Costa (eds.), Role of Vitamin B₆ in Neurobiology. Vol. 4. Advances in Biochemical Psychopharmacology. Raven Press, New York, pp. 171–183.

Cotzias, G. C., and P. S. Papavasiliou. 1971. Blocking the negative effect of pyridoxine on patients receiving levodopa. J. Am. Med. Assoc. *215*:1504–1505.

Cotzias, G. C., M. H. Van Woert, and L. M. Schiffer. 1967. Aromatic amino acids and modification of parkinsonism. New Engl. J. Med. *276*:374–379.

Crane, G. E., I. S. Turek, and A. A. Kurland. 1970. Failure of pyridoxine to reduce drug-induced dyskinesia. J. Neurol. Neurosurg. Psychiatry *33*:511–512.

Davadatta, S., P. R. J. Gangadharam, R. H. Andrews, W. Fox, C. V. Ramakrishman, J. B. Selkon, and S. Velu. 1960. Peripheral neuritis due to isoniazid. Bull. WHO *23*:587–598.

Davanzo, J. P., M. E. Greig, and M. D. Cronin. 1961. Anticonvulsant properties of amino-oxyacetic acid. Am. J. Physiol. *201*:833–837.

Davis, R. E., P. A. Reed, and B. K. Smith. 1975. Serum pyridoxal, folate and vitamin B₁₂ levels in institutionalized epileptics. Epilepsia *16*:463–468.

Davis, V. E., and J. Awapara. 1960. A method for the determination of some amino acid decarboxylase. J. Biol. Chem. *235*:124–127.

Duffy, T. E., S. R. Nelson, and O. H. Lowry. 1972. Cerebral carbohydrate metabolism during acute hypoxia and recovery. J. Neurochem. *19*:959–977.

Duvoisin, R. C. 1973. Pyridoxine as an adjunct in the treatment of parkinsonism. Treatment of Parkinsonism—The role of dopa-decarboxylase inhibitors. Adv. Neurol. *2*:229–247.

Duvoisin, R. C., M. D. Yahr, and L. D. Coté. 1969. Pyridoxine reversal of L-dopa effect in parkinsonism. Trans. Am. Neurol. Assoc. *94*:81–84.

Ebadi, M. S. 1970. Increase in brain pyridoxal phosphate by chlorpromazine. Pharmacology *3*:97–106.

Ebadi, M. S. 1973. The catalytic role of pyridoxal phosphate and the regulatory involvement of pyridoxal kinase in the metabolism of monoamines. Adv. Neurol. *2*:199–227.

Ebadi, M. S. 1975. The pharmacokinetic basis of therapeutics with special reference to drugs used in neurology. Adv. Neurol. *13*:333–380.

Ebadi, M., and E. Costa (eds.). 1972. Role of Vitamin B_6 in Neurobiology. Vol. 4. Advances in Biochemical Psychopharmacology. Raven Press, New York, 238 pp.

Ebadi, M. S., R. L. Russell, and E. E. McCoy. 1968. The inverse relationship between the activity of pyridoxal kinase and the level of biogenic amines in rabbit brain. J. Neurochem. 15:659–665.

Ebadi, M. S., E. E. McCoy, and R. B. Kugel. 1970. Interrelationships between pyridoxal phosphate and pyridoxal kinase in rabbit brain. J. Neurochem. 17:941–948.

Ehringer, H., and O. Hornykiewicz. 1960. Verteilung von Noradrenalin und Dopamin (3 hydroxytyramin) im Gehirn des Menschen und ihr Verhalten bei Erkrankungen des extrapyramidalen Systems. Klin. Wochenschr. 38:1236–1239.

Enna, S. J., and S. H. Snyder. 1975. Properties of γ-aminobutyric acid (GABA) receptor binding in rat brain synaptic membrane fractions. Brain Res. 100:81–97.

Enna, S. J., M. J. Kuhar, and S. H. Snyder. 1975. Regional distribution of postsynaptic receptor binding for gamma-aminobutyric acid (GABA) in monkey brain. Brain Res. 93:168–174.

Enna, S. J., E. D. Bird, J. P. Bennett, D. B. Bylund, H. I. Yamamura, L. L. Iverson, and S. H. Snyder. 1976. Huntington's chorea—Changes in neurotransmitter receptors in the brain. New Engl. J. Med. 294:1305–1309.

Ernsting, W., and T. P. Ferwerda. 1952. Vitamin B_6 in the treatment of epilepsy. J. Am. Med. Assoc. 140:1540–1541.

Essig, C. F. 1968. Possible relation of brain gamma-aminobutyric acid (GABA) to barbiturate abstinence convulsions. Arch. Int. Pharmacodyn. 176:97–103.

Evered, D. F. 1971. L-dopa as a vitamin B_6 antagonist. Lancet 1:914.

Fasella, P. 1967. Pyridoxal phosphate. Ann. Rev. Biochem. 36:185–210.

Fonda, M. L. 1972. Glutamate decarboxylase. Substrate specificity and inhibition by carboxylic acids. Biochemistry 11:1304–1309.

Fonnum, F. 1968. The distribution of glutamate decarboxylase and aspartate transaminase in subcellular fractions of rat and guinea pig brain. Biochem. J. 106:401–412.

Fox, W. 1968. Changing concepts in the chemotherapy of pulmonary tuberculosis. Am. Rev. Respir. Dis. 97:767–790.

Frimpter, G. W., R. J. Andelman, and W. F. George. 1969. Vitamin B_6-dependency syndromes. Am. J. Clin. Nutr. 22:794–805.

Gammon, G. D., E. W. Burge, and G. King. 1953. Neural toxicity in tuberculous patients treated with isoniazid (isonicotinic acid hydrazide). Arch. Neurol. Psychiatr. 70:64–69.

Gey, K. F., and W. P. Burkard. 1969. Chlorpromazine-induced accumulation of pyridoxal-5'-phosphate and activation of the decarboxylase of aromatic amino acids in rat brain. Vitamin B_6 in metabolism of the nervous system. Ann. N.Y. Acad. Sci. 166:213–224.

Gey, K. F., and A. Pletscher. 1968. Acceleration of turnover of ^{14}C-catecholamines in rat brain by chlorpromazine. Experientia 34:335–336.

Goldstein, M. 1966. Inhibition of norepinephrine biosynthesis at the dopamine-β-hydroxylation stage. Pharmacol. Rev. 18:77–82.

Haber, B., K. Kuriyama, and E. Roberts. 1970. L-glutamic acid decarboxylase: A new type in glial cells and human brain gliomas. Science 168:598–599.

Hagberg, B., A. Hamfelt, and O. Hansson. 1966. Tryptophan load tests and pyridoxal phosphate levels in epileptic children. Acta Paediatr. Scand. 55:371–384.

Hansson, O., and B. Hagberg. 1968. Effect of pyridoxine treatment in children with epilepsy. Acta Soc. Med. Ups. 73:35–43.

Harris, R. S., I. G. Wool, and J. A. Loraine. 1964. International symposium on vitamin B_6. Vitam. Horm. 22:359–885.

Hegsted, D. M., and M. N. Rao. 1945. Nutritional studies with the duck. II. Pyridoxine deficiencies. J. Nutr. 30:367–374.

Hiley, C. R., and E. D. Bird. 1974. Decreased muscarinic receptor concentration in postmortem brain in Huntington's chorea. Brain Res. 80:355–358.

Hiley, C. R., and A. S. V. Burgen. 1974. The distribution of muscarinic receptor sites in the nervous system of the dog. J. Neurochem. 22:159–162.

Holtz, P., R. Heise, and K. Lüdke. 1938. Fermentative abbau von L-dioxyphenylalanin (dopa) durch niere. Arch. Exp. Pathol. Pharmakol. 191:87–118.

Holtz, P., and D. Palm. 1964. Pharmacological aspects of vitamin B_6. Pharmacol. Rev. 16:113–178.

Hope, D. B. 1955. Pyridoxal phosphate as the coenzyme of the mammalian decarboxylase for L-cysteine sulphinic and L-cysteic acid. Biochem. J. 59:497–500.

Hornykiewicz, O. 1966. Dopamine (3-hydroxytyramine) and brain function. Pharmacol. Rev. 18:925–964.

Hornykiewicz, O. 1973. Mechanism of action of L-dopa in parkinsonism. Adv. Neurol. 2:1–11.

Hunt, A. D., Jr., J. Stokes, Jr., W. W. McCrory, and H. H. Stroud. 1954. Pyridoxine dependency: Report of a case of intractable convulsions in an infant controlled by pyridoxine. Pediatrics 13:140–145.

Huxtable, R., and A. Barbeau. 1976. Taurine. Raven Press, New York, pp. 275–281.

Iyer, N. T., P. L. McGeer, and E. G. McGeer. 1963. Conversion of tyrosine to catecholamines by rat brain slices. Can. J. Biochem. Physiol. 41:1565–1570.

Jacobsen, J. G., and G. H. Smith. 1968. Biochemistry and physiology of taurine and taurine derivatives. Physiol. Rev. 48:424–511.

Jameson, H. D. 1970. Pyridoxine for levodopa-induced dystonia. J. Am. Med. Assoc. 211:1700.

Janne, J., and H. G. Williams-Ashman. 1971. On the purification of L-ornithine decarboxylase from rat prostate and effects of thiol compounds on the enzyme. J. Biol. Chem. 246:1725–1732.

Jobe, P. C., A. L. Picchioni, and L. Chin. 1973. Role of brain norepinephrine in audiogenic seizure in the rat. J. Pharmacol. Exp. Ther. 184:1–10.

Johnson, B. C., J. A. Pinkos, and K. A. Burke. 1950. Pyridoxine deficiency in the calf. J. Nutr. 40:309–322.

Johnston, G. A. R. 1971. L-dopa and pyridoxal-5'-phosphate: Tetrahydroisoquinoline formation. Lancet 1:1068.

Juchau, M. R., and A. Horita. 1972. Metabolism of hydrazine derivatives of pharmacological interest. Drug Metab. Rev. 1:71–100.

Kahlson, G., and E. Rosingram. 1965. Histamine. Ann. Rev. Pharmacol. 5:305–320.

Kales, A. 1969. Sleep, Physiology and Pathology. J. B. Lippincott Company, Philadelphia, pp. 232–244.

Kalinowski, S. Z., T. W. Lloyd, and E. N. Moyes. 1961. Complications in the chemotherapy of tuberculosis: A review with analysis of the experiences of 3148 patients. Am. Rev. Respir. Dis. 83:359–371.

Karlog, O., and E. Knudsen. 1963. Vitamin B_6 as an antidote against the rodenticide 'Castrix' (2-chloro-4-methyl-6-dimethylamino-pyrimidin). Nature 200:790.

Kaufman, S. 1966. Coenzyme and hydroxylases: Ascorbate and dopamine-β-hydroxylase; tetrahydropteridines and phenylalanine and tyrosine hydroxylases. Pharmacol. Rev. 18:61–69.

Killam, K. F. 1967. Convulsant hydrazides. II. Comparison of electrical changes and enzyme inhibition induced by the administration of thiosemicarbazide. J. Pharmacol. Exp. Ther. *119*:263–271.

Killam, K. F., and J. A. Bain. 1967. Convulsant hydrazides. I. In vitro and in vivo inhibition of vitamin B_6 enzyme by convulsant hydrazides. J. Pharmacol. Exp. Ther. *119*:255–262.

Klawans, H. L., and R. Rubovits. 1972. Central cholinergic-anticholinergic antagonism in Huntington's chorea. Neurology (Minneapolis) *22*:107–116.

Kravitz, E. A. 1967. Acetylcholine, γ-aminobutyric acid and glutamic acid: Physiological and chemical studies related to their roles as neurotransmitter agents. *In* G. C. Quarton, T. Melnechuck, and F. O. Smith (eds.), The Neurosciences. The Rockefeller University Press. New York. pp. 433–444.

Krishnamurthy, D. V., J. B. Selkon, K. Ramachandran, S. Devadatta, D. A. Mitchison, S. Radhakrishna, and H. Stott. 1967. Effect of pyridoxine on vitamin B_6 concentration and glutamic-oxaloacetic transaminase activity in whole blood of tuberculosis patients receiving high-dosage isoniazid. Bull. WHO *38*:853–870.

Kutsky, R. J. 1973. Vitamin B_6. *In* Handbook of Vitamins and Hormones, Van Nostrand Reinhold Co., New York, pp. 60–61.

Langemann, H., and H. Ackermann. 1961. Uber die aktivität der aminosäurendecarboxylasen im gehirn des menschen. Helv. Physiol. Acta *19*:399–406.

Lehmann, B. H., J. D. L. Hansen, and P. J. Warren. 1971. The distribution of copper, zinc, and manganese in various regions of the brain and in other tissues of children with protein-calorie malnutrition. Br. J. Nutr. *26*:197–202.

Lepkovsky, S., and F. H. Kratzer. 1942. Pyridoxine deficiency in chicks. J. Nutr. *24*:515–521.

Lloyd, K., and O. Hornykiewicz. 1970. Occurrence and distribution of L-DOPA decarboxylase in the human brain. Brain Res. *22*:426–428.

Lloyd, K. G., and O. Hornykiewicz. 1973. L-glutamic acid decarboxylase in Parkinson's disease: Effect of L-dopa therapy. Nature *243*:521–523.

Loo, Y. H., and K. Mack. 1971. Subcellular distribution of B_6 vitamers in cerebral cortex. J. Neurochem. *18*:499–502.

Lovell, R. A., S. J. Elliott, and K. A. C. Elliott. 1963. The γ-aminobutyric acid and factor 1 content of the brain. J. Neurochem. *10*:479–488.

Lovenberg, W., H. Weissbach, and S. Udenfriend. 1962. Aromatic L-amino acid decarboxylase. J. Biol. Chem. *237*:89–93.

Mars, H. 1975. Effect of chronic levodopa treatment on pyridoxine metabolism. Neurology *25*:263–266.

Matsuda, T., J. Y. Wu, and E. Roberts. 1973. Electrophoresis of glutamic acid decarboxylase (EC 4.1.1.15) from mouse brain in sodium dodecyl sulphate polyacrylamide gels. J. Neurochem. *21*:167–172.

Maynert, E. W., and H. K. Kaji. 1962. On the relationship of brain γ-aminobutyric acid to convulsions. J. Pharmacol. Exp. Ther. *137*:114–121.

McCormick, D. B., and E. E. Snell. 1959. Pyridoxal kinase of human brain and its inhibition by hydrazine derivatives. Proc. Nat. Acad. Sci. U.S.A., *45*:1371–1379.

McCormick, D. B., M. E. Gregory, and E. E. Snell. 1961. Pyridoxal phosphokinases. I. Assay, distribution, purification, and properties. J. Biol. Chem. *236*:2076–2084.

McCoy, E. E., S. W. Henn, and C. E. Colombini. 1972. The effect of neuropharmacological agents on metabolism of vitamin B_6 in brain. *In* M. S. Ebadi and E. Costa (eds.), Role of Vitamin B_6 in Neurobiology, Vol. 4, Advances in Biochemical Psychopharmacology. Raven Press, New York, pp. 93–104.

McGeer, E. G., P. L. McGeer, J. A. Wada, and E. Jung. 1971. Effects of globus pallidus lesions and Parkinson's disease on brain glutamic acid decarboxylase. Brain Res. *32*:425–431.

McGeer, P. L., S. P. Bagchi, and E. G. McGeer. 1965. Subcellular localization of tyroxine hydroxylase in beef caudate nucleus. Life Sci. *4*:1859–1867.

McGeer, P. L., E. G. McGeer, and J. A. Wada. 1971. Glutamic acid decarboxylase in Parkinson's disease and epilepsy. Neurology (Minneapolis) *21*:1000–1007.

McLaughlin, B. J., J. G. Wood, K. Saito, E. Roberts, and J. Y. Wu. 1975. The fine structural localization of glutamate decarboxylase in developing axonal processes and presynaptic terminals of rodent cerebellum. Brain Res. *85*:355–371.

Meister, A. 1965. Biochemistry of the Amino Acids, Vol. 1. Academic Press, New York, pp. 331–332.

Meldrum, B. S. 1975. Epilepsy and γ-aminobutyric acid mediated inhibition. Int. Rev. Neurobiol. *17*:1–36.

Metzel, E., D. Weinmann, and T. Reichert. 1969. A study of the enzymes of dopa metabolism in parkinsonism from biopsies of the basal ganglia. *In* F. J. Gillingham and I. M. L. Donaldson (eds.), Third Symposium on Parkinson's Disease, Livingstone, Edinburgh, pp. 47–50.

Meyer, H., and H. H. Frey. 1973. Dependence of anticonvulsant drug action on central monoamines. Neuropharmacology *12*:939–947.

Minard, F. N., and I. K. Mushawar. 1966. Synthesis of γ-aminobutyric acid from a pool of glutamic acid in brain after decapitation. Life Sci. *5*:1409–1413.

Mitchell, R. S. 1967. Control of tuberculosis. New Engl. J. Med. *276*:842–848, 905–911.

Money, G. L. 1959. Isoniazid neuropathics in malnourished tuberculosis patients. J. Trop. Med. Hyg. *62*:198–202.

Murakami, Y., and K. Makino. 1973. On the convulsive action of Castrix. Biochem. Pharmacol. *22*:2247–2252.

Murakami, Y., K. Murakami, and K. Makino. 1972. On the convulsive action of Castrix. Biochem. Pharmacol. *21*:277–280.

Myrianthopoulos, N. C. 1966. Huntington's chorea. J. Med. Genet. *3*:298–314.

Nakamura, K., and F. Bernheim. 1962. Transaminase activity of naturally occurring inhibitory substances and effects of some drugs. Jpn. J. Pharmacol. *2*:141–150.

Neary, J. T., R. L. Menelly, M. R. Grever, and W. F. Diven. 1972. The interactions between biogenic amines and pyridoxal, pyridoxal phosphate, and pyridoxal kinase. Arch. Biochem. Biophys. *151*:42–47.

Neff, N. H., and E. Costa. 1966. Effect of tricyclic antidepressants and chlorpromazine in brain catecholamine synthesis. *In* S. Garattini and M. N. G. Dukes (eds.), International Congress Series No. 122, Antidepressant Drugs, Excerpta Medica Foundation, Amsterdam, pp. 28–34.

Nishizawa, Y., T. Kodama, and S. Konishi. 1959. Brain γ-aminobutyric-α-ketoglutaric transaminase. J. Vitaminol. *5*:117–128.

Nyback, H., G. Sedvall, and I. J. Kopin. 1967. Accelerated synthesis of dopamine-C¹⁴ from tyrosine-C¹⁴ in rat brain after chlorpromazine. Life Sci. *6*:2307–2312.

Oates, J. A., and A. Sjoerdsma. 1960. Neurologic effects of tryptophan in patients receiving a monoamine oxidase inhibitor. Neurology *10*:1076–1078.

Obata, K. 1972. The inhibitory action of γ-aminobutyric acid, a profitable synaptic transmitter. Int. Rev. Neurobiol. *15*:167–187.

Ochoa, J. 1970. Isoniazid neuropathy in man: Quantitative electron microscope study. Brain *93*:831–850.

Okada, Y., C. Nitsch-Hasslerc, J. S. Kim, I. J. Bak, and R. Hassler. 1971. Role of γ-aminobutyric acid (GABA) in the extrapyrimidal motor system. Exp. Brain Res. *13*:514–518.

O'Leary, M. H., and J. M. Malik. 1971. Kinetics of the binding of pyridoxal phosphate 5' phosphate to glutamate decarboxylase. J. Biol. Chem. *246*:544–545.

Pelton, E. W., and T. N. Chase. 1975. L-dopa and the treatment of extrapyramidal disease. Adv. Pharmacol. Chemother. *13*:253–304.

Pérez de la Mora, M., A. Feria-Velasco, and R. Tapia. 1973. Pyridoxal phosphate and glutamate decarboxylase in subcellular particles of mouse brain and their relationship to convulsions. J. Neurochem. *20*:1575–1587.

Perry, T. L., S. Hansen, and M. Kloster. 1973. Huntington's chorea—Deficiency of γ-aminobutyric acid in brain. New Engl. J. Med. *288*:337–342.

Pfeiffer, R., and M. S. Ebadi. 1972. On the mechanism of the nullification of CNS effects of L-dopa by pyridoxine in Parkinsonian patients. J. Neurochem. *19*:2175–2181.

Porter, C. C., L. S. Watson, D. C. Titus, J. A. Totaro, and S. S. Byer. 1962. Inhibition of dopa decarboxylase by the hydrazino analog of α methyldopa. Biochem. Pharmacol. *11*:1067–1077.

Rajtar-Leontiew, Z. 1970. Effect of isoniazid on metabolism of pyridoxine in children and experimental study. Sem. Hop. Ann. Pediatr. *17*:150–153.

Roberts, E. 1974. Commentary— γ-aminobutyric acid and nervous system function—a perspective. Biochem. Pharmacol. *23*:2637–2649.

Roberts, E., and S. Frankel. 1950. γ-aminobutyric acid in brain: Its formation from glutamic acid. J. Biol. Chem. *187*:55–63.

Roberts, E., and K. Kuriyama. 1968. Biochemical-physiological correlations in studies of the γ-aminobutyric acid system. Brain Res. *8*:1–35.

Robins, E., J. M. Robins, A. B. Croninger, S. G. Moses, S. J. Spencer, and R. W. Hudgens. 1967. The low level of 5-hydroxytryptophan decarboxylase in human brains. Biochem. Med. *1*:240–251.

Robson, J. M., and F. M. Sullivan. 1963. Antituberculosis drugs. Pharmacol. Rev. *15*:169–223.

Roos, B. E. 1965. Effects of certain tranquilizers on the level of homovanillic acid in the corpus striatum. J. Pharm. Pharmacol. *17*:820–821.

Rosengren, E. 1960. Are dihydroxyphenylalanine decarboxylase and 5-hydroxy-tryptophan decarboxylase individual enzymes? Acta Physiol. Scand. *49*:364–369.

Ross, R. R. 1958. Use of pyridoxine hydrochloride to prevent isoniazid toxicity. J. Am. Med. Assoc. *168*:273–275.

Saito, K., J. Y. Wu, T. Matsuda, and E. Roberts. 1973. Immunochemical studies of glutamic acid decarboxylase from mouse brain. Trans. Am. Soc. Neurochem. *4*:70.

Salganicoff, L., and E. De Robertis. 1965. Subcellular distribution of the enzymes of the glutamic acid, glutamine and γ-aminobutyric acid cycles in rat brain. J. Neurochem. *12*:287–309.

Sandler, M. 1972. Catecholamine synthesis and metabolism in man: Clinical implications (with special reference to parkinsonism). *In* H. Blaschko and E. Muscholl (eds.), Handbook of Experimental Pharmacology, Vol. 33, pp. 845–899.

Sandler, M. 1973. The dopa effect: Possible significance of transamination and tetrahydroisoquinoline formation. Treatment of parkinsonism—The role of dopa-decarboxylase inhibitors. Adv. Neurol. *2*:255–264.

Sauberlich, H. E., J. E. Canham, E. M. Baker, N. Raica, Jr., and Y. F. Herman. 1972. Biochemical assessment of the nutritional status of vitamin B_6 in the human. Am. J. Clin. Nutr. *25*:629–642.

Schayer, R. W., Z. Rothschild, and P. Bizony. 1959. Increase in histidine decarboxylase activity of rat skin following treatment with compound 48/80. Am. J. Physiol. *196*:295–298.

Schlesinger, K., and L. L. Uphouse. 1972. Pyridoxine dependency and central nervous system excitability. *In* M. S. Ebadi and E. Costa (eds.), The Role of Vitamin B₆ in Neurobiology. Vol. 4. Advances in Biochemical Psychopharmacology. Raven Press, New York, pp. 105–140.

Schmidt, M. J., D. E. Schmidt, and G. A. Robinson. 1971. Cyclic adenosine monophosphate in brain areas: Microwave irradiation as a means of tissue fixation. Science *173*:1142–1143.

Schousboe, A., J. Y. Wu, and E. Roberts. 1973. Purification and characterization of the 4-aminobutyrate-2-ketoglutarate transaminase from mouse brain. Biochem. *12*:2968–2873.

Scriver, C. R. 1960. Vitamin B₆—Dependency and infantile convulsions. Pediatrics *26*:62–74.

Scriver, C. R., and J. H. Hutchison. 1963. The vitamin B₆ deficiency syndrome in human infancy: Biochemical and clinical observations. Pediatrics *31*:240–250.

Shank, R. P., and M. H. Aprison. 1971. Post mortem changes in the content and specific radioactivity of several amino acids in four areas of the rat brain. J. Neurobiol. *2*:145–151.

Shaw, R. K., and J. D. Heine. 1965. Ninhydrin positive substances present in different areas of normal rat brain. J. Neurochem. *12*:151–155.

Shoulson, I., and T. N. Chase. 1975. Huntington's disease. Ann. Rev. Med. *26*:419–436.

Smythies, J. R. 1963. Schizophrenia: Chemistry, Metabolism and Treatment. C. C. Thomas, Springfield.

Snell, E. E. 1953. Summary of known metabolic functions of nicotinic acid, riboflavin and vitamin B₆. Physiol. Rev. *33*:509–524.

Snell, E. E. 1958. Chemical structure in relation to biological activities of vitamin B₆. Vitam. Horm. *16*:77–125.

Snell, E. E., P. M. Fasella, A. E. Braunstein, and A. Rossi Fanelli (eds.). 1963. Chemical and Biological Aspects of Pyridoxal Catalysis (International Union of Biochemistry Symposium 30). The Macmillan Company, New York, pp. 1–594.

Snyder, S. H. 1975. Neurotransmitter and drug receptors in the brain. Biochem. Pharmacol. *24*:1371–1374.

Snyder, S. H., and J. P. Bennett, Jr. 1975. Biochemical identification of the postsynaptic serotonin receptor in mammalian brain. *In* E. Usdin and W. E. Bunney, Jr. (eds.), Pre- and Postsynaptic Receptors: Proceedings of a Study Group Held at the Thirteenth Annual Meeting of the American College of Neuropsychopharmacology, San Juan, Puerto Rico. Marcel Decker Incorporated, New York, pp. 191–206.

Sourkes, T. L. 1954. Inhibition of dihydroxyphenylalanine decarboxylase by derivatives of phenylalanine. Arch. Biochem. Biophys. *51*:444–456.

Sourkes, T. L. 1966. DOPA decarboxylase: Substrate, coenzyme, inhibitors. Pharmacol. Rev. *18*:53–60.

Sourkes, T. L., G. F. Murphy, and V. R. Woodford, Jr. 1960. Effect of deficiencies of pyridoxine, riboflavin and thiamine upon the catecholamine content of rat tissue. J. Nutr. *72*:145–152.

Stahl, W. L., and P. D. Swanson. 1974. Biochemical abnormalities in Huntington's chorea brains. Neurology *24*:813–819.

Standal, B. R., S. M. Kao-chen, G. Y. Yang, and D. F. B. Char. 1974. Early changes in pyridoxine status of patients receiving isoniazid therapy. Am. J. Clin. Nutr., *27*:479–484.

Stavinoha, W. B., S. T. Weintraub, and A. T. Modak. 1973. The use of microwave heating to inactivate cholinesterase in the rat brain prior to analysis for acetylcholine. J. Neurochem. 20:361–371.

Stephens, S. M. C., V. Havlicek, and K. Dakshinamurti. 1971. Pyridoxine deficiency and development of the central nervous system in the rat. J. Neurochem. 18:2407–2416.

Sze, P. Y., K. Kuriyama, and E. Roberts. 1971. Thiosemicarbazide and γ-aminobutyric acid metabolism. Brain Res. 25:387–396.

Tapia, R., and J. Awapara. 1967. Formation of gamma aminobutyric acid (GABA) in brain of mice treated with L-glutamic acid-gamma hydrazide and pyridoxal phosphate gamma-glutamyl hydrazone. Proc. Soc. Exp. Biol. Med. 126:218–221.

Tapia, R., and J. Awapara. 1969. Effects of various substituted hydrazones and hydrazines of pyridoxal-5'-phosphate on brain glutamate decarboxylase. Biochem. Pharmacol. 18:145–152.

Tapia, R., and M. E. Sandoval. 1971. Study on the inhibition of brain glutamate decarboxylase by pyridoxal phosphate oxime-o-acetic acid. J. Neurochem. 18:2051–2059.

Tapia, R., H. Pasantes, M. Pérez de la Mora, B. G. Ortega, and G. H. Massiem. 1967. Free amino acids and glutamic decarboxylase activity in brain of mice during drug-induced convulsions. Biochem. Pharmacol. 16:483–496.

Tapia, R., H. Pasantes, and G. Masseur. 1970. Some properties of glutamic decarboxylase and the content of pyridoxal in brains of three vertebrate species. J. Neurochem. 17:921–925.

Tews, J. K., and R. A. Lovell. 1967. The effect of nutritional pyridoxine deficiency on free amino acids and related substances in mouse brain. J. Neurochem. 14:1–7.

Tower, D. B. 1956. Neurochemical aspects of pyridoxine metabolism and function. Am. J. Clin. Nutr. 4:329–345.

Udenfriend, S. 1966. Tyrosine hydroxylase. Pharmacol. Rev. 18:43–51.

Udenfriend, S., and C. R. Creveling. 1959. Localization of dopamine- β-oxidase. J. Neurochem. 4:350–352.

Urquhart, N., T. L. Perry, S. Hansen, and J. Kennedy. 1975. GABA content and glutamic acid decarboxylase activity in brain of Huntington's chorea patients and control subjects. J. Neurochem. 24:1071–1075.

Van Kempen, G. M. J., C. Van Den Berg, H. J. Van Der Helm, and H. Veldstra. 1965. Intracellular localization of glutamate decarboxylase, γ-aminobutyric transaminase and some other enzymes in brain tissue. J. Neurochem. 12:581–588.

Vogel, W. H., H. McFarland, and L. N. Prince. 1970. Decarboxylation of 3,4 dihydroxyphenylalanine in various human adult and fetal tissues. Biochem. Pharmacol. 19:618–620.

Wada, H., and Y. Morino. 1964. Comparative studies on glutamic-oxalacetic transaminases from the mitochondrial and soluble fractions of mammalian tissues. Vitam. Horm. 22:411–444.

Waksman, A., and E. Roberts. 1965. Purification and some properties of mouse brain γ-aminobutyric- α-ketoglutaric acid transaminase. Biochemistry 4:2132–2139.

Waldinger, C. 1964. Pyridoxine deficiency and pyridoxine dependency in infants and children. Postgrad. Med. J. 35:415–422.

Wallach, D. P. 1961. Studies on the GABA pathway. I. The inhibition of γ-aminobutyric acid- α-ketoglutaric acid transaminase in vitro and in vivo by u-7524 (aminooxyacetic acid). Biochem. Pharmacol. 5:323–331.

Weissbach, H., E. F. Bogdanski, B. G. Redfield, and S. Udenfriend. 1957. Studies on the effect of vitamin B$_6$ on 5-hydroxytryptamine (serotonin formation). J. Biol. Chem. 227:617–624.

Wender, P. H. 1971. Minimal Brain Dysfunction in Children. Wiley-Interscience, New York, pp. 163–193.

Werdinius, B. 1966. Effect of probenecid on the level of homovanillic acid in the corpus striatum. J. Pharm. Pharmacol. *18*:546–547.

West, G. B. 1953. Further studies on the formation of adrenaline and noradrenaline in the body. J. Pharm. Pharmacol. *5*:311–316.

Wickner, R. B., C. W. Tabor, and H. Tabor. 1970. Purification of adenosylmethionine decarboxylase from Escherichia coli W: Evidence for covalently bound pyruvate. J. Biol. Chem. *245*:2132–2139.

Williams, M. A., and B. Hata. 1959. Liver coenzyme A levels in the vitamin B₆ deficient rat. Arch. Biochem. Biophys. *80*:367–371.

Wintrobe, M. M., R. H. Follis, Jr., M. H. Miller, H. J. Stein, R. Stein, and S. Alcayaga. 1943. Pyridoxine deficiency in swine with particular reference to anemia, epileptiform convulsions and fatty liver. Bull. Johns Hopkins Hosp. *72*:1–25.

Wood, J. D., and D. E. Abrahams. 1971. The comparative effects of various hydrazides on γ-aminobutyric acid and its metabolism. J. Neurochem. *18*:1017–1025.

Wood, J. D., and S. J. Peesker. 1972. A correlation between changes in GABA metabolism and isonicotinic acid hydrazide-induced seizures. Brain Res. *45*:489–498.

Wood, J. D., and S. J. Peesker. 1975. The anticonvulsant action of GABA elevating agents: A reevaluation. J. Neurochem. *25*:277–282.

Wood, J. D., S. J. Peesker, and J. I. M. Urton. 1972. Development of an anticonvulsant agent based on its effect on γ-aminobutyric acid metabolism. Can. J. Phys. Pharmacol. *50*:1217–1218.

Wu, J. Y., and E. Roberts. 1974. Properties of brain L-glutamic decarboxylase: Inhibition studies. J. Neurochem. *23*:759–767.

Wu, J. Y., T. Matsuda, and E. Roberts. 1973. Purification and characterization of glutamate decarboxylase from mouse brain. J. Biol. Chem. *248*:3029–3034.

Yahr, M. D., R. C. Davoisin, L. Côté, and G. Cohen. 1972. Pyridoxine, Dopa and Parkinsonism. *In* M. Ebadi and E. Costa (eds.), Role of Vitamin B₆ in Neurobiology. Vol. 4. Advances in Biochemical Psychopharmacology. Raven Press, New York, pp. 185–194.

Yamada, K., S. Sawaki, and S. Hayami. 1956. Participation of vitamin B₆ in the biosynthesis of coenzyme A. J. Vitaminol. *2*:296.

Yamamura, H. I., and S. H. Snyder. 1974. Muscarinic cholinergic binding in rat brain. Proc. Nat. Acad. Sci. U.S.A., *71*:1725–1729.

Yamamura, H. I., M. J. Kuhar, D. Greenberg, and S. H. Snyder. 1974. Muscarinic cholinergic receptor binding: Regional distribution in monkey brain. Brain Res. *66*:541–546.

Youatt, J. 1969. A review of the action of isoniazid. Am. Rev. Respir. Dis. *99*:729–749.

Zatz, M., J. W. Kebabian, J. A. Romero, R. J. Lefkowitz, and J. Axelrod. 1976. Pineal β-adrenergic receptor: Correlation of binding of ['H]-(1)-alprenolol with stimulation of adenylate cyclase. J. Pharmacol. Exp. Ther. *196*:714–722.

Zukin, S. R., A. H. Young, and S. H. Snyder. 1974. Gamma-aminobutyric acid binding in receptor sites in the rat central nervous system. Proc. Nat. Acad. Sci. U.S.A., *71*:4802–4807.

9

Vitamin B_6 and Immunity

LINDA C. ROBSON, M. ROY SCHWARZ, *and*
WILLIAM D. PERKINS

It is well accepted that the lymphoid system and consequently the immune system may be influenced adversely by reducing or by eliminating specific nutrients from the diet. In the past 30 years, studies have clearly shown that a dietary deficiency of vitamin B_6 may result in an impairment of both humoral and cell-mediated immune responses. It has been reported that experimental animals deprived of vitamin B_6 for 2 to 10 weeks demonstrated a reduction in the levels of circulating antibodies produced in response to sheep red blood cells (Stoerk and Eisen, 1946; Stoerk *et al.*, 1947), human red blood cells (Axelrod *et al.*, 1947), diphtheria toxoid (Pruzansky and Axelrod, 1955; Axelrod *et al.*, 1961), influenza virus (Axelrod and Hopper, 1960), *B. typhosum* (Agnew and Cook, 1949), *C. kutcheri* (Zucker *et al.*, 1956), murine typhus *Rickettsiae* (Wertman and Sarandria, 1951), *H. pertussis* (Hargis *et al.*, 1960), *Salmonella pullorum* (Harmon *et al.*, 1963), and the synthetic antigen poly $Glu^{52}Lys^{33}Tyr^{15}$ (Gershoff *et al.*, 1968). In vitamin B_6-deficient animals it was noted also that the reduction in the levels of circulating antibodies to sheep red blood cells was accompanied by a reduction in the number of antibody-forming cells in the spleens of such animals. It was demonstrated also that the secondary or anamnestic response to diphtheria toxoid in animals deprived of vitamin B_6 was inhibited to a greater extent than was the primary response to this antigen (Axelrod, 1958).

Axelrod *et al.* (1958), Hargis *et al.* (1960), and Parkes (1959) have reported also that animals deprived of vitamin B_6 rejected foreign or allogeneic tissue grafts more slowly than did normal controls. In addition, vitamin B_6-deficient animals inoculated with *Mycobacterium* BCG vaccine exhibited a reduction in the skin reactions (delayed hypersensitivity) that developed in response to purified protein derivative even though the *in vitro* correlates of sensitization were demonstrable (Trakatellis *et al.*, 1963). In certain strains of mice, Axelrod and Trakatellis (1964) demonstrated that vitamin B_6 deficiency facilitated the development of a specific state of tolerance to foreign antigens. More specifically, allogeneic spleen cells were injected into vitamin B_6-deficient mice. The mice then were returned to a normal diet and subsequently were grafted with allogeneic tissue from the same strain of mouse that donated the spleen cells. Since these allografts survived for long periods of time, the animals were judged to be tolerant of the allogeneic tissue.

In contrast to animals, humans maintained on a vitamin B_6-deficient diet for 5 weeks demonstrated only slightly impaired antibody responses to tetanus and typhoid antigens (Hodges *et al.*, 1962). More recently, it was reported that lymphoid cells from vitamin B_6-deficient, uremic patients exhibited diminished cell-mediated immune responses (Dobbelstein *et al.*, 1974). Since this defect could be corrected by treating such patients with vitamin B_6 orally, it was concluded that suppression of cell-mediated immunity in uremia might be due in part to vitamin B_6 depletion.

On the basis of the above studies, it would appear that an absence of vitamin B_6 from the diets of humans and laboratory animals can lead to a suppression of cellular and humoral immune responses. To explore further the nature of this suppression, experiments that focused on the changes in cell-mediated immunity and on alterations in the structure of the lymphoid organs were conducted. More specifically, efforts were made (1) to determine if the influence of vitamin B_6-deficiency on the capacity of lymphoid cells to participate in cell-mediated immune responses could be monitored *in vitro* by using a well-known cellular immune response, the mixed lymphocyte reaction, and (2) to evaluate the effects of the deficiency on the structure of the thymus by using the electron microscope. In addition, experiments were conducted to determine if a vitamin B_6-deficient diet influenced not only adult animals but also the progeny of such animals. More specifically, these experiments were designed (1) to determine if an absence of vitamin B_6 from the diet of pregnant rats led to reduced immunological competence in the offspring and (2) to evaluate the effects of vitamin B_6 deficiency *in utero* on specific subpopulations of small lymphocytes in the lymphoid organs of the offspring.

INFLUENCE OF VITAMIN B_6 DEFICIENCY ON THE CAPACITY OF SMALL LYMPHOCYTES TO PARTICIPATE IN THE *IN VITRO* MIXED LYMPHOCYTE REACTION (MLR)

It is generally accepted that the proliferation of small lymphocytes in the MLR represents an *in vitro* model of the cell-mediated immune response (Elves, 1969; Häyry and Defendi, 1970; Bach *et al.*, 1973). By using the MLR it has been possible to monitor *in vitro* the capacity of animals to reject foreign skin grafts after the animals had received the immunosuppressive procedures of antilymphocytic serum treatment (Schwarz *et al.*, 1968), X-irradiation (Lamberg and Schwarz, 1970), or thymectomy (Robson and Schwarz, 1971). Since vitamin B_6 deficiency may lead also to a state of immunosuppression, studies were undertaken to determine if the effects of this deficiency could be detected *in vitro* by the MLR (Robson and Schwarz, 1975a).

For these studies, adult Lewis (Lew) strain male rats were fed a vitamin B_6-deficient diet for 2 weeks. The diet consisted of commercially prepared rat chow and drinking water that contained 4-deoxypyridoxine HCl (ICN Nutritional Biochemicals, Cleveland, Ohio). The chow for deficient animals was also purchased from ICN and was *not* the same as that fed to control animals. Chow for pair-fed and pair-weighed control animals was obtained from Ralston Purina Company, St. Louis, Missouri. At the end of 2 weeks, or at a time when the animals had developed skin changes typical of the deficiency (Gross, 1940), lymphocytes were collected from the thoracic duct lymph (TDL) of control and vitamin B_6-deficient animals. These cells then were prepared for the MLR according to the method described previously (Schwarz, 1968). For each MLR, 5×10^6 TDL cells from each Lew rat donor were cultured with an equal number of TDL cells from a normal F_1 (Lew × Brown Norway) hybrid rat. Under these conditions, Lew rat cells, which are immunologically competent, are known to respond to the genetically dissimilar lymphoid cells from the F_1 hybrid by transforming into large blast cells (Dutton, 1965). Since this blastogenesis is accompanied by DNA synthesis, the amount of blast formation may be quantitated by exposing the cultures to tritiated thymidine and then measuring the incorporation of the isotope into DNA (Caffrey *et al.,* 1966).

The results of the MLR test (Figure 9-1) indicated that TDL cells from vitamin B₆-deficient rats had a reduced capacity to respond to foreign lymphoid cells *in vitro.* More specifically, the average amount of ³H-thymidine incorporation in mixed cultures that contained cells from vitamin B₆-deficient donors was approximately 55 percent less than that found in mixed cultures that contained cells from control animals.

To compare the results of the MLR with an *in vivo* correlate of lymphocyte function, TDL cells were tested for their capacity to initiate *in vivo* normal lymphocyte transfer (NLT) reactions. For this test, 10×10^6 TDL cells from each Lew rat donor were injected intradermally into the ventral abdominal wall of an F_1 (Lew × Brown Norway) hybrid rat (Ford, 1967). Five days later, the F_1 animals were injected intravenously with a 1 percent normal saline solution of Evans blue dye. According to this test, Lew rat cells, which are immunologically competent, react against the genetically dissimilar F_1 hybrid by producing a localized graft-versus-host reaction in the skin of the F_1 animal. Because of the dye, such reactions appear as blue, well-defined lesions.

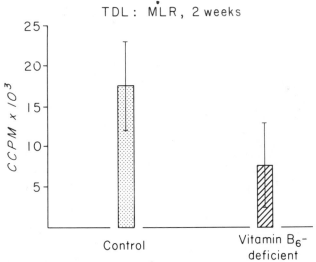

FIGURE 9-1 Response of thoracic duct lymph (TDL) cells in the mixed lymphocyte reaction (MLR). Cells were obtained from adult rats fed either a control diet or a 2-week, vitamin B₆-deficient diet. The amount of blast formation in each MLR has been expressed as corrected counts per minute (CCPM) of ³H-thymidine uptake. Narrow bars represent the range.

The results of the NLT reactions are shown in Figure 9-2. Whereas TDL cells from a control Lew rat produced a distinct reaction which was 8–10 mm in diameter, TDL cells from a vitamin B_6-deficient donor produced a small, poorly defined reaction that was barely visible in the skin of the F_1 hybrid.

From the results of these studies, it was concluded that vitamin B_6 deficiency suppressed cellular immunity in adult animals. It is also significant that the MLR was capable of detecting a significant reduction in lymphocyte function as soon as 2 weeks after the vitamin B_6-deficient diet was begun or at a time when the animals were known to be deficient in vitamin B_6 as judged by the appearance of their skin (Robson and Schwarz, 1975a). Although a reduction in MLR responsiveness by TDL cells probably occurred before the skin changes became evident (unpublished data), the exact time of onset of reduced lymphocyte function in vitamin B_6-deficient animals remains to be determined.

While both the MLR and NLT tests were capable of detecting a reduction in the immunocompetency of TDL cells from vitamin B_6-deficient

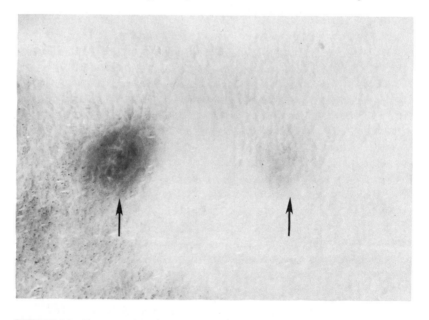

FIGURE 9-2   Two normal lymphocyte transfer reactions produced by 10×10^6 Lew rat cells injected intradermally into the ventral abdominal wall of an F_1 (Lew × Brown Norway) hybrid rat. Left arrow indicates the reaction produced by cells from a rat fed a control diet. Right arrow indicates the reaction produced by cells from a rat fed a vitamin B_6-deficient diet for 2 weeks.

animals, the MLR offered several advantages over the NLT reaction and perhaps over other tests for lymphocyte function. First, it is possible to quantitate the MLR results through the use of a Packard liquid scintillation counting system to determine the ^{3}H-thymidine uptake per culture. Second, the MLR provides results in a relatively short period of time and requires no manipulation of the donor animals beyond the initial collection of cells. Unlike the NLT test, samples can be taken from the MLR at various times during the culture period in order to examine the cells involved in the immune response.

INFLUENCE OF VITAMIN B$_6$ DEFICIENCY ON THE STRUCTURE OF THE THYMUS AS DETERMINED BY ELECTRON MICROSCOPIC OBSERVATION

It is now generally recognized that cell-mediated immune responses such as the MLR involve primarily T cells, i.e., cells derived from or influenced by the thymus (Mosier and Cantor, 1971). It may be suggested, therefore, that the reduction in the capacity of cells from vitamin B$_6$-deficient animals to initiate cellular immune responses should be related to thymic alterations such as those described by Stoerk (1946) and Agnew and Cook (1949). These investigators noted an atrophy of the thymus and a loss of thymic lymphocytes in rats fed a vitamin B$_6$-deficient diet for periods of 2 to 10 weeks. To explore further the influence of vitamin B$_6$ deficiency on thymic tissue, the electron microscope was used to evaluate the ultrastructure of thymuses from animals maintained on a vitamin B$_6$-deficient diet for 2 and 6 weeks.

For these studies, thymuses were taken from control and vitamin B$_6$-deficient animals and were prepared by conventional methods for electron microscopy. From electron micrographs it was determined that thymuses from control animals consisted of a thin connective tissue capsule, a cortex that contained densely packed cells, and a medulla in which the cells were more loosely arranged. As shown in Figure 9-3a, the cells present in the cortical region consisted predominantly of small lymphocytes. In comparison (Figure 9-3b), the thymic cortex of animals fed a vitamin B$_6$-deficient diet for 2 weeks contained a decreased density of small lymphocytes. Also evident in the cortical region of thymuses from deficient animals were numerous plasma cells, macrophages filled with phagocytic debris, and a small number of epithelial cells. Under normal conditions, plasma cells are rarely found in this region.

After a diet period of 6 weeks (Figure 9-3c) the thymus cortex con-

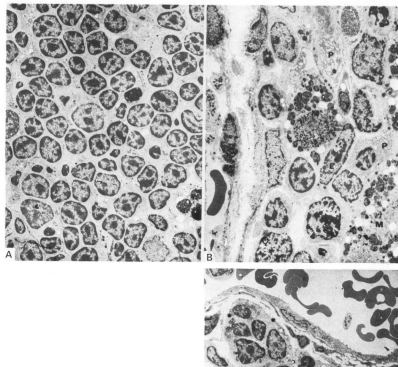

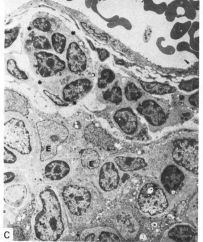

FIGURE 9-3 Electronmicrographs of thymus cortex from vitamin B$_6$ and control rats. (A) Control thymus cortex. Cells are predominantly small lymphocytes. (B) Thymus cortex, 2-week vitamin B$_6$-deficient diet. P is plasma cell. M is macrophage. E is epithelial cell. (C) Thymus cortex, 6-week vitamin B$_6$-deficient diet. E is epithelial cell. An asterisk indicates an aggregate of small lymphocytes.

tained predominantly epithelial cells. Although small lymphocytes, macrophages, and plasma cells were also present in the thymus cortex at this later interval, their numbers were reduced when compared to the 2-week diet period. At 6 weeks, the capsule of thymuses from vitamin B$_6$-deficient rats had increased in thickness and, in contrast to the capsule of control thymuses, contained aggregates of small lymphocytes. Unlike the cortex, the medullary regions of thymuses appeared to be unaltered following either a 2- or 6-week vitamin B_6-deficient diet.

From these observations, it is clear that vitamin B_6 deficiency results in marked alterations in the structure of the thymus. Since the thymus is known to contain predominantly T cells (Perkins *et al.*, 1972), it is reasonable to suggest that the small lymphocytes that are missing from the thymic cortex of vitamin B_6-deficient animals were mainly T cells and that such cells are required for the full expression of cellular immunity as measured by the MLR. It may also be suggested that if the small lymphocytes that remained in the thymic cortex of vitamin B_6-deficient animals were T cells, such cells may have been altered and could not initiate normal cell-mediated immune responses.

This study has also demonstrated that the decreased density of small lymphocytes in the thymic cortex of vitamin B_6-deficient rats was accompanied by an increased proportion of thymic epithelial cells. Recently, Willis and St. Pierre (1976) demonstrated that thymic epithelial cells from vitamin B_6-deficient rats were functionally impaired at the end of a 2-week diet period. Thus, unlike thymic epithelial cells from normal rats, thymic epithelial cells from deficient rats failed to convert incompetent lymphocytes to immunocompetent T cells *in vitro*. It has been suggested that this defect might be due to a failure of the epithelial cells to produce a hormonal substance required for such a maturation of immunologically competent cells (Goldstein *et al.*, 1970). It remains to be determined whether or not a thymic hormone such as thymosin (Goldstein *et al.*, 1970) can restore immunocompetence if administered to vitamin B_6-deficient animals.

INFLUENCE OF VITAMIN B_6 DEFICIENCY DURING PREGNANCY
ON THE IMMUNOLOGICAL COMPETENCE OF THE OFFSPRING

While there is considerable evidence to indicate that laboratory animals that consume diets deficient in vitamin B_6 develop immunological defects, relatively little is known about the immunological competence of the progeny of such animals. In 1970, Davis *et al.* (1970) reported that the spleens and thymuses of fetuses taken from mothers deprived of vitamin B_6 during pregnancy were significantly smaller than those from fetuses taken from control mothers. More recently, Moon and Kirksey (1973) reported that both 19- to 21-day-old fetuses from rats fed a vitamin B_6-deficient diet during pregnancy and 14- to 21-day-old progeny of rats fed a vitamin B_6-deficient diet during pregnancy and lactation had reduced body weights and organ weights. The most severe reduction in organ weight occurred in the thymus. While these studies indicate that vitamin B_6 deficiency *in utero* resulted in grossly observable changes in the lymphoid organs of the offspring, no evidence is available to indicate whether or not the deficiency also altered the capacity of lymphocytes to function in immune responses. A study was undertaken, therefore, to determine whether vitamin B_6 deficiency during pregnancy altered the immune system of the offspring as measured by the MLR and NLT tests (Robson and Schwarz, 1975b).

In this study, pregnant Lew rats were maintained on a vitamin B_6-deficient diet that began on day 4, 5, or 6 of pregnancy. Control mothers were fed a normal diet throughout the study. On day 21 of pregnancy, vitamin B_6-deficient mothers resumed the control diet. When the offspring were approximately 3 months old, TDL cells were collected for use in the MLR and NLT reactions, and cell counts were made of the peripheral blood and TDL.

The peripheral blood cell counts for rats from vitamin B_6-deficient mothers and for rats from control mothers are shown in Figure 9-4. It is clear that the concentrations of peripheral blood lymphocytes and

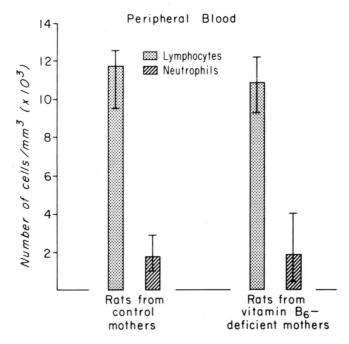

FIGURE 9-4   Concentrations of lymphocytes and neutrophils in the peripheral blood of rats approximately 3 months old and progeny of control mothers or of mothers fed a vitamin B_6-deficient diet during pregnancy. Narrow bars represent the range.

neutrophils were approximately the same in both groups of animals. For the TDL, as denoted in Figure 9-5, the average concentrations of cells for rats from vitamin B$_6$-deficient mothers was 72×10^6 cells/ml of lymph or 16 percent less than that observed in rats from nontreated, control mothers. This difference was not statistically significant.

When the immunocompetency of TDL lymphocytes was assayed by using the MLR (Figure 9-6), the results indicated that TDL cells from rats with vitamin B$_6$-deficient mothers evidenced a decreased response when compared to cells from rats with control mothers. Specifically, cells from rats with vitamin B$_6$-deficient mothers incorporated approximately 48 percent less ^{3}H-thymidine in the MLR than did cells from rats with control mothers.

The results of the *in vivo* NLT test are shown in Figure 9-7. Whereas 10×10^6 TDL cells from a rat with a control mother produced a distinct reaction in the skin of the F$_1$ hybrid, an identical number of TDL cells from a rat with a vitamin B$_6$-deficient mother produced a significantly smaller and less intense reaction.

From the results of these experiments it was concluded that vitamin B$_6$ deficiency during pregnancy in rats influenced the immunological competence of the offspring as young adults. This influence was evi-

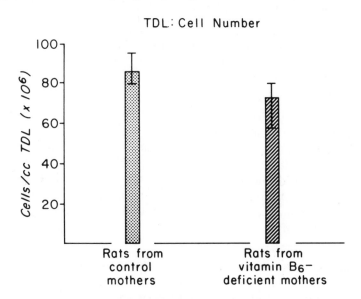

FIGURE 9-5 Concentration of cells in the thoracic duct lymph (TDL) of rats approximately 3 months old and progeny of control mothers or of mothers fed a vitamin B$_6$-deficient diet during pregnancy. Narrow bars represent the range.

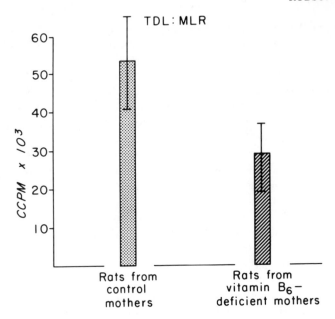

FIGURE 9-6   Response of thoracic duct lymph (TDL) cells in the
mixed lymphocyte reaction (MLR). Cells were obtained from rats
approximately 3 months old and progeny of control mothers or of
mothers fed a vitamin B₆-deficient diet during pregnancy. The
amount of blast formation in each MLR has been expressed as corrected counts per minute (CCPM) of ³H-thymidine uptake. Narrow
bars represent the range.

dent even though the offspring were fed normal diets after birth and
even though the total number of cells in the TDL compartment of rats
with vitamin B₆-deficient mothers was not significantly different from
that in rats with control mothers. These results strongly suggest a
change in the progenitor cell of lymphocytes, which persists for generations of cells. Alternatively, these results may suggest a permanent
change in the microenvironment necessary for the normal functioning
of lymphoid cells.

INFLUENCE OF VITAMIN B₆ DEFICIENCY DURING PREGNANCY ON SPECIFIC SUBPOPULATIONS OF SMALL LYMPHOCYTES IN THE LYMPHOID ORGANS OF THE PROGENY

It is now well known that small lymphocytes of the rat comprise a
heterogeneous population of cells in terms of their tissue distribution,

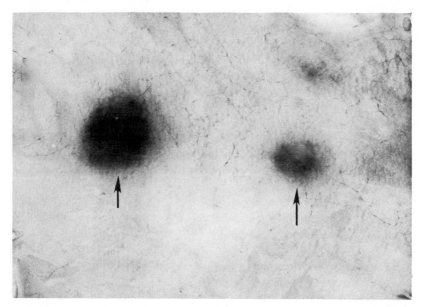

FIGURE 9-7 Two normal lymphocyte transfer reactions produced by 10×10^6 Lew rat cells injected intradermally into the ventral abdominal wall of an F_1 (Lew × Brown Norway) hybrid rat. Left arrow indicates the reaction produced by cells from a rat with a control mother. Right arrow indicates the reaction produced by cells from a rat with a vitamin B₆-deficient mother.

circulating life spans, origins, and functional capacities. It may be suggested, therefore, that the reduced capacity of small lymphocytes to function in cell-mediated immune responses such as the MLR might reflect alterations in the numbers and distribution of specific subpopulations of small lymphocytes within various lymphoid organs. To investigate this possibility, experiments were conducted by using ^{3}H-thymidine to label either (1) populations of small lymphocytes that have a short life span and a rapid rate of proliferation or (2) populations of small lymphocytes that have a long life span and a slow rate of proliferation. The ^{3}H-thymidine was administered to rats with control mothers and to rats with vitamin B₆-deficient mothers according to well-established injection schedules (Caffrey *et al.*, 1962; Everett and Tyler, 1967).

The results of the labeling studies involving populations of small lymphocytes having a short life span and a rapid rate of proliferation are shown in Figures 9-8 and 9-9. In bone marrow, spleen, and TDL, the percentages of labeled cells were approximately the same for both

BM, SPL, TDL: SLSL

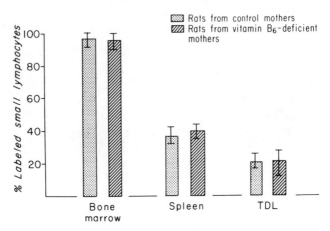

FIGURE 9-8 Percentages of labeled short-lived, small lymphocytes (SLSL) in the bone marrow, spleen, and thoracic duct lymph
(TDL) of rats approximately 3 months old and progeny of control
mothers or of mothers fed a vitamin B$_6$-deficient diet during pregnancy. Narrow bars represent the range.

LN, THY: SLSL

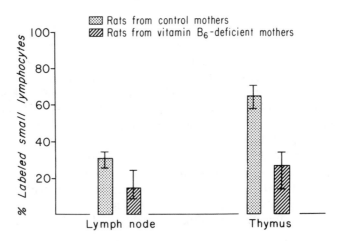

FIGURE 9-9 Percentages of labeled short-lived, small lymphocytes (SLSL) in the lymph nodes and thymuses of rats approximately
3 months old and progeny of control mothers or of mothers fed a
vitamin B$_6$-deficient diet during pregnancy. Narrow bars represent
the range.

groups of animals. However, in lymph nodes and thymuses, the percentages of labeled "short-lived," small lymphocytes were significantly lower in rats with vitamin B_6-deficient mothers than in rats with control mothers. In the case of the thymus, this reduction was approximately 55 percent.

Shown in Figure 9-10 are the results of the labeling studies involving populations of small lymphocytes having a long life span and a slow rate of proliferation. The percentages of labeled cells in the bone marrow and thymus of both groups of rats were nearly equivalent. Similarly, the percentages of labeled "long-lived," small lymphocytes in the spleens and lymph nodes were approximately the same for both animal groups. In contrast, the percentage of labeled long-lived cells in the TDL of offspring with vitamin B_6-deficient mothers was significantly reduced in comparison to rats with normal mothers.

On the basis of the results of these labeling studies, it may be concluded that a reduction in the percentages of either short-lived or long-lived small lymphocytes occurred in certain lymphoid organs of rats with vitamin B_6-deficient mothers. In the case of the short-lived, rapidly proliferating cells, the reduction occurred in lymph nodes and thymuses. This may suggest that a maternal vitamin B_6 deficiency re-

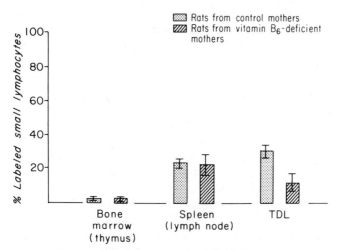

FIGURE 9-10. Percentages of labeled long-lived, small lymphocytes (LLSL) in lymphoid organs of rats approximately 3 months old and progeny of control mothers or of mothers fed a vitamin B_6-deficient diet during pregnancy. Narrow bars represent the range.

sulted in the disappearance of certain lymphoid cells or their precursors *in utero* or that an alteration occurred in the metabolic activity of certain lymphocytes of the offspring. Since the reduction of short-lived small lymphocytes was proportionately smaller in the lymph nodes than in the thymuses, it may be suggested that changes in the lymph nodes reflected the failure of the thymus to produce those cells normally found in thymus-dependent areas of lymph nodes (Parrott *et al.*, 1966). In the case of the long-lived, slowly proliferating, small lymphocyte population, it is recognized that these cells are thymus-derived or T cells involved in cell-mediated immune responses (Everett and Tyler, 1967). It may be suggested, therefore, that the reduction of these cells from the TDL of rats with vitamin B_6-deficient mothers may have accounted, at least in part, for the reduction in MLR competence observed for these animals.

It is evident from these studies that further investigation is required in order to determine the exact nature of the immunological defects that occur in the progeny of deficient mothers. For instance, it remains to be determined whether or not the *in utero* deficiency alters the structure of the thymus and possibly other lymphoid organs of the progeny. A determination should also be made of whether a thymic hormone, such as thymosin (Goldstein *et al.*, 1970), has the capacity to improve immunological competence if administered to the progeny of vitamin B_6-deficient mothers.

Further study is required also to learn whether or not the time at which the deficiency is induced during pregnancy may be a critical factor in determining the effects on the immune system of the offspring. In this regard, it has been reported that when the vitamin B_6-deficient diet was begun on day 0 or 1 of pregnancy, over 40 percent of the fetuses were resorbed (Davis *et al.*, 1970), all live fetuses were small (Davis *et al.*, 1970; Moon and Kirksey, 1973), and many fetuses had grossly observable external anomalies (Davis *et al.*, 1970). The spleen weights and thymus weights in these animals were also significantly less than those in control fetuses. However, when the diet was begun on day 4, 5, or 6 of pregnancy (Robson and Schwarz, 1975b), litter sizes and fetal weights were normal and in most cases thymic weights of the offspring were within the range of control values. While it is not yet possible to explain accurately why the effects of the *in utero* vitamin B_6 deficiency varied according to the time of onset of the diet, it is hoped that the results of forthcoming studies will elucidate the mechanism whereby *in utero* vitamin B_6 deficiency achieves its effects.

SUMMARY

Results of these studies indicated that vitamin B_6 plays an important role in the development and maintenance of a competent immune system. It was demonstrated that (1) vitamin B_6 deficiency in adult animals resulted in a suppression of cellular immune competence and that this suppression could be monitored *in vitro* by the MLR; (2) vitamin B_6 deficiency in adult animals altered the structure of the thymus as determined by electron microscopy; and (3) vitamin B_6 deficiency during pregnancy led to reduced immunological competence in the offspring. For the progeny of vitamin B_6-deficient mothers, it was also demonstrated that alterations in the proportions of short-lived and long-lived small lymphocytes in various lymphoid organs occurred in the progeny of vitamin B_6-deficient mothers, and this correlated with the reduction in cellular immune competence.

ACKNOWLEDGMENTS

The authors wish to thank Miss Sharlene Carlson for her technical assistance and Mrs. Arnita Lawrence for maintaining the animal colony. The critical analysis of this manuscript by Dr. Karen Holbrook is greatly appreciated.

This work was supported by USPHS Grant AI-07509 from the National Institutes of

LITERATURE CITED

Agnew, L. R. C., and R. Cook. 1949. Antibody production in pyridoxin-deficient rats. Br. J. Nutr. *2*:321–329.

Axelrod, A. E. 1958. The role of nutritional factors in the antibody responses of the anamnestic process. Am. J. Clin. Nutr. *6*:119–125.

Axelrod, A. E., and S. Hopper. 1960. Effects of pantothenic acid, pyridoxine and thiamine deficiencies upon antibody formation to influenza virus PR-8 in rats. J. Nutr. *72*:325–330.

Axelrod, A. E., and A. C. Trakatellis. 1964. Induction of tolerance to skin homografts by administering splenic cells to pyridoxine-deficient mice. Proc. Soc. Exp. Biol. Med. *116*:206–210.

Axelrod, A. E., B. B. Carter, R. H. McCoy, and R. Geisinger. 1947. Circulating antibodies in vitamin deficiency states. I. Pyridoxin, riboflavin, and pantothenic acid deficiencies. Proc. Soc. Exp. Biol. Med. *66*:137–140.

Axelrod, A. E., B. Fisher, E. Fisher, Y. C. P. Lee, and P. Walsh. 1958. Effect of a pyridoxine deficiency on skin grafts in the rat. Science *127*:1388–1389.

Axelrod, A. E., S. Hopper, and D. A. Long. 1961. Effects of pyridoxine deficiency upon circulating antibody formation and skin hypersensitivity reactions to diphtheria toxoid in guinea pigs. J. Nutr. *74*:58–64.

Bach, F. H., M. Segall, K. S. Zier, P. M. Sondel, and B. J. Alter. 1973. Cell mediated immunity: Separation of cells involved in recognitive and destructive phases. Science *180*:403–406.

Caffrey, R. W., W. O. Rieke, and N. B. Everett. 1962. Radioautographic studies of small lymphocytes in the thoracic duct of the rat. Acta Haematol. *28*:145–154.

Caffrey, R. W., N. B. Everett,'and W. O. Rieke. 1966. Radioautographic studies of reticular and blast cells in the hemopoietic tissues of the rat. Anat. Rec. *155*:41–57.

Davis, S. D., T. Nelson, and T. H. Shepard. 1970. Teratogenicity of vitamin B₆ deficiency: Omphalocele, skeletal and neural defects, and splenic hypoplasia. Science *169*:1329–1330.

Dobbelstein, H., W. F. Körner, W. Mempel, H. Grosse-Wilde, and H. H. Edel. 1974. Vitamin B₆ deficiency in uremia and its implications for the depression of immune responses. Kidney Int. *5*:233–239.

Dutton, R. W. 1965. Further studies of the stimulation of DNA synthesis in cultures of spleen cell suspensions by homologous cells in inbred strains of mice and rats. J. Exp. Med. *122*:759–770.

Elves, M. W. 1969. The mixed lymphocyte reaction. An *in vitro* model for the homograft reaction. Transplantation *8*:44–50.

Everett, N. B., and R. W. Tyler (Caffrey). 1967. Lymphopoiesis in the thymus and other tissues: Functional implications. Int. Rev. Cytol. *22*:205–237.

Ford, W. L. 1967. A local graft-versus-host reaction following intradermal injection of lymphocytes in the rat. Br. J. Exp. Pathol. *48*:335–345.

Gershoff, S. N., T. J. Gill, S. J. Simonian, and A. I. Steinberg. 1968. Some effects of amino acid deficiencies on antibody formation in the rat. J. Nutr. *95*:184–190.

Goldstein, A. L., Y. Asanuma, J. R. Battisto, M. A. Hardy, J. Quint, and A. White. 1970. Influence of thymosin on cell-mediated and humoral responses in normal and immunologically deficient mice. J. Immunol. *104*:359–366.

Gross, P. 1940. The role of the unsaturated fatty acids in the acrodynia (vitamin B₆ deficiency) of the albino rat. J. Invest. Dermatol. *3*:505–521.

Hargis, B. J., L. C. Wyman, and S. Malkiel. 1960. Skin transplantation in pyridoxine-deficient mice. Int. Arch. Allergy Appl. Immunol. *16*:276–287.

Harmon, B. G., E. R. Miller, J. A. Hoefer, D. E. Ullrey, and R. W. Luecke. 1963. Relationship of specific nutrient deficiencies to antibody production in swine. II. Pantothenic acid, pyridoxine or riboflavin. J. Nutr. *79*:269–275.

Häyry, P., and V. Defendi. 1970. Mixed lymphocyte cultures produce effector cells: Model *in vitro* for allograft rejection. Science *168*:133–135.

Hodges, R. E., W. B. Bean, M. A. Ohlson, and R. E. Bleiler. 1962. Factors affecting human antibody response. IV. Pyridoxine deficiency. Am. J. Clin. Nutr. *11*:180–186.

Lamberg, J. D., and M. R. Schwarz. 1970. The recovery of immunological competence following sublethal irradiation as monitored by the mixed lymphocyte reaction. *In* O. R. McIntyre (ed.), Proceedings of the Fourth Leucocyte Culture Conference Appleton-Century-Crofts, New York, pp. 173–182.

Moon, W.-H. Y., and A. Kirksey. 1973. Cellular growth during prenatal and early postnatal periods in progeny of pyridoxine-deficient rats. J. Nutr. *103*:123–133.

Mosier, D., and H. Cantor. 1971. Functional maturation of mouse thymic lymphocytes. Eur. J. Immunol. *1*:459–461.

Parkes, A. S. 1959. Dietary factors in the homograft reaction. Nature *184*:699–701.

Parrott, D. M. V., M. A. B. deSousa, and J. East. 1966. Thymus-dependent areas in the lymphoid organs of neonatally thymectomized mice. J. Exp. Med. *123*:191–204.

Perkins, W. D., M. J. Karnovsky, and E. R. Unanue. 1972. An ultrastructural study of lymphocytes with surface-bound immunoglobulin. J. Exp. Med. *135*:267–276.

Pruzansky, J., and A. E. Axelrod. 1955. Antibody production to diphtheria toxoid in vitamin deficiency states. Proc. Soc. Exp. Biol. Med. *89*:323–325.

Robson, L. C., and M. R. Schwarz. 1971. The influence of adult thymectomy on immunological competence as measured by the mixed lymphocyte reaction. Transplantation *11*:465–470.

Robson, L. C., and M. R. Schwarz. 1975a. Vitamin B₆ deficiency and the lymphoid system. I. Effects on cellular immunity and *in vitro* incorporation of ³H-uridine by small lymphocytes. Cell. Immunol. *16*:135–144.

Robson, L. C., and M. R. Schwarz. 1975b. Vitamin B₆ deficiency and the lymphoid system. II. Effects of vitamin B₆ deficiency *in utero* on the immunological competence of the offspring. Cell. Immunol. *16*:145–152.

Schwarz, M. R. 1968. The mixed lymphocyte reaction: An *in vitro* test for tolerance. J. Exp. Med. *127*:879–890.

Schwarz, M. R., R. W. Tyler, and N. B. Everett. 1968. Mixed lymphocyte reaction: An *in vitro* test for antilymphocytic serum activity. Science *160*:1014–1017.

Stoerk, H. C. 1946. Effects of calcium deficiency and pyridoxin deficiency on thymic atrophy (accidental involution). Proc. Soc. Exp. Biol. Med. *62*:90–96.

Stoerk, H. C., and H. N. Eisen. 1946. Suppression of circulating antibodies in pyridoxin deficiency. Proc. Soc. Exp. Biol. Med. *62*:88–89.

Stoerk, H. C., H. N. Eisen, and H. M. John. 1947. Impairment of antibody response in pyridoxine-deficient rats. J. Exp. Med. *85*:365–371.

Trakatellis, A. C., W. R. Stinebring, and A. E. Axelrod. 1963. Studies on systemic reactivity to purified protein derivative (PPD) and endotoxin. I. Systemic reactivity to PPD in pyridoxine-deficient guinea pigs. J. Immunol. *91*:39–45.

Wertman, K., and J. L. Sarandria. 1951. Complement-fixing murine typhus antibodies in vitamin deficiency states. II. Pyridoxine, and nicotinic acid deficiencies. Proc. Soc. Exp. Biol. Med. *78*:332–335.

Willis, J. I., and R. L. St. Pierre. 1976. Vitamin B₆ deficiency: Impairment of thymic epithelial cell function. Anat. Rec. *184*:564.

Zucker, T. F., L. M. Zucker, and J. Seronde. 1956. Antibody formation and natural resistance in nutritional deficiencies. J. Nutr. *59*:299–308.

10

Vitamin B_6 Nutriture in Patients with Uremia and with Liver Disease

C. L. SPANNUTH, D. MITCHELL, W. J. STONE,
S. SCHENKER, *and* C. WAGNER

During the past several years we have been concerned with an evaluation of vitamin B_6 status in certain disease states. We would like to review some data obtained in our laboratories that indicate that a functional vitamin B_6 deficiency may be present in humans with uremia and with liver disease.

STUDIES WITH UREMIA

The first indication that the uremic patient may be suffering from a vitamin B_6 deficiency came as a result of an observation made regarding the serum aspartate aminotransferase (GOT) measuremets performed in the clinical laboratory of the VA Hospital, Nashville, Tennessee. Elevated serum GOT values are found in patients with hepatitis and with myocardial infarction. Figure 10-1 (Warnock *et al.,* 1974) shows the results of all the serum GOT and creatinine measurements performed in a single day by the SMA-12. Uremic patients have serum creatinine levels greater than 4 mg per 100 ml. The normal range for serum GOT values is 10 to 40 international units (IU) per liter. It can be seen from Figure 10-1 that there is an inverse relationship between the serum creatinine and serum GOT values. Some of the serum GOT values

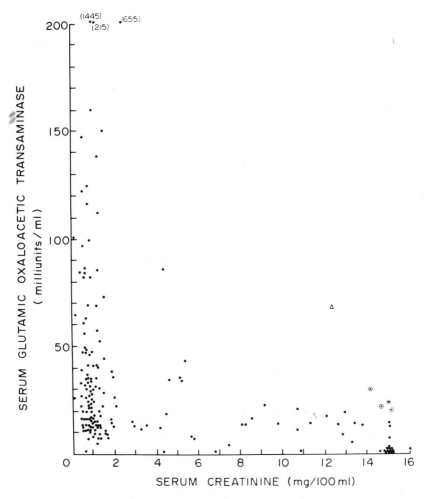

FIGURE 10-1   Comparison of serum glutamate-oxaloacetate transaminase activity and serum creatinine values as measured by SMA 12/60. Δ and * are uremic patients with hepatitis. ⊙ are values for a uremic patient after myocardial infarction. Units are those routinely used for SMA 12/60.

obtained with the uremic patients were so low as to be unreadable. In addition, two uremic patients with early acute active hepatitis were included in this sample. One had a serum GOT in the normal range; the other had a value of about 70 units. One would normally expect these values to fall in the range of 500–1000. Figure 10-2 shows values obtained with a patient having recurrent cardiac infarcts. These values were also in the normal range but should have been much higher.

SPANNUTH *et al.*

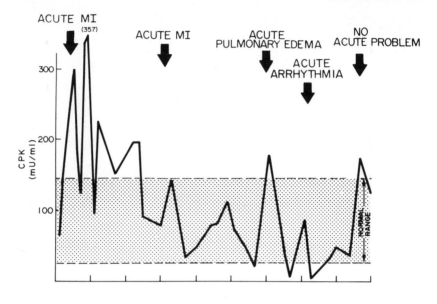

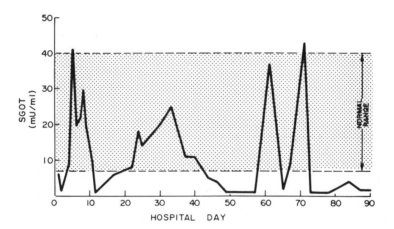

FIGURE 10-2 Comparison of serum glutamate-oxaloacetate (SGOT) activity and creatine kinase activity for a patient with severe cardiac episodes. MI is myocardial infarction. Note the extremely low baseline for SGOT activity.

We went on to show that part of the reason for the depressed serum GOT values obtained for uremic patients was due to the method of measurement by the SMA-12, which tends to exaggerate the low values in uremic serum. The decreased level of serum GOT activity in both dialyzed and nondialyzed uremic patients has been confirmed by other independent assays (Babson *et al.*, 1962; Karmen, 1955) and in other laboratories (Dobbelstein *et al.*, 1974; Cohen *et al.*, 1976).

We have listed below some defects that have been cited to be common to both uremia and vitamin B$_6$ deficiency:

- Depression of central nervous system
- Convulsions
- Skin and mucous membrane changes
- Anemia
- Peripheral neuropathy
- Improvement on low protein diet
- Increased oxalate production
- Low serum aspartate aminotransferase
- Changes in plasma amino acids
- Depression of immune responses

It seemed possible, therefore, that some of the problems experienced by the uremic patient might be secondary to a deficiency in vitamin B$_6$, which accompanies the uremia.

Further evidence for vitamin B$_6$ deficiency in uremic patients was provided by measurement of erythrocyte (EGOT) levels (Stone *et al.*, 1975). Assays were performed in the absence of and in the presence of added pyridoxal phosphate (PLP). The data are shown in Figure 10-3. It may be seen that erythrocyte GOT activity is significantly lower in both dialyzed and nondialyzed uremic patients than in the control group. Values obtained in the presence of added PLP were greater in all groups. The amount of stimulation produced by the added PLP, however, varied. The ratio of erythrocyte GOT activity measured in the presence and absence of added PLP is the EGOT index. In the non-dialyzed uremic patients, the EGOT index was greater than 2.0, indicating a large amount of unsaturated apoenzyme, a mark of vitamin B$_6$ deficiency. The EGOT index decreased, however, in the group of uremic patients undergoing dialysis. This indicates less unsaturated apoenzyme in these patients and would normally signify that the patients were not deficient. The uremic patients undergoing dialysis had been uremic much longer than the other group. Decreased EGOT indices in prolonged vitamin B$_6$ deficiency have been cited by other work-

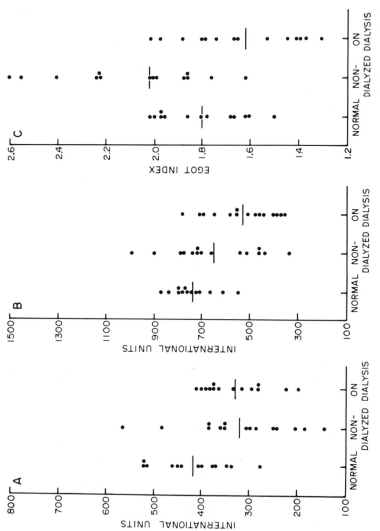

FIGURE 10-3 A, EGOT activity in normal and uremic patients. B, EGOT activity following preincubation with pyridoxal 5'-phosphate (note change in ordinate scale). C, EGOT index of normal and uremic patients.

ers (Shane and Contractor, 1975). It has been suggested that the apoenzyme portion of many PLP-requiring enzymes is less stable (more susceptible to protease action) than the holoenzyme (Kominami *et al.,* 1972). This results in a decreased EGOT index, and therefore the use of this as a sole criterion of vitamin B_6 deficiency should be viewed with caution.

A more reliable indication of vitamin B_6 status has recently been shown to be the measurement of plasma PLP by the enzymatic method of Hamfelt (1967). The validity of this method has been documented by Li and his associates (Ryan *et al.,* 1976). Application of this method to the study of the plasma PLP values in uremic patients is complicated by the fact that the plasmas of these patients contain material that affects the recovery of added PLP. Although recovery of PLP added to plasma of normal individuals is normally greater than 90 percent, the recovery of PLP added to plasma of uremic individuals averages about 69 percent. If PLP is added to the deproteinized filtrate of uremic plasma, the recovery is over 90 percent, and there is no difference between recoveries of PLP added to uremic and control plasma. The identity of this inhibitor in uremic plasma is unknown. It may be related to one of the many putative uremic toxins (Black, 1970). If it is assumed that measurement of the endogenous PLP in the plasma is inhibited to the same extent as that of the added PLP, then a correction can be made. "Normalized" values obtained in this way show a significant difference in the level of PLP between a control group and both dialyzed ($p < 0.02$) and nondialyzed ($p < 0.04$) uremics. The control group had a mean plasma PLP of 10.1 ng/ml $\pm$ 0.9 [standard error of mean (SE)] ($n = 13$), while the dialyzed uremics had values of 7.8 ng/ml $\pm$ 0.6 ($n = 13$) and the nondialyzed uremics had 7.6 ng/ml $\pm$ 0.5 ($n = 16$).

We have also measured the disposition of administered pyridoxine and PLP in both normal and uremic man. These data will be published shortly. Briefly, 50 mg of pyridoxine were administered intravenously to groups of normal and uremic subjects. Blood samples were taken at intervals and assayed for plasma PLP. Even when correction was made for decreased recovery of PLP in the uremic plasma, the formation of PLP from the administered pyridoxine by the uremic group of subjects was only one half that found in normal subjects.

Decreased levels of PLP following administration of pyridoxine could be due either to reduced synthesis of the coenzyme or to a more rapid removal of PLP from the circulation. In order to evaluate the latter possibility, 5 mg of PLP were administered intravenously to groups of uremic and control subjects. Blood samples were collected and assayed as before. The results obtained from these studies showed that injected PLP was cleared from the plasma twice as rapidly in uremic patients as in normal subjects. Pharmacokinetic analysis of the data showed that disappearance from the plasma was biexponential. Control studies in which binding of PLP to plasma proteins was measured showed no detectable difference between the two groups.

Whether vitamin B_6 status is measured by the activities of PLP transaminase in plasma or erythrocytes, by the stimulation of transaminase activity in the presence of added PLP, or by the PLP content of plasma, uremic patients appear deficient in this vitamin. In addition, PLP is cleared more rapidly from the blood of uremic patients, which may be a reflection of increased destruction of the coenzyme. A decreased recovery of PLP added to the uremic plasma is seen, also. The substances in the uremic plasma that cause the lowered recovery may be responsible, in part, for the decreased levels of transaminase in plasma and erythrocytes of these patients. Such an interference in the activity of a variety of PLP-dependent enzymes may occur in other tissues of the body and contribute to the symptoms of the uremic conditions described above.

STUDIES WITH LIVER DISEASE

The studies of Li and his associates have shown that the liver is the primary source of the plasma PLP in dogs (Lumeng *et al.*, 1974). This group has also shown that chronic alcohol abuse results in lower plasma PLP levels in man (Lumeng and Li, 1974) and that this effect is probably due to the formation of acetaldehyde as the responsible agent (Veitch *et al.*, 1975).

We were, therefore, interested in learning whether patients with liver disease might also have decreased levels of plasma PLP as a result of decreased liver function. Experiments were carried out with three groups of patients suffering from various forms of liver disease: cirrhosis, acute viral hepatitis, and extrahepatic obstruction. These data have recently been published (Mitchell *et al.*, 1976) and are included in Table 10-1. They show that baseline values of plasma PLP are significantly lower in cirrhotic patients. Those with extrahepatic obstruction also have lower PLP levels, but the differences are not significant probably because of the small numbers of patients studied.

Since baseline values represent only single determinations and may be affected by dietary intake and absorption of pyridoxine, as well as by regulation of PLP content in the plasma, a more extensive study was undertaken. In the first series of studies, 50 mg of pyridoxine was administered intravenously as a bolus to subjects and the PLP levels in

TABLE 10-1　Pharmacokinetic Characteristics of Pyridoxal 5′ Phosphate (PLP) in Normal Subjects and in Patients with Liver Disease

Parameter[a]	Normal (n = 5)	Alcoholic Cirrhosis (n = 5)	Acute Viral Hepatitis (n = 3)	Extrahepatic Obstruction[b]
$t_{\frac{1}{2}(\alpha)}$ h	1.06 ± 0.09[c]	0.48 ± 0.15[d]	0.14[e]	
			0.4	0.1
			0.15	0.5
$t_{\frac{1}{2}(\beta)}$ h	8.0　± 1.6	2.4　± 0.6[d]	0.57[e]	
			1.6	0.4
			0.8	2.3
V_1, l	4.47 ± 0.53	4.49 ± 1.05	3.2	
			2.8	3.7
			4.1	3.4
V_1, l/kg	0.06 ± 0.007	0.07 ± 0.015	0.05	
			0.06	0.08
			0.05	0.05
$V_{d(ss)}$, l	10.3　± 1.8	7.9　± 1.6	5.1	
			4.4	5.5
			6.7	4.4
$V_{d(ss)}$, l/kg	0.15 ± 0.02	0.11 ± 0.02	0.08	
			0.1	0.1
			0.08	0.06
Plasma clearance, ml/min	31.7　± 2.7	63.0　± 7.4	148.8[e]	
			54.6	200.2
			115.2	64.7
Plasma binding, %	99.5　± 0.05 (n = 5)	99.4　± 0.07 (n = 6)		
Plasma PLP	11.8　± 1.6 (n = 9)	7.1　± 1.3[d] (n = 12)	11.4 ± 1.8 (n = 6)	6.8 ± 2.1 (n = 4)

[a] $t_{\frac{1}{2}}$ is the half-life; V_1 refers to the initial volume of distribution and $V_{d(ss)}$ to volume of distribution at steady state.
[b] Extrahepatic obstruction secondary to malignant disease—diagnosis established at operation.
[c] Each value is the mean ± SE.
[d] Comparison of cirrhotic patients to normal controls, $p \leq 0.01$. All other comparisons in this column not statistically significant.
[e] Comparison of hepatitis patients to normal controls, $p \leq 0.01$. All other comparisons in this column not statistically significant. Individual values given for the hepatitis patients because of the small number of cases.

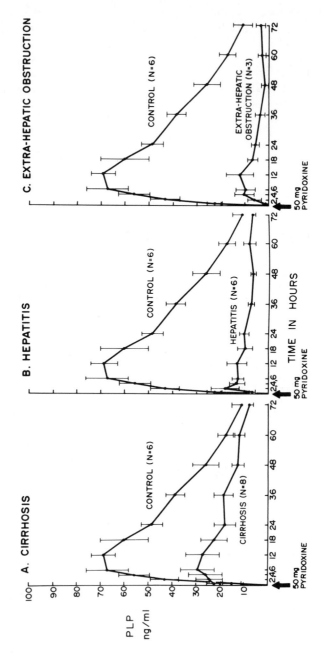

FIGURE 10-4 Plasma PLP levels following i. v. administration of 50 mg of pyridoxine to control subjects and to patients with various types of liver disease.

plasma were determined after various intervals. These results are shown in Figure 10-4. It may be seen that there is a striking decrease in the level of PLP achieved after pyridoxine administration. The patients curve (mean ± SE) was 2631 ± 260 for the normal controls and in patients with cirrhosis, acute viral hepatitis, and extrahepatic obstruction the area was 1232 ± 256, 638 ± 118, and 351 ± 144, respectively. The values obtained for the controls were significantly greater than in any liver disease group.

Because the decreased level of PLP appearing in the plasma of liver disease patients could be a result of a variety of factors, the clearance of PLP from the plasma was studied directly.

Five mg of PLP was administered intravenously and plasma samples were obtained at intervals following PLP injection. Figure 10-5 shows typical curves of PLP decay for the patients with three types of liver disease compared to the normal curve. In each case the data fit a biphasic exponential decay curve (Klotz *et al.,* 1975). In each case of liver disease the clearance of PLP from the plasma was more rapid than in normal control subjects. Various pharmacokinetic parameters have been calculated as a result of fitting the data to this biexponential model. These are presented in Table 10-1. It may be seen that clearance of PLP from the plasma is more rapid in liver disease patients than in normal subjects. The calculated parameters indicate that the more rapid clearance is a result of a decreased half-life of the PLP rather than a change in the volume of distribution of the administered coenzyme. Control experiments showed that there was no difference in binding of PLP to plasma protein between normal subjects and those with liver diseases. In contrast to the uremic patients, recoveries of PLP added to plasma of the patients with liver disease were all greater than 90 percent.

CONCLUSIONS

We believe that the data presented here are consistent with the existence of a vitamin B_6 deficiency state in both uremic patients and in patients with various forms of liver disease. This deficiency appears to result as a consequence of the particular disease and is secondary to the pathologic condition. The vitamin deficiency may therefore be thought of as a functional deficiency, since the patients were on an adequate diet and there was no evidence of malabsorption. In both conditions, uremia and liver malfunction, the decreased PLP levels appeared to be a result of increased clearance of the coenzyme from the circulation.

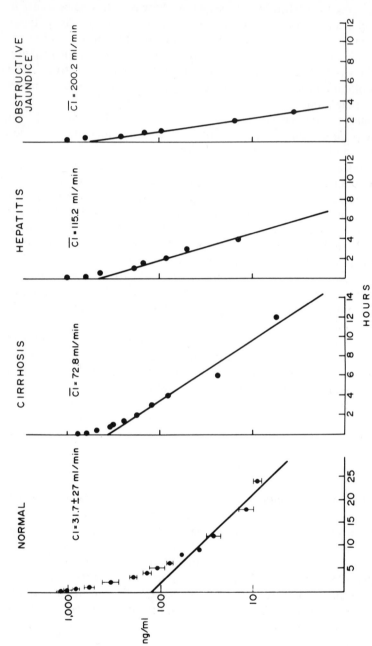

FIGURE 10-5 Plasma PLP levels following I.V. administration of 5 mg of PLP to normal control subjects and patients with various types of liver disease. Values for the normals are means of five subjects. Values plotted for the liver disease patients are typical for a single patient. The line is the $t_{1/2(\beta)}$ calculated from the biexponential model by computer analysis.

In the case of uremia, it is tempting to speculate that some of the symptoms exhibited by these patients, such as peripheral neuropathy, anemia, and depression of the immune response, may result in part from the associated vitamin B_6 deficiency. In this regard, administration of oral pyridoxine (50 mg) to uremic patients returned the plasma PLP and erythrocyte GOT values to normal levels. In a related study, Kopple *et al.* (1975) used the erythrocyte alanine aminotransferase (EGPT) measurement as an index of vitamin B_6 status in uremic patients. They found that supplementation of the diet with 5 mg of pyridoxine per day was sufficient to return the EGPT values to normal levels. It has been our experience that the addition of 50 mg of pyridoxine per day did not improve the clinical well-being nor the anemia of the patients even though the plasma PLP levels were normalized. The peripheral neuropathy and the immune responsiveness of these patients were not quantified. It is possible that symptoms of uremia such as peripheral neuropathy may be the result of a prolonged deficiency that is not easily reversible by the administration of pyridoxine over a period of a few months.

LITERATURE CITED

Babson, A. L., P. O. Shapiro, P. A. R. Williams, and G. E. Phillips. 1962. The use of a diazonium salt for the determination of glutamic oxaloacetic transaminase in serum. Clin. Chem. Acta 7:199–205.

Black, D. A. K. 1970. A perspective on uremic toxins. Arch. Int. Med. *126*:905–909.

Cohen, G. A., J. A. Goffinet, R. K. Donabedian, and H. O. Conn. 1976. Observations on decreased serum glutamic oxaloacetic transaminase (SGOT) activity in azotemic patients. Ann. Int. Med. *84*:275–280.

Dobbelstein, H., W. F. Koener, W. Mempel, H. Grosse-Wilde, and H. H. Edel. 1974. Vitamin B_6 deficiency in uremia and its implications for the depression of immune responses. Kidney Int. *5*:233–239.

Hamfelt, A. 1967. Enzymatic determination of pyridoxal phosphate in plasma by decarboxylation of L-tyrosine-¹⁴C (U) and a comparison with the tryptophan load test. Scand. J. Clin. Lab. Invest. *20*:1–10.

Karmen, A. 1955. A note on the spectrophotometric assay of glutamic oxaloacetic transaminase in human blood serum. J. Clin. Invest. *34*:131–133.

Klotz, U., G. R. Avant, A. Hoyumpa, S. Schenker, and G. T. Wilkinson. 1975. The effects of age and liver disease on the disposition and elimination of diazepam in adult man. J. Clin. Invest. *55*:347–359.

Kominami, E., K. Kobayashi, S. Kominami, and N. Kotunuma. 1972. Properties of a specific protease for pyridoxal enzymes and its biological role. J. Biol. Chem. *247*:6848–6855.

Kopple, J. D., K. C. Mercurio, R. Saltzman, B. K. Card, M. R. Jones, J. A. Tallos, and M. E. Swendseid. 1975. Vitamin B_6 requirement in uremia. *In* Abstracts of the American Society of Nephrology, November 25–26, Washington, D.C., p. 32 (Abstract).

Lumeng, L., and T.-K. Li. 1974. Vitamin B_6 metabolism in chronic alcohol abuse. Pyridoxal phosphate levels in plasma and the effect of acetaldehyde on pyridoxal phosphate synthesis and degradation in human erythrocytes. J. Clin. Invest. *53*:693–704.

Lumeng, L., R. E. Brashear, and T.-K. Li. 1974. Pyridoxal-5'-phosphate in plasma: Source, protein-binding, and cellular transport. J. Lab. Clin. Med. *84*:334–343.

Mitchell, D., C. Wagner, W. J. Stone, G. R. Wilkinson, and S. Schenker. 1976. Abnormal regulation of plasma pyridoxal 5'-phosphate in patients with liver disease. Gastroenterology *71*:1043–1049.

Ryan, M. P., L. Lumeng, and T.-K. Li. 1976. Validation of plasma pyridoxal-5'-phosphate measurements as an indicator of vitamin B_6 nutritional status. Fed. Proc. *35*:660.

Shane, B., and S. F. Contractor. 1975. Assessment of vitamin B_6 status. Studies on pregnant women and oral contraceptive users. Am. J. Clin. Nutr. *28*:739–747.

Stone, W. J., L. G. Warnock, and C. Wagner. 1975. Vitamin B_6 deficiency in uremia. Am. J. Clin. Nutr. *28*:950–957.

Veitch, R. L., L. Lumeng, and T.-K. Li. 1975. Vitamin B_6 metabolism in chronic alcohol abuse. The effect of ethanol oxidation on hepatic pyridoxal-5'-phosphate metabolism. J. Clin. Invest. *55*:1026–1032.

Warnock, L. G., W. J. Stone, and C. Wagner. 1974. Decreased aspartate aminotransferase ("SGOT") activity in serum of uremic patients. Clin. Chem. *20*:1213–1216.

11

Oral Contraceptives and Vitamin B₆

DAVID P. ROSE

The first report that women using estrogen-containing oral contraceptives exhibit an abnormality of tryptophan metabolism similar to that present in vitamin B_6 deficiency was published over 10 years ago (Rose, 1965). Despite a great deal of research effort since that time, there remains uncertainty as to whether oral contraceptives produce a true vitamin B_6 deficiency, and, if they do, whether it is of sufficient clinical importance to merit routine supplementation with pyridoxine.

The metabolic pathway by which L-tryptophan is converted to nicotinic acid ribonucleotide has been described in detail elsewhere in this monograph. In dietary vitamin B_6 deficiency an increased excretion of xanthurenic acid, 3-hydroxykynurenine, kynurenine, and, to a lesser extent, kynurenic acid occurs after an oral tryptophan load. This is considered to occur because there is a loss of activity of the pyridoxal phosphate-requiring supernatant kynureninase, whereas the mitochondrial kynurenine aminotransferase remains relatively intact (Ogasawara *et al.*, 1962; Ueda, 1967).

Although the majority of oral contraceptive users have abnormal tryptophan metabolism, the incidence is influenced by the composition

193

of the various preparations, both with respect to the dose of estrogen and the chemical nature of the progestogen (Rose *et al.,* 1973a; Leklem *et al.,* 1973). As is the case with most of the metabolic side effects of oral contraception, it is the estrogenic component that is responsible for changes in tryptophan metabolism. Thus, administration of ethinyl estradiol alone produces an identical abnormality (Rose, 1966), but the progestogen megestrol acetate is without effect (Rose and Adams, 1972). Nevertheless, there are differences in the excretion of tryptophan metabolites by women using oral contraceptives that contain an identical dose of the same estrogen but a different progestogen. These differences appear to arise because some progestogens are more efficient than others in impeding the action of estrogens on the tryptophan-nicotinic acid ribonucleotide pathway.

When the altered tryptophan metabolism of oral contraceptive users was first described, it appeared that there was a readily acceptable biochemical explanation. Mason and Gullekson (1960) had shown earlier that estrogen conjugates can inhibit pyridoxal phosphate-dependent enzymes by competing with the coenzyme for the apoprotein, and it seemed likely that the estrogenic component of the oral contraceptives, after conjugation in the liver, could inhibit hepatic kynureninase by a similar mechanism.

Further studies, however, showed that this could not be the entire explanation. It was found that, in addition to those metabolites that are formed prior to the kynureninase reaction, oral contraceptive users also excrete elevated levels of urinary 3-hydroxyanthranilic acid (Rose, 1966; Price *et al.,* 1972), quinolinic acid (Rose and Toseland, 1973), and N^1-methylnicotinamide (Rose *et al.,* 1968). These findings led to the postulate that estrogens increase the turnover of the tryptophan-nicotinic acid metabolic pathway, perhaps because they cause an elevation in circulating corticosteroids with consequent induction of tryptophan oxygenase. As a result, it was suggested that an increased amount of tryptophan enters the metabolic pathway, the yield of nicotinyl derivatives is increased, and this is reflected by an elevated urinary N^1-methylnicotinamide excretion. But, under the artificial conditions of tryptophan loading, more substrate may be presented to the partially inhibited kynureninase than can be metabolized; in consequence, intermediates that are formed proximally to this point on the metabolic sequence accumulate and appear in the urine (Rose and Braidman, 1971; Rose *et al.,* 1972).

Later, it was shown in the rat that treatment with estrogens does cause increased activity of tryptophan oxygenase, and of two other glucocorticoid-inducible enzymes, tyrosine aminotransferase and alanine aminotransferase (Braidman and Rose, 1971). In parallel with these enzymological investigations, oral contraceptives were found to affect both plasma tyrosine and alanine; indirect evidence suggests that in both instances, induction of the corresponding vitamin B_6-dependent aminotransferase is responsible (Rose and Cramp, 1970; Rose *et al.*, 1976).

Although these various observations indicated that contraceptive steroids may increase the requirement for vitamin B_6, none of them addressed the crucial question of whether a true deficiency of the vitamin can develop in women employing this form of contraception.

The first approach to this problem employed erythrocyte alanine aminotransferase assays, with and without the *in vitro* addition of pyridoxal phosphate, as an index of vitamin B_6 nutritional status. In vitamin B_6 deficiency the enzyme activity is reduced, but the stimulation obtained when pyridoxal phosphate is added to the assay medium is increased.

Doberenz *et al.* (1971) studied 13 women using oral contraceptives and 11 female controls. Although the number in each group was small, they did find that the mean basal enzyme activity was significantly lower, and the percentage of stimulation by pyridoxal phosphate greater, in the oral contraceptive-treated women.

Rose *et al.* (1973b), in a much larger study involving 80 oral contraceptive users and 50 untreated women, could detect no difference in basal alanine aminotransferase activity. As a group, the oral contraceptive users did show a higher stimulation *in vitro* of the enzyme by pyridoxal phosphate, but this indicator of vitamin B_6 deficiency was only present in 12 of the 80 women (15 percent), although most of them had abnormal tryptophan metabolism.

Salkeld *et al.* (1973) chose to use the stimulation *in vitro* of erythrocyte aspartate aminotransferase by pyridoxal phosphate as an index of vitamin B_6 deficiency. They reported a frankly abnormal degree of stimulation in 37 percent of oral contraceptive-treated women but in only 13 percent of controls. The interpretation of these results is difficult because contraceptive steroids increase the basal activity of erythrocyte aspartate aminotransferase (Aly *et al.*, 1971; Rose *et al.*, 1973b).

Plasma pyridoxal phosphate concentrations were assayed by Lumeng *et al.* (1974). They found that 20 percent of 55 women who had been taking an oral contraceptive for at least 6 months had levels of less than 5 ng/ml, the lowest value observed in 77 female controls of similar age. In a separate experiment, 10 women were studied in a prospective manner. Significant decreases in plasma pyridoxal phosphate, compared with pretreatment levels, occurred in 9 of these subjects during the first 3 months of oral contraception. But, in the majority the plasma pyridoxal phosphate concentrations increased again and were frequently back to pretreatment values by the sixth month. It appears from these results that the effect of contraceptive steroids on plasma pyridoxal phosphate is usually a temporary one and is then corrected, perhaps by a redistribution of the vitamer among the various tissue compartments. On the other hand, in a minority of women the subnormal level is maintained beyond the initial period of treatment, perhaps because other factors, for example, a low dietary intake, are operative in producing a true vitamin B_6 deficiency. Supporting evidence for this conclusion is provided by a report that after more than 6 months of oral contraceptive use, 11 of 40 (27 percent) women had low urinary 4-pyridoxic acid excretions (Rose et al., 1972). This abnormality is usually associated with a dietary deficiency of the vitamin.

Leklem and co-workers performed a dietary study of tryptophan metabolism and vitamin B_6 nutrition in groups of oral contraceptive users and matched controls. The results have been summarized in a review article (Leklem et al., 1975). This investigation was designed to compare the rates at which the two groups became depleted of vitamin B_6 when they consumed a diet providing only 0.19 mg of pyridoxine equivalents per day. Rates of repletion were then studied with different supplemental doses of pyridoxine hydrochloride (0.8 mg, 2.0 mg, and 20 mg).

A number of indices were measured, including urinary tryptophan metabolite excretions, urinary 4-pyridoxic acid, the excretion of cystathionine after a methionine load, and the plasma pyridoxal phosphate concentrations. As was expected, the oral contraceptive users had abnormal tryptophan metabolism before commencing the vitamin B_6 deficient diet. Urinary cystathionine excretion, which is abnormal in dietary vitamin B_6 deficiency (Park and Linkswiler, 1970), was unaffected by the use of oral contraceptives. During the 4-week period of low vitamin B_6 intake the excretion of tryptophan metabolites and cystathionine increased in both groups of subjects, but the rates at which the abnormalities progressed were greater in the contraceptive steroid-treated women. Plasma pyridoxal phosphate concentrations were similar in controls and oral contraceptive users before the induction of vitamin B_6 deficiency, but again, the latter showed a more rapid decline during the depletion period.

Supplementation of the deficient diet with 0.8 mg of pyridoxine hydrochloride daily reversed promptly the abnormalities of tryptophan and methionine metabolism in the control group, whereas the oral contraceptive users showed a somewhat slower, and incomplete, response. This dose of the vitamin was insufficient to restore plasma pyridoxal phosphate concentrations to normal in either group, but nevertheless, concentrations were higher in the controls.

When the dietary vitamin B_6 intake was supplemented with 2.0 mg of pyridoxine hydrochloride a day, the oral contraceptive users showed a rapid reduction in tryptophan metabolite excretions to levels below those present prior to the depletion period. They remained, however, above those of the controls. Plasma pyridoxal phosphate concentrations in the oral contraceptive users were higher after the 2.0-mg daily supplement than at the start of the study; in the controls this dose of pyridoxine was just sufficient to restore plasma pyridoxal phosphate to the predeficiency level.

Apart from abnormal tryptophan metabolism, the 15 oral contraceptive users included in this study had no evidence of vitamin B_6 deficiency before they began the depletion period. Specifically, their mean plasma pyridoxal phosphate concentration, erythrocyte aminotransferase activities, urinary 4-pyridoxic acid excretion, and cystathionine excretion after methionine loading were all similar to those of the nine controls. However, published evidence suggests that abnormalities of these direct measures of vitamin B_6 nutritional status may be expected in only 15 to 20 percent of oral contraceptive-treated women.

Thus it must be stressed that, because of the small number of subjects involved, this study in no way excludes the possibility that vitamin B_6 deficiency may develop in some women when taking an oral contraceptive. The differences between the two groups in the rates at which the various indices changed during the vitamin B_6 depletion and repletion periods were frequently small and not statistically significant. They did, however, suggest that contraceptive steroids increase the requirement for vitamin B_6.

The crucial question from a practical viewpoint is whether the biochemical abnormalities that have been described are of clinical significance; only then should supplementation of the dietary vitamin B_6 intake receive serious consideration. Thus far, attention has focused on two areas: carbohydrate tolerance and mental depression.

Impaired glucose tolerance occurs in some women taking estrogen-containing oral contraceptives. In one study 78 percent of women showed a deterioration in glucose tolerance compared with their pre-contraception test; in 13 percent the tests became frankly abnormal and were classified as indicating the presence of subclinical ("chemical") diabetes (Wynn and Doar, 1969). The significance of impaired glucose tolerance in oral contraceptive users remains to be established. Concern arises from fear that long-term exposure to contraceptive steroids may, in some women, result in exhaustion of the capacity of the pancreatic islets to secrete insulin. Should this occur, clinical diabetes mellitus would follow.

An association between altered carbohydrate metabolism and vitamin B_6 in oral contraceptive users was postulated because of the work published by Kotake and his co-workers (Kotake, 1955; Kotake et al., 1968). They found that a high tryptophan-low vitamin B_6 diet caused a diabetic state to develop in rats. A similar effect was obtained by the administration of xanthurenic acid, and the formation of a complex between this tryptophan metabolite and insulin was demonstrated, which markedly reduced insulin activity.

Spellacy et al. (1972) published a preliminary report of the effect of pyridoxine treatment in 12 women whose oral glucose tolerance had deteriorated while taking oral contraceptives. On the whole, a significant improvement in glucose tolerance was achieved by giving pyridoxine in a dose of 25 mg daily for 4 weeks.

Adams et al. (1976) studied 46 oral contraceptive users and classified them according to the presence or absence of biochemical evidence of vitamin B_6 deficiency. Glucose tolerance was improved by pyridoxine supplementation, 20 mg twice daily for 4 weeks, only in the 18 who were considered to be deficient in the vitamin.

There is a body of evidence that subnormal levels of 5-hydroxytryptamine (serotonin) in the brain are involved in the cause of mental depression. Depression has also been recognized as a complication of oral contraception; the incidence is disputed, but it probably occurs in about 6 percent of women (Herzberg et al., 1970). Three possible mechanisms may be postulated by which contraceptive steroids could reduce brain 5-hydroxytryptamine because of their known effects on tryptophan metabolism: divergence of the amino acid away from synthesis of the amine due to increased tryptophan oxygenase activity, interference with brain uptake of tryptophan by kynurenine and other metabolites of the tryptophan-nicotinic acid pathway (Green and Curzon, 1970), and vitamin B_6 deficiency with resulting loss of 5-hydroxytryptophan decarboxylase activity (Winston, 1969).

These considerations led to attempts to treat oral contraceptive-induced depression with pyridoxine. Baumblatt and Winston (1970) were the first to report success, but their study was criticized because it was uncontrolled. Adams et al. (1973, 1974), however, performed a double-blind crossover clinical trial that established the benefit of treatment with large doses of pyridoxine (20 mg twice daily) in those oral contraceptive users with biochemical evidence of vitamin B_6 deficiency.

In addition to alleviating carbohydrate intolerance and depression, some recent work suggests another beneficial effect of pyridoxine administration to oral contraceptive users: the reversal of estrogen-induced hypertriglyceridemia. One serious complication of oral contraception is the increased risk of thromboembolic disease and myocardial infarction. In other clinical situations, elevated plasma lipid levels are associated with these diseases, and hypertriglyceridemia is a recognized side effect of the oral contraceptives (Wynn *et al.*, 1969). Rose *et al.*, (1977), have found that in oral contraceptive users, but not in controls, there is a marked rise in the serum triglycerides after an oral alanine load. Treatment with pyridoxine hydrochloride, 25 mg daily for 4 weeks, not only reduced this effect but also decreased previously elevated fasting serum triglycerides in oral contraceptive-treated women. A large-scale clinical trial is now underway in an attempt to confirm this preliminary observation.

SUMMARY AND CONCLUSIONS

The majority of women taking estrogen-progestogen preparations for contraceptive purposes excrete abnormally elevated amounts of xanthurenic acid and other tryptophan metabolites after an oral load of the amino acid. This disturbance of tryptophan metabolism is similar to that seen in vitamin B$_6$ deficiency, and it is reversible by treatment with large doses of pyridoxine. Although 25 mg of pyridoxine hydrochloride, or more, may be required to prevent increased xanthurenic acid excretion after a tryptophan load, such supplementation is not necessary to maintain normal levels of metabolites derived from dietary sources of the amino acid.

Despite the frequency with which abnormal tryptophan metabolism occurs in oral contraceptive users, only 15 to 20 percent have direct biochemical evidence of vitamin B$_6$ deficiency.

The available evidence does not justify the routine supplementation of dietary vitamin B$_6$ intake with pyridoxine. In pharmacological doses, the vitamin does appear of value in the management of oral contraceptive-related mental depression and in correcting impaired glucose tolerance.

LITERATURE CITED

Adams, P. W., V. Wynn, D. P. Rose, M. Seed, J. Folkard, and R. Strong. 1973. Effect of pyridoxine hydrochloride (vitamin B$_6$) upon depression associated with oral contraception. Lancet *1*:897–904.
Adams, P. W., V. Wynn, M. Seed, and J. Folkard. 1974. Vitamin B$_6$, depression and oral contraception. Lancet *2*:516–517.

Adams, P. W., V. Wynn, J. Folkard, and M. Seed. 1976. Influence of oral contraceptives, pyridoxine (vitamin B_6), and tryptophan on carbohydrate metabolism. Lancet 1:759–764.

Aly, H. E., E. A. Donald, and M. H. W. Simpson. 1971. Oral contraceptives and vitamin B_6 metabolism. Am. J. Clin. Nutr. 24:297–303.

Baumblatt, M. J., and F. Winston. 1970. Pyridoxine and the pill. Lancet 2:832–833.

Braidman, I. P., and D. P. Rose. 1971. Effects of sex hormones on the glucocorticoid-inducible enzymes concerned with amino acid metabolism in rat liver. Endocrinology 89:1250–1255.

Doberenz, A. R., J. P. Van Miller, J. R. Green, and J. R. Beaton. 1971. Vitamin B_6 depletion in women using oral contraceptives as determined by erythrocyte glutamic-pyruvic transaminase activities. Proc. Soc. Exp. Biol. Med. 137:1100–1103.

Green, A. R., and G. Curzon. 1970. The effect of tryptophan metabolites on brain 5-hydroxytryptamine metabolism. Biochem. Pharmacol. 19:2061–2068.

Herzberg, B. N., A. L. Johnson, and S. Brown. 1970. Depressive symptoms and oral contraceptives. Br. Med. J. 4:142–145.

Kotake, Y. 1955. Xanthurenic acid, an abnormal metabolite of tryptophan and the diabetic symptoms caused in albino rats by its production. J. Biochem. (Tokyo) 2:157–171.

Kotake, Y., T. Sotokawa, E. Murakami, A. Hisatake, M. Abe, and Y. Ikeda. 1968. Studies on the xanthurenic acid-insulin complex. II. Physiological activities. J. Biochem. (Tokyo) 63:578–581.

Leklem, J. E., D. P. Rose, and R. R. Brown. 1973. Effect of oral contraceptives on urinary metabolite excretions after administration of L-tryptophan or L-kynurenine sulfate. Metabolism 22:1499–1505.

Leklem, J. E., R. R. Brown, D. P. Rose, and H. M. Linkswiler. 1975. Vitamin B_6 requirements of women using oral contraceptives. Am. J. Clin. Nutr. 28:535–541.

Lumeng, L., R. E. Cleary, and T.-K. Li. 1974. Effect of oral contraceptives on the plasma concentration of pyridoxal phosphate. Am. J. Clin. Nutr. 27:326–333.

Mason, M., and E. Gullekson. 1960. Estrogen-enzyme interactions: Inhibition and protection of kynurenine transaminase by the sulfate esters of diethylstilbestrol, estradiol, and estrone. J. Biol. Chem. 235:1312–1316.

Ogasawara, N., Y. Hagino, and Y. Kotake. 1962. Kynurenine transaminase, kynureninase and the increase of xanthurenic acid excretion. J. Biochem. (Tokyo) 52:162–166.

Park, Y. K., and H. Linkswiler. 1970. Effect of vitamin B_6 depletion in adult men on the excretion of cystathionine and other methionine metabolites. J. Nutr. 100:110–116.

Price, S. A., D. P. Rose, and P. A. Toseland. 1972. Effects of dietary vitamin B_6 deficiency and oral contraceptives on the spontaneous urinary excretion of 3-hydroxyanthranilic acid. Am. J. Clin. Nutr. 25:494–498.

Rose, D. P. 1965. Cited in Report of a conference on tryptophan metabolism in relation to cancer research. Br. Med. J. 1:1432.

Rose, D. P. 1966. The influence of oestrogens upon tryptophan metabolism in man. Clin. Sci. 31:265–272.

Rose, D. P., and P. W. Adams. 1972. Oral contraceptives and tryptophan metabolism: Effects of oestrogen in low dose combined with a progestogen and of a low-dose progestogen (megestrol acetate) given alone. J. Clin. Path. 25:252–258.

Rose, D. P., and I. P. Braidman. 1971. Excretion of tryptophan metabolites as affected by pregnancy, contraceptive steroids, and steroid hormones. Am. J. Clin. Nutr. 24:673–683.

Rose, D. P., and D. G. Cramp. 1970. Reduction of plasma tyrosine by oral contraceptives and oestrogens: A possible consequence of tyrosine aminotransferase induction. Clin. Chim. Acta 29:49–53.

Rose, D. P., and P. A. Toseland. 1973. Urinary excretion of quinolinic acid and other tryptophan metabolites after deoxypyridoxine or oral contraceptive administration. Metabolism 22:165–171.

Rose, D. P., and J. E. Leklem, R. R. Brown, and C. Potera. 1976. Effect of oral contraceptives and vitamin B₆ supplements on alanine and glycine metabolism. Am. J. Clin. Nutr. 29:956–960.

Rose, D. P., J. E. Leklem, L. Fardal, R. B. Baron, and E. Shrago. 1977. Effect of oral alanine loads on the serum triglycerides of oral contraceptive users and normal subjects. Am. J. Clin. Nutr. 30:691–694.

Rose, D. P., R. R. Brown, and J. M. Price. 1968. Metabolism of tryptophan to nicotinic acid derivatives by women taking oestrogen-progestogen preparations. Nature (London) 291:1259–1260.

Rose, D. P., R. Strong, P. W. Adams, and P. E. Harding. 1972. Experimental vitamin B₆ deficiency and the effect of oestrogen-containing oral contraceptives on tryptophan metabolism and vitamin B₆ requirements. Clin. Sci. 42:465–477.

Rose, D. P., P. W. Adams, and R. Strong. 1973a. Influence of the progestogenic component of oral contraceptives on tryptophan metabolism. Br. J. Obstet. Gynecol. 80:82–85.

Rose, D. P., R. Strong, J. Folkard, and P. W. Adams. 1973b. Erythrocyte aminotransferase activities in women using oral contraceptives and the effect of vitamin B₆ supplementation. Am. J. Clin. Nutr. 26:48–52.

Salkeld, R. M., K. Knorr, and W. F. Korner. 1973. The effect of oral contraceptives on vitamin B₆ status. Clin. Chim. Acta 49:195–199.

Spellacy, W. N., W. C. Buhi, and S. A. Birk. 1972. The effects of vitamin B₆ on carbohydrate metabolism in women taking steroid contraceptives: Preliminary report. Contraception 6:265–273.

Ueda, T. 1967. Studies on the intracellular change of vitamin B₆ content and kynurenine aminotransferase activity in the vitamin B₆ deficient rat. Nagoya J. Med. Sci. 30:259–268.

Winston, F. 1969. Oral contraceptives and depression. Lancet 2:377.

Wynn, V., and J. W. H. Doar. 1969. Longitudinal studies of the effects of oral contraceptive therapy on plasma glucose, non-esterified fatty acid, insulin and blood pyruvate levels during oral and intravenous tolerance tests. In H. A. Salhanick, D. M. Kipnis, and R. L. Vande Wiele (eds.), Metabolic Effects of Gonadal Hormones and Contraceptive Steroids. Plenum Press, New York, pp. 157–177.

Wynn, V., J. W. H. Doar, G. L. Mills, and T. Stokes. 1969. Fasting serum triglyceride, cholesterol, and lipoprotein levels during oral-contraceptive therapy. Lancet 2:756–760.

12

Vitamin B$_6$ and Pregnancy

WALTER B. DEMPSEY

The current recommended dietary allowance of vitamin B$_6$ for pregnant women was set at 2.5 mg/day (Food and Nutrition Board, 1974). It seems appropriate to consider evidence for and against the adequacy of this recommendation in view of recent data.

Pyridoxine deficiency in pregnancy has been suspected since 1942 (Willis *et al.*, 1942). This has been based on the following observations:

(1) Pregnant women have significantly lower plasma PLP levels than nonpregnant women (Brin, 1971; Brophy and Siiteri, 1975; Cleary *et al.*, 1975; Hamfelt and Tuvemo, 1972; Shane and Contractor, 1975; Wachstein *et al.*, 1960) and exhibit abnormal response to the tryptophan load test.

(2) Supplementation at a level of 2.5 mg/day of pyridoxine or at 4 mg/day of pyridoxine does not bring the plasma value for PLP in the average pregnant woman to the levels seen in nonpregnant women, nor does 2.5 mg/day return the tryptophan load test to normal. It does, however, restore serum aminotransferases to activities found in non-pregnant women (Cleary *et al.*, 1975; Lumeng *et al.*, 1976).

(3) Supplementation at 10 mg/day brings both plasma PLP level and

202

tryptophan load test close to those values found in nonpregnant women (Cleary *et al.*, 1975; Lumeng *et al.*, 1976).

Many specific investigations in this area have been made by several laboratories over the last 10 years. Among recent reports, Shane and Contractor show the mean value of blood PLP for 12 nonpregnant women as 9.63 ± 1.67 ng/ml and the value for 10 third trimester pregnant women as 5.06 ± 1.32 ng/ml (Shane and Contractor, 1975). Cleary *et al.* (1975) report normal values for 58 nonpregnant women as 10.5 ± 4.1 ng/ml and for 13 pregnant women receiving 2–2.5 mg/day of pyridoxine as 3.7 ± 1.5 ng/ml. Eleven other pregnant women receiving 10 mg pyridoxine per day had mean plasma values of 7.5 ± 4.5 ng/ml. At least four other groups have reported similar differences. These and other data are summarized in Table 12-1. The table shows clearly that blood PLP values are lower in pregnant women than in nonpregnant women. Neither the recommended allowance of 2.5 mg of vitamin B_6 nor supplementation at 4 mg/day is adequate to raise blood levels of PLP in pregnant women to those found in nonpregnant women (Cleary *et al.*, 1975).

It is worth considering whether vitamin B_6 supplementation of pregnant women should be given in sufficient amounts to return their average blood PLP values to those of nonpregnant women. Instead, should such supplementation be given only to bring blood values up to those found in average pregnant women? Basically, there are insufficient data to support either position. It seems possible that these phenomena observed with regard to vitamin B_6 nutritional status are normal physiological phenomena not requiring a maximum response. In fact, it seems reasonable to relate values obtained from individual pregnant

TABLE 12-1   Average Plasma PLP Concentration in Nonpregnant and Pregnant Women, ng/ml

Nonpregnant		Pregnant	
No. of Samples	Value	No. of Samples	Value
19	8.4 ± 2.5	19	4.3^a
		20	3.09 ± 0.324^a
		20	2.43^a
9	11.7 ± 3.2		
77	9.4 ± 4.2		
12	9.63 ± 1.67	10	5.06 ± 1.32
58	10.5 ± 4.1	13	3.7 ± 1.5^b
4	16.9	9	4.3

[a]Mothers at term.
[b]This group was receiving 2–2.5 mg/day pyridoxine.

females to those observed in populations of pregnant females rather than to norms for nonpregnant women.

The problem can perhaps be stated a little more clearly as follows: (1) Although blood PLP levels definitely decrease in pregnant women, there are limited data to support the hypothesis that these observations reflect a real clinical insufficiency of vitamin B_6. (2) There are no data to show that pregnant humans would profit by having all the parameters used for measuring vitamin B_6 nutrition, including the tryptophan load test, restored to the nonpregnant levels by pyridoxine supplementation. Indeed it is clearly impossible to establish normality by supplementation, because supplementation sufficient to raise the tryptophan load test to normal would raise blood PLP levels to unusually high values. The question then arises as to whether supplementation should be provided in amounts adequate to return vitamin B_6 status to levels of normal nonpregnant women or to those of normal pregnant women. Some insight can be gained from investigations in three related areas. From studies with women on oral contraceptives who received 2.0 mg/day of pyridoxine, all parameters used for measuring vitamin B_6 nutrition are normal except the tryptophan load test (Leklem et al., 1975). From studies with pregnant rats, high levels of vitamin B_6 apparently are not harmful (Khera, 1975). Most important, studies with preeclamptic women indicate that levels of blood PLP are close to the lowest acceptable level observed in normal pregnant women (Brophy and Siiteri, 1975).

Recent studies on plasma PLP levels in users of oral contraceptives are contradictory. Shane and Contractor (1975) reported that blood PLP levels were significantly lower for contraceptive users than for nonusers. Their values were 7.6 ± 1.1 ng/ml for the former versus 9.6 ± 1.7 ng/ml for the latter. Other workers report no significant differences for the two groups (Haspels et al., 1975).

A rather comprehensive analysis of vitamin B_6 nutrition in a group of women was published last year by D. P. Rose and his co-workers (Brown et al., 1975; Leklem et al., 1975). They first depleted of pyridoxine 15 oral contraceptive users and nine nonusers and then compared the rapidity and extent to which the blood PLP levels were restored to normal values on 0.8 mg/day of pyridoxine and on 2.0 mg/day of pyridoxine. Both groups reached normal levels in a few days on 2.0 mg/day pyridoxine but not on 0.8 mg/day.

The contraceptive users, however, had noticeably altered tryptophan metabolism, which was not restored to normal at 2.0 mg/day supplementation. At 20 mg/day, tryptophan metabolism was normal.

Studies with users of oral contraceptives indicate that the tryptophan load test is the only vitamin B_6 related function that consistently appears to be seriously lowered by estrogen therapy. The ease with which this metabolic alteration develops suggests that it is a normal response that does not need correction rather than an abnormality that must be forced into normal range by massive doses of the vitamin.

A second set of observations bears on the problem of vitamin B_6 nutrition, although not so directly as those quoted above. Khera (1975) reported no evidence of maternal toxicity or an increased number of dead or resorbed fetuses in rats fed 20 mg of pyridoxine per kilogram of body weight from the sixth to the fifteenth day of pregnancy.

Other studies with rats showed that the vitamin B_6 levels in fetal brains responded directly to the amount in the maternal diet (Lumeng *et al.*, 1976). These results and the results reported previously at this meeting (see Bauernfeind and Miller) suggest that a small increase in the recommended intake of vitamin B_6 for pregnant women is unlikely to be harmful.

Finally, data from preeclamptic patients provide some guidance as to whether the apparently low blood PLP values in pregnancy are significant. Preeclampsia or toxemia of pregnancy is a hypertensive disorder of pregnancy that is usually found only in very young primagravidas. In addition to hypertension, it is characterized by proteinuria and edema. In severe cases, oliguria and cerebral or visual disturbances are seen. A number of reports have suggested that pyridoxine insufficiency is related to this disease, but a cause-effect relationship has not been established.

Several measurements have been made of enzyme and metabolite concentrations in preeclamptic placentae and clearly abnormal values obtained for some components. This should not be construed as evidence that the placenta is necessarily the cause of the problem. A number of cases would, in fact, point away from the placenta *per se* as the cause of preeclampsia. Among these are cases in which preeclamptic symptoms were removed by amniocentesis and cases in which preeclampsia developed a week or so after fetal death (Sophian, 1972).

Preeclamptic placentae have higher than normal amounts of 5-hydroxytryptamine (Sophian, 1972), one-third normal cholineacetyltransferase (Harbison *et al.*, 1975), and levels of both pyridoxine vitamers and pyridoxal kinase that are 40 percent those of normal (Klieger *et al.*, 1969). We have examined the pyridoxine phosphate oxidase content of normal and preeclamptic placentae and found this enzyme also to be lower than in nonpreeclamptic placentae (Gaynor and Dempsey, 1972). Several individuals had barely detectable amounts of the enzyme (Figure 12-1).

206

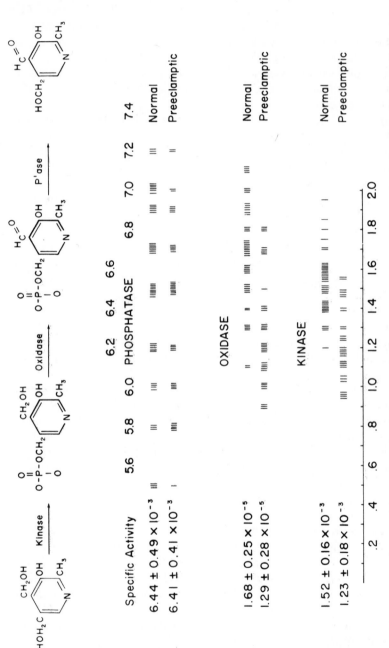

FIGURE 12-1 Values of specific activities for three enzymes of vitamin B₆ metabolism in normal and preeclamptic placentae. The numbers are specific activities in units of μM/min/mg of protein. Small vertical bars represent values for individual placentae. Methodology and mean values from Gaynor and Dempsey (1972).

The blood PLP values in preeclamptic mothers and the cord blood PLP values of their newborns have only recently been measured for the first time. Brophy and Siiteri (1975) reported the average blood PLP was 4.3 ng/ml in nonpreeclamptic women and 3.3 ng/ml in preeclamptic ones. Although these differences were not significant, the differences in the cord blood values were. These values were 28.4 ng/ml for normal newborns and 12.2 for preeclamptic newborns. Slightly higher values for normal cord blood have been recently reported by Lumeng *et al.* (1976).

Contradictory reports of the efficacy of pyridoxine therapy to preeclamptics have appeared (Hillman *et al.*, 1963; Wachstein and Graffeo, 1956). To the present time, data in this area remain, at best, inconclusive. The finding that cord blood values are halved in preeclamptics, however, seems to argue that vitamin B₆ therapy is indicated at least to an extent sufficient to raise the level to normal cord blood values.

In view of the reduction in pyridoxine phosphate oxidase in toxemic placentae and the high concentration of pyridoxine phosphate, supplementation with pyridoxal instead of pyridoxine is indicated. The aldehyde form would bypass the need for the oxidase and might be much more efficient at relieving the apparent deficiency of pyridoxine.

Available evidence demonstrates unequivocally that blood PLP values are significantly lower in pregnant women than in nonpregnant women. Moreover, blood PLP levels are, in general, even lower in preeclamptic women than in normal pregnant women. Even without rigorous proof, it seems probable that preeclampsia is, in part at least, related to low blood PLP values and that the range of blood PLP values observed in preeclamptic women represents the lower levels of acceptability.

To expand the above, one can interpret the facts two ways: (1) The levels found in pregnant women are normal for pregnancy. (2) The levels found in pregnant women are low and abnormal. Unfortunately, there are no conclusive data which clearly point to the proper interpretation, but there are arguments that suggest that the second of the two interpretations is more likely the correct one.

The strongest argument that can be made in favor of the interpretation that the observed low blood PLP values should be considered normal is an evolutionary one. This argument says that man has evolved successfully for millions of years without vitamin B₆ supplementation during pregnancy. In fact, every human conceived before 1934 was conceived before vitamin B₆ was discovered and consequently underwent embryogenesis without vitamin B₆ supplementation. Our experience tells us that these people are normal regardless of vitamin B₆. This evolutionary argument cannot be dismissed easily. It can be reconciled, however, if dietary conditions today are significantly different than those of earlier days because the protein composition of the diet has a major effect upon vitamin B_6 requirements. If we eat more meat and fish today, then our vitamin B_6 needs will change.

Increased dietary protein increases the vitamin B_6 requirement presumably because the amino acid catabolic pathways induced by the dietary protein almost all contain at least one PLP-requiring enzyme. This increase in the number of enzymes requiring PLP raises the number of molecules of PLP required for normal metabolism in the individual. Thus, the minimum daily requirement for pyridoxine varies with the protein content of the diet.

It can be argued that blood PLP levels in pregnant women on diets much less rich in protein than the average American diet but of the same average vitamin B_6 content would be higher than that of modern American women. Indeed, a diet high in cereals and low in animal protein should easily provide adequate vitamin B_6.

SUMMARY

The present recommended vitamin B_6 allowance for pregnant women appears to be inadequate. The allowance should be sufficient to raise the blood PLP concentration to values at least equal to low, normal nonpregnant levels. The limited information available suggests that the vitamin B_6 intake during pregnancy should be between 4 and 10 mg/ day. Further research may establish more precisely the vitamin B_6 need during pregnancy.

ACKNOWLEDGMENTS

The work reported was supported by the U.S. Veterans Administration and by U.S. Public Health Service Grant AM 14157.

LITERATURE CITED

Brin, M. 1971. Abnormal tryptophan metabolism in pregnancy and with the oral contraceptive pill. II. Relative levels of vitamin B_6-vitamers in cord and maternal blood. Am. J. Clin. Nutr. *24*:704–708.

Brophy, M. H., and P. K. Siiteri. 1975. Pyridoxal phosphate and hypertensive disorders of pregnancy. Am. J. Obstet. Gynecol. *121*:1075–1079.

Brown, R. R., D. P. Rose, J. E. Leklem, H. Linkswiler, and R. Anand. 1975. Urinary 4-pyridoxic acid, plasma pyridoxal phosphate, and erythrocyte aminotransferase levels in oral contraceptive users receiving controlled intakes of vitamin B_6. Am. J. Clin. Nutr. *28*:10–19.

Cleary, R. E., L. Lumeng, and T.-K. Li. 1975. Maternal and fetal plasma levels of pyridoxal phosphate at term: Adequacy of vitamin B_6 supplementation during pregnancy. Am. J. Obstet. Gynecol. *121*:25–28.

Food and Nutrition Board. 1974. Recommended Dietary Allowances, 8th ed. National Academy of Sciences, Washington, D.C., 129 pp.

Gaynor, R., and W. B. Dempsey. 1972. Vitamin B_6 enzymes in normal and preeclamptic human placentae. Clin. Chim. Acta *37*:411–416.

Hamfelt, A., and T. Tuvemo. 1972. Pyridoxal phosphate and folic acid concentration in blood and erythrocyte aspartate aminotransferase activity during pregnancy. Clin. Chim. Acta *41*:287–298.

Harbison, R. D., J. Olubadewo, C. Divivedi, and B. V. Rama Sastry. 1975. *In* P. L. Morselli, S. Garattini, and F. Serini (eds.), Basic and Therapeutic Aspects of Perinatal Pharmacology, Raven Press, New York, p. 107.

Haspels, A. A., H. J. T. Coelingh Bennik, P. A. Van Keep, and W. H. P. Schreurs. 1975. Estrogens and vitamin B_6. Front. Horm. Res. *3*:199–207.

Hillman, R. W., P. B. Cabaud, D. E. Nilsson, P. D. Arpin, and R. J. Tufano. 1963. Pyridoxine supplementation during pregnancy. Clinical and laboratory observations. Am. J. Clin. Nutr. *12*:427–430.

Khera, K. S. 1975. Teratogenicity study in rats given high doses of pyridoxine during organogenesis. Experientia *31*:469–470.

Klieger, J. A., C. H. Altshuler, G. Krakow, and C. Hollister. 1969. Abnormal pyridoxine metabolism in toxemia of pregnancy. Ann. N.Y. Acad. Sci. *166*:288–296.

Leklem, J. E., R. R. Brown, D. P. Rose, and H. M. Linkswiler. 1975. Vitamin B_6 requirements of women using oral contraceptives. Am. J. Clin. Nutr. *28*:535–541.

Lumeng, L., R. E. Cleary, and T.-K. Li. 1974. Effect of oral contraceptives on the plasma concentration of pyridoxal phosphate. Am. J. Clin. Nutr. *27*:326–333.

Lumeng, L., R. E. Cleary, R. Wagner, P.-L. Yu, and T.-K. Li. 1976. Adequacy of vitamin B_6 supplementation during pregnancy: A prospective study. Am. J. Clin. Nutr. *29*:1376–1383.

Shane, B., and S. F. Contractor. 1975. Assessment of vitamin B_6 status. Studies on pregnant women and oral contraceptive users. Am. J. Clin. Nutr. *28*:739–747.

Sophian, J. 1972. Pregnancy Nephropathy, Vol. I. Appleton-Century-Crofts, New York, p. 82.

Wachstein, M., and L. Graffeo. 1956. The influence of vitamin B_6 on the incidence of preeclampsia. Obstet. Gynecol. *8*:177–180.

Wachstein, M., J. D. Kellner, and J. M. Ortiz. 1960. Pyridoxal phosphate in plasma and leukocytes of normal and pregnant subjects following B_6 load tests. Proc. Soc. Exp. Biol. Med. *103*:350–353.

Willis, R. S., W. W. Winn, A. T. Morris, A. A. Newsom, and W. E. Massey. 1942. Clinical observations in treatment of nausea and vomiting in pregnancy with vitamins B_1 and B_6. Am. J. Obstet. Gynecol. *44*:265–271.

13

Factors Influencing Vitamin B_6 Requirement in Alcoholism

TING-KAI LI

Alcoholism is a disease characterized by a pathological dependency on alcohol, the result of which is the impairment of health and social functioning (Criteria Committee, National Council on Alcoholism, 1972). It is estimated that 8–9 million Americans abuse alcohol and that the consequent economic loss to the country exceeds 8 billion dollars annually. The medical consequences of alcoholism have been recently reviewed (Seixas *et al.*, 1975).

It is well known that alcoholic beverages are a good source of calories. The oxidation of 1 g of ethanol to CO_2 and H_2O yields 7 kcal. Hence alcoholic beverages, when taken in excessive amounts, can contribute substantially to total energy intake and impair nutritional balance. As an example, 1 pint of whiskey or its equivalent provides approximately 1,400 kcal. This amount, or 10 standard-sized drinks, is not infrequently consumed during the course of 12 h by many individuals without obvious manifestations of intoxication. Let us assume that the dietary intake of a subject to stay in caloric balance is 2,400 kcal, divided into 48 percent carbohydrates, 40 percent fats, and 12 percent protein. If this subject does not alter his eating habits, an unusual circumstance, he would be consuming 3,800 kcal, and rapid weight gain

210

would ensue. If, on the other hand, he desires to remain in energy balance, food intake must be reduced by at least 50 percent. As a result, a curtailment in amount and a severe imbalance in the proportion of normal dietary nutrients would be produced. In practice, probably a situation between these two extremes prevails in the majority of instances, and the typical alcoholic, more often than not, ingests an inadequate diet. Over a prolonged period of time, a variety of nutritional deficiences can develop·on this basis alone, i.e., inadequate intake.

The deficiency diseases most commonly encountered in chronic alcoholism are those of protein; the water soluble vitamins, thiamin, niacin, riboflavin, pyridoxine, and folic acid; and the minerals, magnesium, potassium, and zinc. In the case of vitamin B_6, two factors would facilitate the early development of a primary deficiency state. One is that alcoholic beverages, i.e., all the distilled spirits, beer, and most wines, contain immeasurably small amounts of vitamin B_6 (Leevy *et al.*, 1965). The other is that recent dietary record analyses indicate that a high percentage of Americans actually ingest less vitamin B_6 than the 1974 recommended dietary allowance (Driskell *et al.*, 1976). Moreover, chronic alcohol abuse also produces impairment or alteration in the metabolism of vitamin B_6 (*vide infra*), thus leading to an increased requirement. In the face of an already marginal intake, these conditioning factors can become crucial determinants.

APPROACHES TO THE EVALUATION OF VITAMIN B_6 NUTRITION IN CHRONIC ALCOHOLISM

It is unfortunate that in the clinical evaluation of vitamin B_6 deficiency, the findings tend to be rather nonspecific and to occur only when the deficiency is already severe. In infants, vitamin B_6 deficiency produces convulsions. In the adult, the most specific clinical manifestation is probably the sideroblastic abnormality of bone marrow, reversed by vitamin B_6 administration (Hines and Grasso, 1970). The incidence of this finding in populations of chronic alcoholics has been estimated to be 20 to 30 percent. However, even the development of this abnormality is probably the end result of multiple contributing factors (Horrigan and Harris, 1968; Hines and Cowan, 1970; Eichner and Hillman, 1971; Pierce *et al.*, 1976). Therefore, the clinical evaluation of vitamin B_6 deficiency in the alcoholic is imprecise and insensitive. More accurate assessment must rely either on the determination of the functional integrity of vitamin B_6-dependent pathways or the measurement of the content of the vitamin in tissues and body fluids.

One of the first attempts to determine the prevalence of vitamin B_6 deficiency or undernutrition in alcoholics by specific testing was the examination of the tryptophan metabolic pathway. Initially, it was reported that a significant percentage of alcoholics exhibited increased xanthurenic acid excretion after tryptophan administration (Lerner et al., 1958). However, this observation could not be consistently confirmed. More often than not, it was found that chronic alcoholics exhibited decreased excretion of xanthurenic acid, kynurenine, and 3-hydroxy-kynurenine after tryptophan loading and not increased excretion (Walsh et al., 1966). The basis for this variation has not been elucidated, but two factors may have been contributory. One is that the patients studied may have had variable amounts of liver disease. The other is that alcoholics may have an increased requirement for nicotinamide and hence increased nicotinic acid synthesis (Gabuzda and Davidson, 1962).

Because of these uncertainties, which affect the tryptophan metabolic pathway, more recent studies have employed the measurement of the concentration of vitamin B_6 compounds in blood plasma as a more reliable indicator. The predominant form of the vitamin B_6 compounds in plasma is pyridoxal phosphate (PLP). It is derived almost entirely from hepatic synthesis and behaves as a relatively stable, albeit small, circulating storage pool of the vitamin B_6 compounds in the body (Lumeng et al., 1974). It is firmly bound to albumin, and its concentration correlates with a high degree of certainty with the intake of vitamin B_6 in animals (Ryan et al., 1976) and in man (Lumeng et al., 1974; Brown et al., 1975).

Figure 13-1 shows the results of a recent study in which weanling rats were fed diets containing 0–100 μg of pyridoxine daily for 9 weeks. Growth curve analysis indicated that 12–24 μg/day is an optimal intake for these animals. Plasma PLP content increased as a function of the dietary intake of vitamin B_6 over the entire range examined. In tissues, PLP, and, to a lesser extent, pyridoxamine phosphate (PMP), are the stable storage forms of the vitamin. Skeletal muscle, by virtue of its total mass, is by far the largest tissue storage depot of this vitamin. As is apparent, plasma PLP concentration exhibited a very high degree of correlation with muscle PLP content. On the other hand, the PLP content of brain and of liver had already reached saturating levels at relatively low levels of pyridoxine intake, 4 and 12 μg/day, respectively (Ryan et al., 1976). These results demonstrate that the measurement of plasma PLP is a reliable and sensitive indicator of the state of vitamin B_6 nutrition, since its concentration reflects not only the degree of undernutrition but also of storage. The postulated interrelationship of PLP in

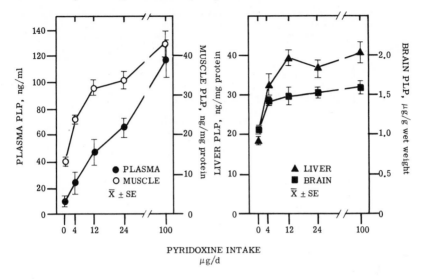

FIGURE 13-1 The PLP content of plasma, muscle, liver, and brain from rats fed varying amounts of vitamin B₆.

plasma to that in other tissues and organs and the role of protein binding in the body economy of this coenzyme (*vide infra*) is depicted in Figure 13-2.

PREVALENCE OF VITAMIN B₆ UNDERNUTRITION IN CHRONIC ALCOHOLISM

The problem of vitamin B₆ deficiency in alcoholics has been studied by measurement of blood concentrations of the vitamin (Baker *et al.*, 1964; Leevy *et al.*, 1965). They studied 172 hospitalized alcoholics and measured the circulating concentration of a number of vitamins and correlated the incidence of hypovitaminemia with the degree of liver disease. It was found that an abnormality in circulating folic acid was the most prevalent, followed by vitamin B₆ and then thiamin. For these studies, the total vitamin B₆ content of serum was measured by means of the protozoan assay. The incidence of decreased serum vitamin B₆ concentration was almost 40 percent in patients with alcoholic cirrhosis, 30 percent in those with fatty liver, and about 20 percent in those with normal liver histology.

Since that time, a number of studies have firmly established that a high percentage of chronic alcoholics, whether with or without hepatic disease, exhibits abnormally lowered plasma PLP levels (Pierce *et al.*,

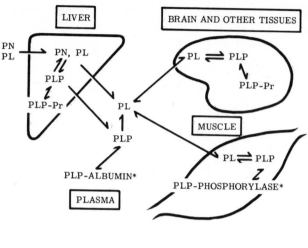

*storage

FIGURE 13-2   Postulated interrelationships of the vitamin B₆ compounds in various body compartments. Binding of PLP and PMP by proteins (Pr) protects the coenzyme against hydrolysis. The principal PLP-binding protein in plasma is albumin (Lumeng et al., 1974), and in muscle, it is glycogen phosphorylase. Phosphorylase, alanine aminotransferase, and aspartate aminotransferase are major PLP-binding proteins in liver (Veitch et al., 1976).

1976; Walsh et al., 1966; Hines and Love, 1969; Lumeng and Li, 1974; Davis and Smith, 1974; Mitchell et al., 1976). Figure 13-3 shows the results of one of these studies designed specifically to examine the incidence of vitamin B₆ abnormality in acknowledged alcoholics who were free of liver disease (Lumeng and Li, 1974). The plasma PLP content of 66 alcoholic subjects and 94 control subjects was measured by the tyrosine apodecarboxylase method. As shown by the regression lines, the mean plasma PLP concentration of the alcoholic population was significantly lower than that of the control group. This relationship held true for all the age groups examined, even though plasma PLP concentrations in healthy individuals normally show a decline with age. Plasma PLP values below 5 ng/ml, the lower limit of normal, were found in 35 of the 66 alcoholic subjects. Thus, depending on the population surveyed, the incidence of abnormally lowered plasma PLP levels in alcoholic subjects may be as high as 50 percent, even when they are devoid of liver disease. This finding has since been confirmed by Davis and Smith (1974) in a similar study. However, in agreement with the studies of Leevy et al. (1965), these investigators, as well as Hines and

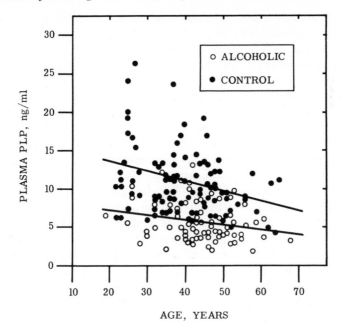

FIGURE 13-3   Plasma PLP concentration of alcoholic and nonalcoholic men, plotted as a function of age. The upper line is the regression line of the control group, and the lower, of the alcoholic group.

Love (1969), have shown that the incidence of reduced plasma PLP levels in alcoholics with liver disease is higher and may be as high as 80–100 percent.

Because decreased serum PLP levels tend to occur more frequently in the setting of prolonged and severe alcohol abuse and to correlate with other manifestations of malnutrition, it is probable that inadequate dietary intake of vitamin B$_6$ is a major cause of this abnormality. However, there is now good evidence that the process of alcohol oxidation, and also liver disease, can profoundly alter the metabolism of vitamin B$_6$ and PLP and thus contribute to the development of a deficiency state. The mechanism by which alcohol produces this abnormality has been elucidated and is described in the following section.

DERANGEMENT OF VITAMIN B$_6$ METABOLISM WITH ETHANOL OXIDATION

Hines and Cowan (1970) observed during their investigation of the pathogenesis of the anemia of alcoholism that the conversion of intravenously administered pyridoxine to PLP in the plasma is impaired in heavily drinking alcoholic subjects. Although the effect of liver disease was not ruled out in that study, the findings suggested that alcohol itself or its oxidation products may interfere directly with the metabolism of vitamin B_6.

To study this phenomenon, we began investigations first with human red blood cells (Lumeng and Li, 1974). Erythrocytes possess the full complement of enzymes for the synthesis of PLP as well as for its degradation, and hence the entire metabolic cycle can be studied. Moreover, because erythrocytes do not metabolize ethanol, the effects of ethanol and its oxidation product, acetaldehyde, can be examined separately. As is shown in Figure 13-4, the incubation of intact erythrocytes with pyridoxine (PN) resulted in the accumulation of substantial quantities of PLP. The time course was nonlinear, because concurrent with synthesis, there was also degradation of PLP, catalyzed by a membrane-bound phosphatase. Ethanol, in concentrations as high as 70 mM, was found not to affect the net formation of PLP at all. However, acetaldehyde, in concentrations as low as 0.05 mM, significantly lowered the accumulation of PLP in the erythrocyte. Similar results

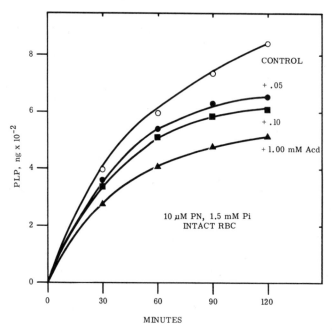

FIGURE 13-4   The effect of acetaldehyde (Acd) on the net synthesis of PLP from pyridoxine (PN) by human erythrocytes.

were obtained when pyridoxal (PL) or pyridoxine phosphate (PNP) served as the substrate.

The effect of acetaldehyde can be due to either inhibition of PLP synthesis or accelerated degradation. In order to separate these events, the experiment was repeated with hemolyzed erythrocytes. Because the phosphatase that hydrolyzes PLP is bound to the erythrocyte cell membrane, it can be removed by centrifugation. PLP synthesis can then be examined in the hemolysate supernatant, unhampered by degradation. However, it was found that the synthesis of PLP from PL, PN, and PNP was not affected by acetaldehyde. The same phenomenon was observed also with intact cells, when the phosphatase activity was inhibited by 80 mM phosphate (Lumeng and Li, 1974). Hence, acetaldehyde does not inhibit PLP synthesis.

We, therefore, arrived at the hypothesis that acetaldehyde mediates the derangement in vitamin B₆ metabolism associated with ethanol abuse by accelerating the degradation of PLP. However, because the liver is the principal organ responsible for the oxidation of ethanol as well as for the synthesis of PLP from dietary precursors, validation of the hypothesis requires that the effect of acetaldehyde be demonstrable in this organ. It must also be demonstrated that the effect is independent of the nutritional status of vitamin B₆ and that it can be blocked when ethanol oxidation by the liver is inhibited. Moreover, the effect should be observed both chronically and acutely.

To test the above hypothesis, experiments were then performed in rats (Veitch *et al.*, 1975). One group was fed a liquid diet containing an excess of vitamin B₆, and another, a diet that was deficient in vitamin B₆ (Figure 13-5). In each group, the experimental animals received 36 percent of their calories as alcohol, while the control animals were pair-fed diets with ethanol isocalorically replaced by dextrin-maltose. After 6–7 weeks, liver PLP content was measured. The experimental, alcohol-fed animals in both groups exhibited significantly lower liver PLP levels than those of their corresponding controls. Therefore, chronic alcohol ingestion lowers liver PLP content, irrespective of whether the diet is sufficient or deficient in vitamin B₆.

The effect of ethanol oxidation should also be demonstrable acutely. This was accomplished with the use of isolated perfused livers (Figure 13-6). When livers isolated from vitamin B₆-sufficient animals were perfused in the absence of ethanol, little or no change in liver PLP content occurred during 3 h of isolated perfusion. By contrast, when the livers were perfused with 18 mM of ethanol in the medium, a mean decrease in liver PLP content of more than 3 μg per 200 mg of protein was observed. A deleterious effect of alcohol upon PLP metabolism was

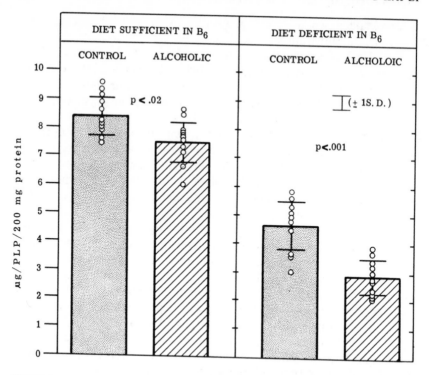

FIGURE 13-5   The effect of chronic ethanol ingestion on the hepatic PLP content of
pair-fed rats. Animals fed the vitamin B$_6$-sufficient diets consumed 50 μg of pyridoxine
daily. The vitamin B$_6$-deficient diet contained no pyridoxine. The liver PLP content of the
vitamin B$_6$-sufficient animals was measured after 52 days, and that for the vitamin B$_6$-
deficient group, after 42 days.

also demonstrated in perfused livers isolated from vitamin B$_6$-deficient
rats. With these animals, it was experimentally more convenient to
measure PLP formation by the liver in the presence of a vitamin precursor. Thus perfusion with 1.2 mg percent pyridoxine increased liver PLP
content by more than 4 μg per 200 mg of protein in 2 h. When 18 mM of
ethanol was added to the perfusate, liver PLP accumulation was significantly reduced (Figure 13-6). It had been reported previously that the
administration of ethanol to rats increases the urinary excretion of
nonphosphorylated vitamin B$_6$ compounds (Oura et al., 1963) and that
the perfusion of rat livers with ethanol increases the amount of nonphosphorylated vitamin B$_6$ compounds that appear in the perfusate
(Sorrell et al., 1974). The findings in Figure 13-6 are consistent with and
provide an explanation for these observations.

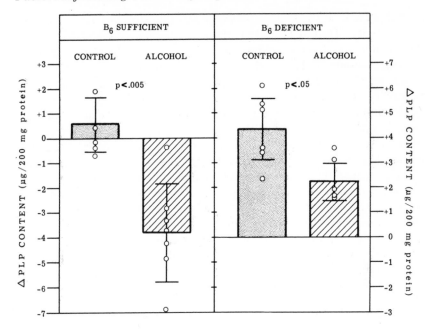

FIGURE 13-6   The effect of ethanol (18 mM) on the hepatic PLP content of isolated perfused livers from vitamin B₆-sufficient and B₆-deficient rats. The livers from vitamin B₆-sufficient animals were perfused without pyridoxine in the medium. The livers from vitamin B₆-deficient animals were perfused with 1.2 mg of pyridoxine added to each 100 ml of medium. Results are expressed as mean ± 1 SD.

In order to demonstrate that it was the oxidation product of ethanol and not ethanol itself that was the active principle, the effect of 4-methylpyrazole was examined. This compound is a very potent inhibitor of alcohol dehydrogenase and prevents the oxidation of ethanol to acetaldehyde. Whereas 4-methylpyrazole itself had no effect on PLP formation in the control situation, it effectively abolished the actions of ethanol on PLP metabolism (Veitch *et al.*, 1975). Therefore, when alcohol oxidation was inhibited, PLP metabolism was restored to normal. These data substantiate the results with the human erythrocytes (Figure 13-4) and indicate that it is acetaldehyde, not ethanol, that mediates the deleterious action of ethanol oxidation on PLP metabolism.

As was already noted, the action of acetaldehyde appeared to be one of stimulation of PLP degradation and not of inhibition of synthesis. How this might occur has recently been elucidated. The enzyme principally responsible for the degradation of PLP in liver is the plasma membrane-bound alkaline phosphatase (Lumeng and Li, 1974). Studies with this enzyme showed that acetaldehyde does not increase its specific activity. Thus it appeared that the stimulatory effect of acetaldehyde must be to increase the availability of PLP for hydrolysis by this enzyme. About one half of the PLP in liver cytosol is tightly bound to proteins. The other half is either free or loosely bound, since this portion can be removed by dialysis or gel filtration. Whether or not PLP is protein-bound, and how it is bound, greatly affects its susceptibility to hydrolytic cleavage (Li *et al.*, 1974). It was found that PLP existing freely in solution was rapidly hydrolyzed by alkaline phosphatase present in the liver plasma membranes (Figure 13-7). In contrast, PLP that was tightly bound to cytosolic proteins, and, therefore, not removed by dialysis, was virtually unhydrolyzed. Therefore, protein binding of PLP protects it against degradation. Moreover, a considerable degree of protection against degradation appeared to be extended also to that fraction of PLP in cytosol that was only loosely bound to proteins and removable by dialysis. These and other studies have led us to believe that protein binding and the hydrolysis of unbound PLP are important mechanisms for the regulation of the body content of PLP. In the nor-

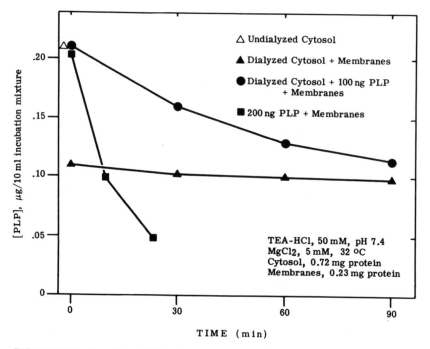

FIGURE 13-7   The effect of dialysis and plasma membrane-associated phosphatase on the PLP content of hepatic cytosol.

mal state, the tissue content of PLP is determined to a large extent by protein binding. PLP synthesized in excess of this binding capacity is rapidly hydrolyzed by alkaline phosphatase. Thus, there is a dynamic equilibrium between synthesis and degradation, with protein binding serving as an intracellular buffer and the modifier of the rate of PLP degradation (Li *et al.*, 1974).

The manner in which acetaldehyde acts to increase the availability of PLP for hydrolysis is demonstrated in Figure 13-8. When rat liver cytosol was dialyzed against 30 volumes of buffer for 24 hours, only about 20 percent of the PLP was removed. In the presence of 7.5 and 15 mM acetaldehyde, considerably more PLP was removed in dialysis. Similar results have been obtained with PLP and erythrocyte hemolysates. Thus acetaldehyde displaces or facilitates the dissociation of PLP from protein binding and in this manner promotes PLP degradation. In agreement with this interpretation, we have also demonstrated that acetaldehyde inhibits the activation of purified tyrosine aminotransferase apoenzyme by PLP. The kinetics of the inhibition shows a mixed competitive-noncompetitive pattern. The activation of ornithine decarboxylase apoenzyme by PLP is similarly inhibited by acetaldehyde. We infer from these studies that not only does alcohol oxida-

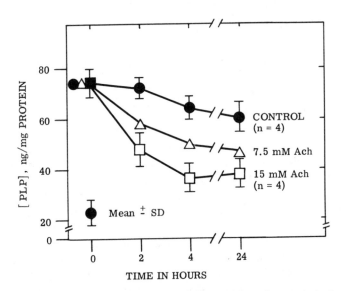

FIGURE 13-8   The effect of acetaldehyde (Acd) on the PLP content of rat liver cytosol. Cytosol was dialyzed against 30 volumes of buffer containing different concentrations of Acd, and the PLP remaining in the dialysis bags was measured as a function of time of dialysis.

tion itself accelerate the degradation of PLP, but that with chronic, excessive alcohol ingestion, the body storage capacity for vitamin B_6 is also lowered. Both processes would contribute to the development of vitamin B_6 deficiency.

Chronic alcohol ingestion can result also in other abnormalities of vitamin B_6 metabolism. Hines (1975) reported that heavy alcohol consumption may cause an impairment of erythrocyte pyridoxal kinase activity. When alcoholic subjects were given 900 ml of 86-proof whiskey per day for 2–9 weeks, a progressive decline in the pyridoxal kinase activity of erythrocyte hemolysates was noted. Furthermore, he reported the appearance of a large molecular weight substance in the serum of these drinking alcoholics that inhibits erythrocyte and hepatic pyridoxal kinase activity. The significance of these findings to the development of vitamin B_6 undernutrition in chronic alcohol abuse is difficult to define at this point because (1) the origin of the serum inhibitor and its relationship to pyridoxal kinase, which is an intracellular enzyme, are unknown and (2) it is unknown to what extent the level of pyridoxal kinase activity in erythrocytes and other tissues contributes to the regulation of the cellular and body economy of PLP. It is known, however, that the total and specific activities of pyridoxal kinase of erythrocytes can vary widely from individual to individual (Chern and Beutler, 1975).

IMPAIRMENT OF VITAMIN B_6 METABOLISM WITH LIVER DISEASE

As was noted previously, the incidence of vitamin B_6 deficiency is higher in alcoholic patients with liver disease than in those without liver disease. There is now evidence that liver disease itself will impose additional stresses on vitamin B_6 metabolism, by mechanisms other than those already discussed. Thus Baker et al. (1975) recently reported that chronic alcoholics with liver disease exhibit an abnormality in their ability to use food as a source of folate, thiamin, and vitamin B_6. Whereas alcoholics with liver disease are able to absorb synthetic vitamin B_6 normally, absorption of vitamin B_6 from food, as exemplified by brewers yeast, is significantly impaired. Such an abnormality would, of course, aggravate the already marginal or inadequate intake of vitamin B_6 in the alcoholic and contribute to the development of deficiency. Moreover, Mitchell et al. (1976) have recently reported that PLP degradation is accelerated in liver disease. Experimentally, this is manifest as a marked curtailment in the rise of plasma PLP levels after intravenous pyridoxine administration. This abnormality is, therefore, identical to that previously reported by Hines and Cowan (1970) in the heavily drinking alcoholic. However, they have found that there is also a striking increase in PLP clearance, when PLP is injected intravenously. Importantly, these phenomena were observed not only in patients with alcoholic cirrhosis but also in patients with hepatitis and biliary obstruction. They interpret these findings to indicate that there is increased degradation of PLP by diseased livers.

SUMMARY AND CONCLUSION

The different mechanisms by which the excessive use of alcohol can produce stress upon dietary intake and nutritional balance and upon vitamin B₆ metabolism have been reviewed. Because alcoholic beverages have high energy value but are empty in nutritional value, the excessive use of alcohol promotes the development of primary nutritional deficiency by preempting food intake. Furthermore, alcohol ingestion and alcoholic liver disease can interfere with the normal processes of vitamin B₆ metabolism, e.g., absorption, storage, conversion to biologically active forms, degradation, or excretion. These conditioning factors can occur concurrently, thereby accelerating the development of vitamin B₆ deficiency. Evidence has been presented that acetaldehyde, the oxidation product of ethanol, interferes with the metabolism of vitamin B₆ by promoting the degradation of PLP. It may also lower the tissue storage capacity for vitamin B₆. In patients with alcoholic liver disease, there is impairment of the intestinal absorption of vitamin B₆ from food sources, and PLP degradation is accelerated. Liver disease may also impair the ability of the liver to synthesize PLP. Because of these conditioning factors, discontinuation of excessive alcohol ingestion is a necessary step in treatment.

The incidence of vitamin B₆ undernutrition, as measured by the concentration of vitamin B₆ compounds or PLP in blood plasma, may be as high as 30–50 percent in alcoholics without liver disease and 80–100 percent in those with liver disease. Viewed in the light that the dietary intake of vitamin B₆ of normal individuals is, at best, only slightly in excess of the RDA for this vitamin, these findings are not surprising. However, the clinical manifestations of vitamin B₆ deficiency tend to occur only when the deficiency is severe, and most are nonspecific. As measured by the ring sideroblastic change in bone marrow, the incidence of vitamin B₆ deficiency in alcoholic populations may be as high as 20–30 percent. It is well known that PLP participates as an essential cofactor in many metabolic pathways. However, because the PLP-dependent enzymes have widely different affinities for PLP and have different adaptive responses to PLP deficiency (Ryan et al., 1976), the search for enzymatic abnormalities that are most readily and seriously affected by chronic and excessive alcohol ingestion should be the direction for future research in this area. These abnormalities should also represent the most sensitive and specific functional indicators for the diagnosis of vitamin B_6 deficiency.

ACKNOWLEDGMENT

The work reported was supported in part by a grant from the Veterans Administration (MRIS 5363).

LITERATURE CITED

Baker, H., O. Frank, R. K. Zetterman, K. S. Rajan, W. TenHove, and C. M. Leevy. 1975. Inability of chronic alcoholics with liver disease to use food as a source of folates, thiamin and vitamin B_6. Am. J. Clin. Nutr. 28:1377–1380.

Baker, H., O. Frank, H. Zitter, S. Goldfarb, C. M. Leevy, and H. Sobotka. 1964. Effect of hepatic disease on liver B-complex vitamin titers. Am. J. Clin. Nutr. 14:1–6.

Brown, R. R., D. P. Rose, J. E. Leklem, H. Linkswiler, and R. Anand. 1975. Urinary 4-pyridoxic acid, plasma pyridoxal phosphate, and erythrocyte aminotransferase levels in oral contraceptive users receiving controlled intakes of vitamin B_6. Am. J. Clin. Nutr. 28:10–19.

Chern, C. J., and E. Beutler. 1975. Pyridoxal kinase: Decreased activity in red blood cells of Afro-Americans. Science 187:1084–1086.

Criteria Committee, National Council on Alcoholism. 1972. Criteria for the diagnosis of alcoholism. Ann. Int. Med. 77:249–258.

Davis, R. E., and B. K. Smith. 1974. Pyridoxal and folate deficiency in alcoholics. Med. J. Aust. 2:357–360.

Driskell, J. A., J. M. Geders, and M. C. Urban. 1976. Vitamin B_6 status of young men, women and women using oral contraceptives. J. Lab. Clin. Med. 87:813–821.

Eichner, E. R., and R. S. Hillman. 1971. The evolution of anemia in alcoholic patients. Am. J. Med. 50:218–232.

Gabuzda, G. J., and C. S. Davidson. 1962. Tryptophan and nicotinic acid metabolism in patients with cirrhosis of the liver. Am. J. Clin. Nutr. 11:502–508.

Hines, J. D. 1975. Hematologic abnormalities involving vitamin B_6 and folate metabolism in alcoholic subjects. Ann. N.Y. Acad. Sci. 252:316–326.

Hines, J. D., and D. H. Cowan. 1970. Studies on the pathogenesis of alcohol-induced sideroblastic bone marrow abnormalities. New Engl. J. Med. 283:441–446.

Hines, J. D., and J. A. Grasso. 1970. The sideroblastic anemias. Semin. Hematol. 7:86–106.

Hines, J. D., and D. S. Love. 1969. Determination of serum and blood pyridoxal phosphate concentrations with purified rabbit skeletal muscle apophosphorylase b. J. Lab. Clin. Med. 73:343–349.

Horrigan, D. L., and J. W. Harris. 1968. Pyridoxine-responsive anemias in man. Vitam. Horm. 26:549–567.

Leevy, C. M., H. Baker, W. TenHove, O. Frank, and G. R. Cherrick. 1965. B-complex vitamins in liver disease of the alcoholic. Am. J. Clin. Nutr. *16*:339–346.

Lerner, A. M., L. M. DeCarli, and C. S. Davidson. 1958. Association of pyridoxine deficiency and convulsions in alcoholics. Proc. Soc. Exp. Biol. Med. *98*:841–843.

Li, T.-K., L. Lumeng, and R. L. Veitch. 1974. Regulation of pyridoxal 5'-phosphate metabolism in liver. Biochem. Biophys. Res. Commun. *61*:677–684.

Lumeng, L., and T.-K. Li. 1974. Vitamin B₆ metabolism in chronic alcohol abuse: Pyridoxal 5'-phosphate levels in plasma and the effects of acetaldehyde on pyridoxal phosphate synthesis and degradation in human erythrocytes. J. Clin. Invest. *53*:693–704.

Lumeng, L., and T.-K. Li. 1975. Characterization of the pyridoxal 5'-phosphate and pyridoxamine 5'-phosphate hydrolase activity in rat liver. J. Biol. Chem. *250*:8126–8131.

Lumeng, L., R. E. Brashear, and T.-K. Li. 1974. Pyridoxal 5'-phosphate in plasma: Source, protein-binding and cellular transport. J. Lab. Clin. Med. *84*:334–343.

Mitchell, D., C. Wagner, W. J. Stone, G. R. Wilkinson, and S. Schenker. 1976. Abnormal regulation of plasma pyridoxal 5'-phosphate in patients with liver disease. Gastroenterology *70*:988.

Oura, E., K. Konttinen, and H. Suomalainen. 1963. The influence of alcohol intake on vitamin excretion in the rat. Acta Physiol. Scand. *59*:119.

Pierce, H. I., R. G. McGuffin, and R. S. Hillman. 1976. Clinical studies in alcoholic sideroblastosis. Arch. Int. Med. *136*:283–289.

Ryan, M. P., L. Lumeng, and T.-K. Li. 1976. Validation of plasma pyridoxal 5'-phosphate measurements as an indicator of vitamin B₆ nutritional status. Fed. Proc. *35*:660.

Seixas, F. A., K. Williams, and S. Eggleston (eds.). 1975. Medical consequences of alcoholism. Ann. N.Y. Acad. Sci. *252*:399 pp.

Sorrell, M. F., H. Baker, A. J. Barak, and O. Frank. 1974. Release by ethanol of vitamins into rat liver perfusates. Am. J. Clin. Nutr. *27*:743–745.

Veitch, R. L., L. Lumeng, and T.-K. Li. 1975. Vitamin B₆ metabolism in chronic alcohol abuse: The effect of ethanol oxidation on hepatic pyridoxal 5'-phosphate metabolism. J. Clin. Invest. *55*:1026–1032.

Veitch, R. L., W. F. Bosron, and T.-K. Li. 1976. Distribution of pyridoxal 5'-phosphate binding proteins in rat liver. Fed. Proc. *35*:1545.

Walsh, M. P., P. J. N. Howarth, and V. Marks. 1966. Pyridoxine deficiency and tryptophan metabolism in chronic alcoholics. Am. J. Clin. Nutr. *19*:379–383.

14

Vitamin B$_6$ Requirement
of Young Women

ELIZABETH A. DONALD

Only two studies have been conducted to specifically study the vitamin B$_6$ needs of "normal" young women. One study was conducted at Cornell University and reported in 1971 (Donald et al., 1971), the second at the University of Wisconsin and reported in 1974 (Shin and Linkswiler, 1974). Data from young women used as control subjects in a study of the effect of oral contraceptives on the needs for vitamin B$_6$ were reported in 1975 (Brown et al., 1975; Leklem et al., 1975). This study was also done at Wisconsin. Data from these four reports will be considered in this paper.

Descriptions of subjects and protein and vitamin B$_6$ levels in the diet and duration of each study are outlined in Table 14-1. A total of 23 young women, of similar age and approximately similar body weight, participated in the studies. In all cases they were given a basic food diet, low in vitamin B$_6$ but adequate in all other nutrients except energy. To meet body needs for energy, each subject consumed enough fat and sugar to maintain her initial body weight.

The Wisconsin studies included a short predepletion period; the Cornell study did not. The length of the depletion period varied among studies, from 14 to 43 days (Table 14-1). The regimen for the repletion period also varied. In the Cornell study (Donald *et al.*, 1971), the basic diet was supplemented with 0.6, 1.2, and 30.0 mg of pyridoxine hydrochloride (PN-HCl) for 7, 3, and 1 days, respectively. The total intake of vitamin B_6 was 0.9 mg and 1.5 mg for the first two phases of the repletion period. The diet was supplemented with 2.0 mg of PN-HCl, for a total intake of 2.2 mg of vitamin B_6, in the first Wisconsin study (Shin and Linkswiler, 1974). Four of the 10 subjects received this same level in the second study (Brown *et al.*, 1975; Leklem *et al.*, 1975), whereas, the other six subjects received 0.8 mg of PN-HCl for a total vitamin B_6 intake of 1.0 mg.

The usual criterion used to judge nutrient requirement is restoration of one or more biochemical parameters to original levels. In these studies, a number of parameters were measured in blood and urine to assess the need for vitamin B_6 in young women.

BLOOD LEVELS

Pyridoxal phosphate (PLP) levels in plasma were used in the second Wisconsin study (Brown *et al.*, 1975). Levels rapidly decreased during depletion, and original levels were restored after an intake of 2.2 mg of vitamin B_6 for approximately 10 days (Figure 14-1). One mg/day of the vitamin was not sufficient to restore the original levels.

TABLE 14-1   Description of Studies

Study	Cornell 1971[a]	Wisconsin 1974[b]	Wisconsin 1975[c]
Subjects			
Number	8	5	10
Mean age, yr	24.7	23.2	22.3
Mean weight, kg	56.3	49.1	59.8
Diet			
Protein, g	57	109	78
Vitamin B_6, mg	0.34	0.16	0.19
Duration of study			
Adjustment period, days	—	7	4
Depletion period, days	43	14	28
Repletion period, days	11	14	28

[a]Donald *et al.* (1971).
[b]Shin and Linkswiler (1974).
[c]Brown *et al.* (1975) and Leklem *et al.* (1975).

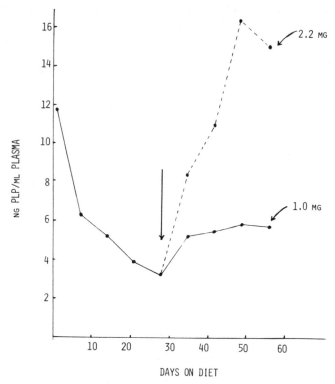

FIGURE 14-1   Plasma pyridoxal phosphate levels (Brown *et al.*, 1975).

Transferase activity in erythrocytes was studied in both the Cornell and Wisconsin studies (Brown *et al.*, 1975). A method utilizing commercially prepared solutions was used in the Cornell study (Donald *et al.*, 1971). Aspartate aminotransferase (ASP-AT) activity decreased during depletion, but supplementation with PN-HCl failed to restore original levels. Alanine aminotransferase (ALA-AT) levels did not respond to either depletion or repletion. The method of Woodring and Storvick (1970) was used in the Wisconsin study. These investigators also found that the levels of ASP-AT decreased with depletion, but intakes of neither 1.0 nor 2.2 mg of vitamin B₆ restored original levels (Figure 14-2). *In vitro* stimulation of the enzymatic system with pyridoxal phosphate (PLP) resulted in an increase in the ASP-AT activity during depletion and a decrease with repletion. However, original levels were not reached (Figure 14-3).

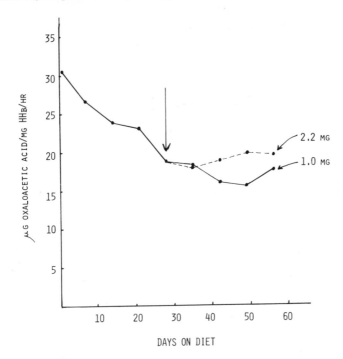

FIGURE 14-2   Aspartate aminotransferase activity in erythrocytes
(Brown *et al.*, 1975).

Erythrocyte ALA-AT levels decreased with depletion. An intake of 1
mg of vitamin B₆ was not sufficient to restore activity to normal, but 2.2
mg was (Figure 14-4). Results of the activation of this system with PLP
were inconclusive (Figure 14-5).

In the Cornell study (Donald *et al.*, 1971), the vitamin B₆ level in
erythrocytes was determined by using the microbiological method proposed by Baker *et al.* (1966). A vitamin B₆ intake of 1.5–1.6 mg/day
was enough to restore levels to normal (Figure 14-6).

EXCRETION OF METABOLITES IN URINE

The excretion of 4-pyridoxic acid (4-PDA) was followed in both the
Cornell study (Donald *et al.*, 1971) and the second Wisconsin study
(Brown *et al.*, 1975). A vitamin B₆ intake of 0.9–1.0 mg/day was not
sufficient to restore original levels; 1.5 mg/day was borderline;
whereas, 2.2 mg/day was overly generous, since a high proportion of
intake was excreted (Figure 14-7).

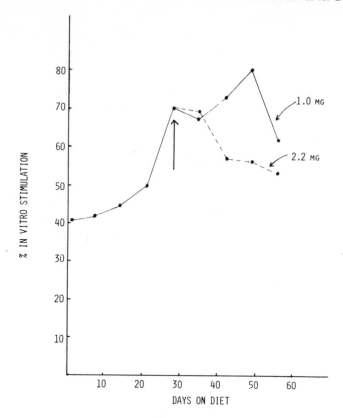

FIGURE 14-3   Percent of *in vitro* stimulation of erythrocyte aspartate aminotransferase (Brown *et al.*, 1975).

Urinary excretion of a number of tryptophan metabolites was determined in both studies conducted at Wisconsin (Shin and Linkswiler, 1974; Leklem *et al.*, 1975). Following a 2-g L-tryptophan load dose, the levels of kynurenine, acetyl kynurenine, kynurenic acid, 3-OH kynurenine, and xanthurenic acid markedly increased with vitamin depletion and rapidly decreased to original levels with either a 1.0-mg or 2.2-mg intake of vitamin B_6. A loading dose of 3.0 g of L-methionine caused variable results in the excretion of methionine metabolites (Shin and Linkswiler, 1974). The excretion of methionine did not change significantly either during depletion or repletion phases of the study. Homocystine levels in two of five subjects increased during depletion and quickly returned to the original zero levels with repletion. Levels of cystathionine and L-cysteine sulfinic acid were significantly in-

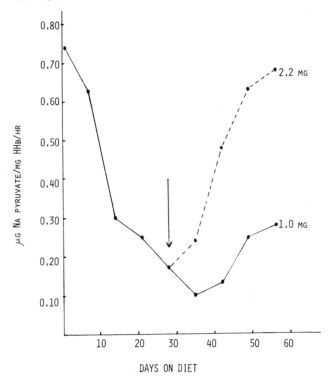

FIGURE 14-4   Alanine aminotransferase activity in erythrocytes
(Brown *et al.*, 1975).

creased with depletion and returned to original levels with an intake of
2.2 mg of the vitamin within 1 week. Taurine levels decreased during
the depletion phase and remained depressed during repletion. The reasons for and significance of this finding have not been determined.

Levels of N^1 methyl nicotinamide (N^1 MeN) in urine were determined
both before and after loading with tryptophan (Leklem *et al.*, 1975).
The post-tryptophan levels of N^1 MeN increased with depletion and
decreased to normal following intakes of 2.2 mg of the vitamin (Figure
14-8). Urinary excretion of 2-pyridone decreased with depletion and
increased to original levels with either 1.0 mg or 2.2 mg of vitamin B_6
(Figure 14-9).

The limited data available would tend to support the conclusion that
a vitamin B_6 intake of 1.0 mg/day is not sufficient to meet the needs of a
population. An intake of 2.2 mg may be overly generous, since this
amount more than restored many of the parameters studied to normal.

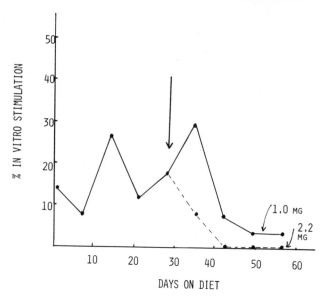

FIGURE 14-5   Percent *in vitro* stimulation of erythrocyte alanine aminotransferase (Brown *et al.*, 1975).

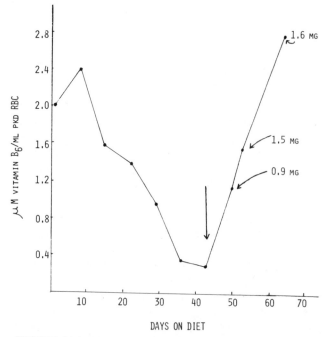

FIGURE 14-6   Vitamin B₆ levels in erythrocytes (Donald *et al.*, 1971).

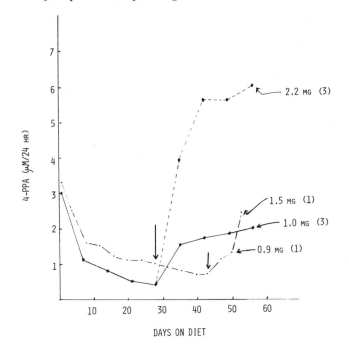

FIGURE 14-7   4-Pyridoxic acid excretion in urine (Donald *et al.*, 1971; Brown *et al.*, 1975).

Unfortunately, data are available from only one study pertaining to the efficiency of levels between these two extremes to meet the vitamin B_6 needs of women (Donald *et al.*, 1971). Data from this study indicates that 1.5 mg/day may be sufficient.

Because of the lack of data describing the vitamin B_6 needs of the human, an alternate approach should be considered. In 1973, when the latest revision of the Dietary Standard for Canada was being written (Bureau of Nutritional Sciences, 1975), data from only the Cornell study were available on the vitamin B_6 needs of young women (Donald *et al.*, 1971). The committee revising the standards decided to relate vitamin B_6 needs to the amount of protein consumed, thus recognizing the metabolic interrelationships of the vitamin and protein.

In the 1975 version of the Dietary Standard for Canada (Bureau of Nutritional Sciences, 1975) this statement appears: "An intake of 0.02 mg of vitamin per gram of protein eaten is recommended as the basis for an adult allowance." This ratio was calculated by using data from studies reporting both the intake of vitamin B_6 and protein (Donald *et al.*, 1971; Harding *et al.*, 1959; Swan *et al.*, 1964; Baker *et al.*, 1964;

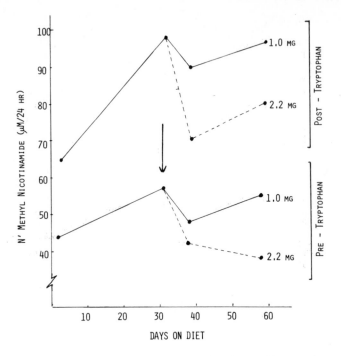

FIGURE 14-8   N¹ methyl nicotinamide in urine (Leklem *et al.*, 1975).

Canham *et al.*, 1969). These studies had been conducted with the use of either men or women and are summarized in Table 14-2. The authors of each paper had also expressed their opinions as to the "adequacy" or "inadequacy" of the vitamin B_6 intakes. Using these data, a ratio of milligrams of vitamin B_6 to grams of protein consumed was calculated. A ratio of 0.017 was considered "inadequate," whereas, one of 0.019 was "adequate." Thus, a ratio of 0.02 mg of vitamin B_6 per gram of protein eaten was arrived at and was used to calculate the vitamin B_6 allowance for the Dietary Standard for Canada (Bureau of Nutritional Standards, 1975). These calculations are summarized in Table 14-3.

SUMMARY

Using the ratio of 0.02 mg of vitamin B_6 per gram of protein consumed, the recommended allowance for young women would be 1.5 mg of vitamin B_6 per day. This value is similar to the amount suggested by requirement studies.

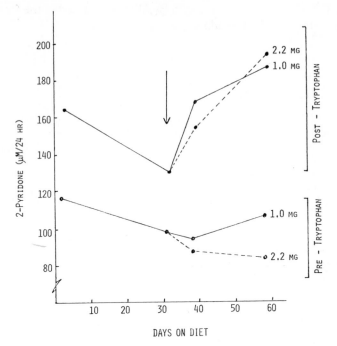

FIGURE 14-9   2-Pyridone in urine (Leklem *et al.*, 1975).

TABLE 14-2   Vitamin B₆/Protein Interrelationships for the Adult

		B₆ Intake[a], mg	
References	Protein Intake, g	Inadequate	Adequate
Harding *et al.*, 1959	165	1.93	2.76
Swan *et al.*, 1964	100	1.06	—
Baker *et al.*, 1964	30	1.25	—
	100	1.50	1.75
	—	—	2.00
Canham *et al.*, 1969	80	1.0	—
	100	1.3	1.5
Donald *et al.*, 1971	57	—	1.5

[a]Vitamin B₆ intake was considered to be "adequate" or "inadequate" to meet the needs of the group studied according to the judgment of the authors.

TABLE 14-3 Calculated Vitamin B_6 Allowance Used in the Revised Dietary Standard for Canada

Age Group, yr	Approximate Protein Intake[a]		Vitamin B_6[b]		Vitamin B_6 Values to Appear in Table, mg/day	
	Male	Female	Male	Female	Male	Female
1-3	47		0.84		0.8	
4-6	64		1.28		1.3	
7-9	79	70	1.58	1.40	1.6	1.4
10-12	89	73	1.78	1.46	1.8	1.5
13-15	96	74	1.96	1.48	2.0	1.5
16-18	100	74	2.0	1.48	2.0	1.5
19-35	109	71	2.18	1.42	2.0	1.5
36-50	102	64	2.04	1.28	2.0	1.5
51+	86	58	1.72	1.06	2.0	1.5

SOURCE: Bureau of Nutritional Sciences, 1975.
[a]Approximate protein intake of Canadians (private communication).
[b]Factor is 0.02 mg of vitamin B_6 per gram of protein.

LITERATURE CITED

Baker, E. M., J. E. Canham, W. T. Nunes, H. E. Sauberlich, and M. E. McDowell. 1964. Vitamin B_6 requirement for adult men. Am. J. Clin. Nutr. *15*:59–64.

Baker, H., O. Frank, M. Ning, R. A. Gelene, S. H. Hutner, and C. M. Leevy. 1966. A protozoological method for detecting clinical vitamin B_6 deficiency. Am. J. Clin. Nutr. *18*:123–133.

Brown, R. R., D. P. Rose, J. E. Leklem, H. Linkswiler, and R. Anand. 1975. Urinary 4-pyridoxic acid, plasma pyridoxal phosphate, and erythrocyte aminotransferase levels in oral contraceptive users receiving controlled intakes of vitamin B_6. Am. J. Clin. Nutr. *28*:10–19.

Bureau of Nutritional Sciences. 1975. Dietary Standard for Canada, revised ed., Food Directorate, Health Protection Branch, Department of National Health and Welfare, Ottawa, 110 pp.

Canham, J. E., E. M. Baker, R. S. Harding, H. E. Sauberlich, and I. C. Plough. 1969. Dietary protein—Its relationship to vitamin B_6 requirements and function. N.Y. Acad. Sci. *166*:16–29.

Donald, E. A., L. D. McBean, M. H. W. Simpson, M. F. Sun, and H. E. Aly. 1971. Vitamin B_6 requirement of young adult women. Am. J. Clin. Nutr. *24*:1028–1041.

Harding, R. S., I. C. Plough, and T. E. Friedmann. 1959. The effect of storage on the vitamin B_6 content of a packaged army ration, with a note on the human requirement for the vitamin. J. Nutr. *68*:323–332.

Leklem, J. E., R. R. Brown, D. P. Rose, H. Linkswiler, and R. A. Arend. 1975. Metabolism of tryptophan and niacin in oral contraceptive users receiving controlled intakes of vitamin B_6. Am. J. Clin. Nutr. *28*:146–156.

Shin, H. K., and H. Linkswiler. 1974. Tryptophan and methionine metabolism of adult females as affected by vitamin B_6 deficiency. J. Nutr. *104*:1348–1355.

Swan, P., J. Wentworth, and H. Linkswiler. 1964. Vitamin B_6 depletion in man: Urinary taurine and sulfate excretion and nitrogen balance. J. Nutr. *84*:220–228.

Woodring, M. J., and C. A. Storvick. 1970. Effect of pyridoxine supplementation of glutamic-pyruvic transaminase and *in vitro* stimulation in erythrocytes of normal women. Am. J. Clin. Nutr. *23*:1385–1395.

15

Relationship Between Vitamin B$_6$ Intake and the Content of the Vitamin in Human Milk

AVANELLE KIRKSEY and KERSTIN D. WEST

The content of vitamin B$_6$ in milk appears to reflect the nutritional state of the mother with respect to the vitamin. Support for this view has come recently from animal studies in our laboratory (Pang and Kirksey, 1974; Thomas and Kirksey, 1976), in which the vitamin B$_6$ content in milk of the rat was reduced to trace amounts by feeding a low level of vitamin in the diet. Increments in the vitamin B$_6$ content in the diet resulted in parallel increases in the vitamin content in milk until a peak level was reached. After the peak was reached, further increases in the dietary level of the vitamin had no effect on the level in milk. At low levels of vitamin B$_6$ intake the priority of mammary gland tissue for the vitamin was less than liver or muscle tissue.

Karlin (1959) found that a single, large dose of vitamin B$_6$ administered orally or intramuscularly to women during the second and seventh months of lactation caused a rapid increase in the concentration of the vitamin in milk. She found that daily administration of large oral doses of vitamin B$_6$ resulted in even greater increases in the concentration of the vitamin in milk, which were maintained for several days following the treatment.

238

Vitamin B_6 is known to be a critical dietary factor, especially during the early stages of central nervous system development in the human infant from the seventh month of gestation to several months after birth (Snyderman *et al.,* 1953; Coursin, 1954, 1955a; Molony and Parmelee, 1954). Recently, in this laboratory, Pang and Kirksey (1974) found that a low level of vitamin B_6 fed to rats during pregnancy and lactation resulted in a pyridoxine deficiency syndrome in the offspring and changes in the composition of cerebrosides in brain during the early postnatal period. The changes were also associated with adverse effects on myelination.

Information is limited concerning the level of vitamin B_6 in human milk and the effect of the dietary level of the vitamin on milk composition. Therefore, this study was concerned with the influence of the amount of vitamin B_6 ingested by lactating women on the level of the vitamin in milk and the adequacy of the vitamin B_6/protein ratio. Also, the vitamin B_6 content in milk was examined in relation to different stages of lactation as well as to diurnal, daily, and weekly patterns.

MATERIALS AND METHODS

Selection and Description of Subjects

Nineteen healthy, lactating women volunteered to participate in the study. All subjects were members of the Lafayette chapter of La Leche League International, an organization whose purpose is to encourage breast feeding. Subjects participating in the study represented a college-educated, middle income, professional group.

Initially, the subjects were grouped according to three different stages of lactation: early (<3 months), middle (3–7 months), and late (>7 months). Five of the subjects who were in the early months of lactation participated in a phase of the study concerned with diurnal patterns on the level of vitamin B_6 in milk.

The subjects ranged in age from 24 to 42 years and had successfully established lactation practices. Each of 12 multiparas had had previous breast feeding experience; seven of the subjects were primiparas. All women reported having good appetites and normal eating habits.

Collection of Milk Samples

Subjects collected samples of fore milk before the first morning feeding for 3 consecutive days during 1 week and for 1 day in each of the following 2 weeks. A preliminary experiment conducted with two individuals indicated that the vitamin B_6 content in a fore sample of early morning milk was representative of milk expressed completely from the breast. Subjects were instructed to collect samples from the breast to be used for the particular feeding and to collect all subsequent samples from the same breast. Approximately 5 ml of milk were expressed manually into plastic vials before nursing, and the samples were frozen immediately in the home. All samples were collected in insulated ice chests and were taken to the laboratory for storage at $-20°C$ until analyzed for vitamin B_6 and protein content.

For the study of diurnal patterns, five subjects collected fore milk, as described previously, for five or six 4-h intervals during an approximate 18-h period on 2 consecutive days. A total of 10 to 12 samples was collected from each subject.

Dietary Analysis

A modified version of Burke's dietary record form was used to obtain dietary information (Burke, 1947). Diet records were kept by each subject on each of the 3 consecutive days during the first week of milk sample collection. The importance of collecting dietary information representative of their usual intakes was explained individually to the subjects. Prior to collecting the data, a dietetic scale was provided each subject for weighing food portions. The use of the scale and of other household measuring equipment was emphasized. Subjects participating in the study of diurnal patterns recorded dietary intakes on the day previous to sample collection and during the 2 days of milk sampling. The vitamin B_6 content of the diet was estimated by use of Home Economics Research Report No. 36 (Orr, 1969) and other nutrients by use of Home and Garden Bulletin No. 72 (U.S. Department of Agriculture, 1964). The computer was used for the dietary analyses. Additional information regarding intake of vitamin, mineral, or other nutrient supplements was obtained from each participant by means of an interview form.

Biochemical Analysis

Total vitamin B_6 content of milk samples was measured by a *Saccharomyces carlsbergensis* microbiological assay based on the methods of Storvick *et al.* (1964), Thiele and Brin (1966), Brin and Thiele (1967), and Toepfer and Polansky (1970). A modification of the original method of Lowry *et al.* (1951) was used for the determination of the total protein of milk samples.

Methods of Statistical Analysis

All data were analyzed by computer. A one-way analysis of variance program was used to determine any significant differences among group means. Group means with a significant F-value were further tested by the Newman-Keuls Sequential Range Test to determine differences ($p < 0.05$ or $p < 0.01$) among individual means. Correlation coefficients were obtained between certain variables and were compared with r-values according to the degrees of freedom ($n - 2$) and two significance levels, $p < 0.05$ and $p < 0.01$ (Steel and Torrie, 1960).

RESULTS AND DISCUSSION

Dietary Intakes

Group means of the 19 subjects either met or exceeded the recommended dietary allowances (Food and Nutrition Board, 1974) for lactating women for kilocalories, protein, calcium, thiamin, riboflavin, niacin, vitamin B_{12}, ascorbic acid, and vitamin A. However, dietary intakes of iron and vitamin B_6 for most subjects were less than the allowances. Iron intakes ranged from 8.0–16.8 mg/day with a group mean of 14.3 ± 2.5 mg; none of the subjects met the 18-mg allowance. Vitamin B_6 intakes ranged from 1.2 to 2.7 mg/day with a group mean of 2.0 ± 0.6 mg. Sixteen women had dietary intakes of vitamin B_6 that were less than 2.5 mg/day, the recommendation for lactation. However, the inclusion of extra dietary sources of vitamin B_6 in the form of pyridoxine • HCl in vitamin and vitamin-mineral supplements increased the total intakes so that only six subjects had intakes of the vitamin that did not meet the allowance.

Protein and Vitamin B₆ Content in Milk at Different Stages of Lactation

Thirteen subjects were grouped according to three different stages of lactation, <3.0, 3.0–7.0, and >7.0 months, in order to study the effects of the stage of lactation on the protein and vitamin B_6 content in milk (Table 15-1). Each subject who participated in this part of the study had an intake of vitamin B_6 that was equal to or greater than 2.5 mg/day, the recommended allowance for lactation. Means for protein content, vitamin B_6 content, and the vitamin B_6/protein ratio in milk were not significantly different statistically for the three stages of lactation. Because the stage of lactation did not influence either the protein or the

TABLE 15-1   Protein and Vitamin B_6 Content in Milk at Different
Stages of Lactation

Subject	Lactation Stage, months	Milk[a] Protein, g/100 ml	Vitamin B_6, μg/l	B_6/Protein, μg/g
Less than 3.0 months				
A.N.	1.00	1.12 ± 0.38	270 ± 119	23
S.S.	1.50	1.01 ± 0.13	258 ± 44	26
J.L.	1.75	0.87 ± 0.18	246 ± 64	28
P.L.	1.75	0.84 ± 0.13	212 ± 45	25
B.H.	2.00	1.05 ± 0.10	298 ± 106	28
Mean ± SD		0.98 ± 0.12	257 ± 31	26 ± 2
3.0 – 7.0 months				
L.K.	3.00	1.29 ± 0.38	221 ± 56	17
M.F.	3.50	0.94 ± 0.13	233 ± 48	25
C.M.	5.00	1.05 ± 0.20	454 ± 105	43
C.D.	6.00	1.29 ± 0.19	214 ± 55	17
E.G.	7.00	1.16 ± 0.09	348 ± 121	30
Mean ± SD		1.15 ± 0.15	294 ± 105	26 ± 11
More than 7.0 months				
L.F.	15.50	1.05 ± 0.19	247 ± 25	24
E.B.	15.80	1.10 ± 0.51	189 ± 41	17
M.A.	20.00	1.64 ± 0.07	307 ± 121	19
Mean ± SD		1.26 ± 0.33	248 ± 59	20 ± 3
		NS[b]	NS[b]	NS[b]

[a]Means ± SD of five or more samples per subject.
[b]Means in columns are not significantly different.

vitamin B_6 content of milk, stage of lactation was eliminated as a variable in the classification of subjects for other aspects of the study.

Vitamin B_6 Intake and Levels of the Vitamin in Milk

Nineteen subjects were grouped according to three levels of vitamin B_6 intake, <2.5, 2.5–5.0, and >5.0 mg/day, in order to determine whether the level of vitamin B_6 intake influenced the content of the vitamin in milk (Table 15-2). As estimated from 3-day records of both food intake and extradietary supplements, six subjects had vitamin B_6 intakes less than 2.5 mg/day; eight had intakes ranging from 2.5 to 4.2 mg/day, and the remaining five subjects had intakes ranging from 7.1 to 12.5 mg/day. The vitamin B_6 intake of the latter group was significantly higher ($p < 0.01$) than that of the other two groups.

TABLE 15-2   Vitamin B_6 Intake and Levels of Vitamin B_6 in Milk

Subjects	Vitamin B_6 Intake,[a] mg/day	Milk[b]	
		Vitamin B_6, μg/l	Vitamin B_6/Protein, μg/g
Less than 2.5 mg/day			
K.J.	1.3 ± 0.2	142 ± 15	13
P.Y.	1.4 ± 0.0	67 ± 22	5
B.M.	1.5 ± 0.4	177 ± 36	18
M.P.	2.1 ± 0.6	136 ± 17	11
J.O.	2.2 ± 0.0	148 ± 56	17
J.G.	2.0 ± 0.4	101 ± 27	12
Mean ± SD	1.8 ± 0.4[c]	129 ± 39[c,d]	13 ± 5[c,d]
2.5–5.0 mg/day			
C.D.	2.5 ± 1.1	214 ± 55	17
P.L.	2.5 ± 0.3	212 ± 45	25
M.F.	2.6 ± 0.5	233 ± 48	25
L.K.	2.7 ± 0.8	221 ± 56	17
L.F.	2.7 ± 0.9	247 ± 25	24
E.B.	2.8 ± 0.4	189 ± 41	17
E.G.	3.4 ± 1.9	348 ± 121	30
J.L.	4.2 ± 0.6	246 ± 64	28
Mean ± SD	2.9 ± 0.6[c]	239 ± 51	23 ± 5
More than 5.0 mg/day			
A.N.	7.1 ± 1.0	256 ± 117	23
M.A.	11.6 ± 0.2	307 ± 121	19
B.H.	12.0 ± 0.5	298 ± 106	28
S.S.	12.3 ± 0.4	258 ± 44	26
C.M.	12.5 ± 0.5	454 ± 105	43
Mean ± SD	11.1 ± 2.0	314 ± 52	28 ± 8

[a]Mean ± SD of at least 3 days per subject and includes both dietary and extra-dietary sources of vitamin B_6.
[b]Mean ± SD of five or more milk samples per subject.
[c]Means significantly different ($p < 0.01$) from those of subjects with vitamin B_6 intakes > 5.0 mg/day.
[d]Means significantly different ($p < 0.01$) from those of subjects with vitamin B_6 intakes of 2.5 to 5.0 mg/day.

Changes in the level of vitamin B_6 intake had a marked influence on the vitamin B_6 content in milk. Subjects consuming the lowest intake of vitamin B_6 (<2.5 mg/day) had the lowest mean level of vitamin B_6 in milk, 129 ± 37 μg/l. This level was significantly lower ($p < 0.01$) than the means of the other two groups but was slightly higher than the average level for human milk, 100 μg/l of vitamin B_6 reported by some investigators (Karlin, 1959; Coursin, 1955b). However, investigators are not in agreement regarding the average level of the vitamin in human milk or the vitamin B_6 needs of the young infant. Hassinen *et al.* (1954) reported that the average level of vitamin B_6 in human milk was 130 $\mu g/l$ and that this level of vitamin appeared adequate for metabolism in the infant. Two subjects in this study had levels less than 130 $\mu g/l$; one of these had a level of only 67 $\mu g/l$. Bessey (1957) reported that the infant needs an intake of not less than 200 μg of vitamin B_6 daily and that infants receiving milk containing less than 100 μg of vitamin B_6 per liter may develop convulsions. The vitamin B_6 allowance (Food and Nutrition Board, 1974) for the infant 0–6 months of age is 300 μg daily and for infants 6–12 months of age, 400 μg daily. In this study, the vitamin B_6 content in milk of subjects with low intakes of vitamin B_6 (<2.5 mg/day) did not provide the level of vitamin B_6 recommended for the infant by Bessey (1957) or by the Food and Nutrition Board (1974). However, in this study the six infants who possibly received low or inadequate levels of vitamin B_6 from their mother's milk were consuming additional foods that would have contributed to the total vitamin B_6 intake.

The groups consuming 2.5–5.0 mg/day or greater than 5.0 mg/day of vitamin B_6 had mean levels of 239 ± 51 and 314 ± 52 μg of vitamin B_6 per liter of milk, respectively. Values of these two groups were not significantly different statistically but were approximately 2 times that of the group consuming the low level of vitamin B_6 intake. The findings indicated that intakes of vitamin B_6 2 to 5 times the RDA did not result in a significant increase in the level of the vitamin in milk compared to values for subjects whose intakes approximated the allowance. However, the individual (C.M.) with the highest vitamin B_6 intake among the subjects in this study also had the highest level of vitamin B_6 in milk, 454 $\mu g/l$.

The mean vitamin B_6/protein ratio of 13 ± 5 $\mu g/g$ for the group of subjects with the lowest intake of vitamin B_6 was significantly lower ($p < 0.01$) than values for the groups with higher intakes. Ratios of 23 ± 5 and 28 ± 8 $\mu g/g$ observed for groups receiving 2.5–5.0 and greater than 5.0 μg of vitamin B_6 daily, respectively, were not significantly different (Table 15-2). In order to satisfy the metabolic requirements of infants a vitamin B_6/protein ratio of 15 $\mu g/g$ has been recommended. In this study four of the six subjects consuming less than 2.5 μg of vitamin B_6 had ratios of vitamin B_6/protein in milk of less than 15 $\mu g/g$.

A significant ($p < 0.01$) correlation ($r = 0.65$) was observed between the level of vitamin B_6 intake (milligrams per day) and the level of the vitamin in milk (micrograms per liter). Because the levels of vitamin B_6 in milk plateaued at levels of intake exceeding 5.0 mg/day, the correlation was also determined for vitamin B_6 intakes ranging from 1.3 to 4.2 mg/day and the content of the vitamin in milk. The correlation coefficient ($r = 0.74$) was statistically significant ($p < 0.01$) and was slightly greater than that obtained when the higher levels of vitamin B_6 intake were included in the computation.

Vitamin B₆ Content in Milk on Different Days and Weeks

Milk samples collected by 13 subjects prior to the early morning feeding were also analyzed for vitamin B_6 content (Table 15-3). Subjects were divided into supplemented and unsupplemented groups, depending on whether or not an extra-dietary source of vitamin B_6 was taken. The mean intake of vitamin B_6 per day for the supplemented subjects was 7.5 ± 1.1 mg and was significantly greater ($p < 0.05$) than that for the unsupplemented group, 2.2 ± 0.47 mg/day.

No significant differences were found among the mean levels of vitamin B_6 in milk on different days and weeks for either the supplemented or unsupplemented groups. The results indicated that day-to-day and week-to-week variations of the vitamin B_6 content in milk were small for milk collected prior to the first feeding in early morning. However, means for the supplemented groups for daily, weekly, and daily and weekly combined values were significantly higher ($p < 0.01$) than values for unsupplemented subjects. These findings are consistent with other observations made in this study, i.e., the total amount of vitamin B_6 consumed daily markedly influenced the level of the vitamin in milk.

Diurnal Patterns of Vitamin B₆ Content in Milk

The diurnal patterns of vitamin B_6 content in milk for five women in the early stages of lactation (3 weeks to 3½ months) were also determined. The mean vitamin B_6 content in 50 samples of milk from the five subjects was 207 ± 99 µg/l. No significant differences were observed in the mean values of vitamin B_6 content in milk of these five subjects, grouped according to six different times of feeding on 2 consecutive days (Figure 15-1). Hytten (1954) made similar observations in the constancy in protein levels in human milk. However, individual variation was observed in the vitamin B_6 content in milk during the day. Subjects A.N. and J.L., who were taking vitamin B_6 supplements, demonstrated marked diurnal changes in the vitamin B_6 content in milk (Figure 15-2). Minimal and maximal values ranged from 100 to 447 and 172 to 340 µg of vitamin B_6 per liter of milk for subjects A.N. and J.L.,

TABLE 15-3 Vitamin B_6 Content in Milk from the Early Morning Feeding on Different Days and Weeks of Vitamin B_6 Supplemented and Unsupplemented Subjects

| | Vitamin B_6 Intake | | | Vitamin B_6, $\mu g/l$ | | | | | | | | Days + Weeks |
| | | | | Day | | | | Week | | | | |
Subjects	Diet	Supplement, mg/day	Total	1	2	3	Mean ± SD	1	2	3	Mean ± SD	Mean ± SD
Supplemented												
C.M.	1.5	11.0	12.5	522	314	556	464 ± 131	522	504	372	466 ± 82	454 ± 105
S.S.	2.3	10.0	12.3	250	236	304	263 ± 36	250	300	200	250 ± 50	258 ± 44
B.H.	2.0	10.0	12.0	266	184	309	253 ± 64	266	263	470	333 ± 118	298 ± 106
M.A.	1.6	10.0	11.6	212	189	337	246 ± 80	212	302	493	335 ± 143	307 ± 121
E.G.	2.6	0.9	3.5	248	451	197	299 ± 134	248	375	469	364 ± 111	348 ± 121
E.B.	1.8	1.0	2.8	210	193	230	211 ± 19	210	150	157	172 ± 33	188 ± 34
L.K.	1.7	1.0	2.7	143	210	220	191 ± 42	143	233	300	225 ± 79	221 ± 56
J.O.	1.2	1.0	2.2	82	136	127	115 ± 29	82	163	233	159 ± 75	148 ± 56
Mean			7.5[a]	242[b,c]	239[b]	285[b]	257 ± 115[b]	242[b,c]	286[b]	338[b]	288 ± 127[b]	278 ± 121[b]
± SD			4.5	129	100	129		129	115	133		
Unsupplemented												
L.F.	2.7	—	2.7	242	275	269	262 ± 18	242	213	236	230 ± 15	247 ± 25
C.D.	2.5	—	2.5	131	159	209	166 ± 40	131	156	242	176 ± 58	179 ± 45
J.G.	2.2	—	2.2	68	91	131	97 ± 32	68	127	86	94 ± 30	101 ± 27
M.P.	2.0	—	2.0	156	128	124	136 ± 17	—	—	—		136 ± 17
B.M.	1.5	—	1.5	120	180	213	171 ± 47	120	200	172	164 ± 41	177 ± 36
Mean			2.2	143[c]	167	189	168 ± 64	140[c]	174	184	166 ± 61	170 ± 59
± SD			0.5	64	69	61		73	40	73		

[a]Means significantly different from those of unsupplemented subjects, $p < 0.05$.
[b]Means significantly different from those of unsupplemented subjects, $p < 0.01$.
[c]Means in rows are not significantly different.

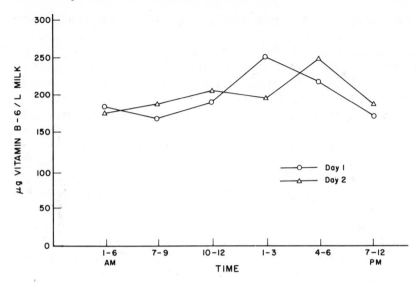

FIGURE 15-1   Mean diurnal patterns of vitamin B_6 content in milk from five subjects.

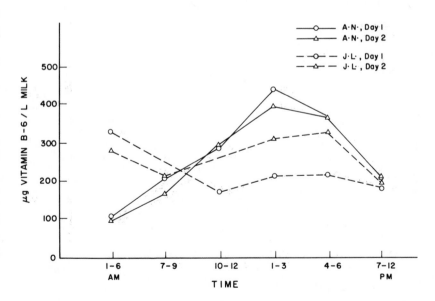

FIGURE 15-2   Diurnal patterns of vitamin B_6 content in milk from subjects A.N. and J.L.

respectively. The changes in levels of vitamin B_6 content in milk were associated with the time elapsed between vitamin ingestion and its appearance in the milk. This is in agreement with the findings of Karlin (1959) that high levels of orally and intramuscularly administered vitamin B_6 produced rapid increases in the vitamin B_6 content in the milk within 3 h after the administration.

Two subjects, M.F. and P.Y., who were not taking vitamin B_6 supplements, also showed some diurnal fluctuation in the vitamin B_6 content in milk (Figure 15-3), but the peak in vitamin content in midafternoon did not occur as was observed in the subjects taking vitamin B_6 supplements (Figure 15-4). Values for subject P.Y. ranged from 38 to 111 μg of vitamin B_6 per liter milk (Figure 15-3) with a mean of 67 μg and a mean vitamin B_6/protein ratio of only 5 μg/g. This subject's dietary intake of vitamin B_6 was only 1.5 mg/day, and she was not taking any extra-dietary sources of the vitamin. The infant of subject P.Y. was reported by the mother to have suffered mild periodic seizures at birth, diagnosed as resulting from hypoglycemia. The mother had used oral contraceptives for a period of 3½ years prior to pregnancy, and this in addition to the low level of dietary pyridoxine could have interfered with the coenzyme functions of pyridoxal phosphate (Miller *et al.*, 1974; Leklem *et al.*, 1975) resulting in a pyridoxine deficiency that was reflected in milk.

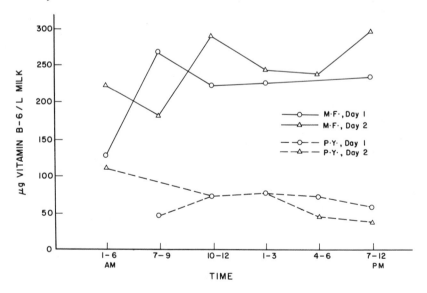

FIGURE 15-3   Diurnal patterns of vitamin B_6 content in milk from subjects M.F. and P.Y.

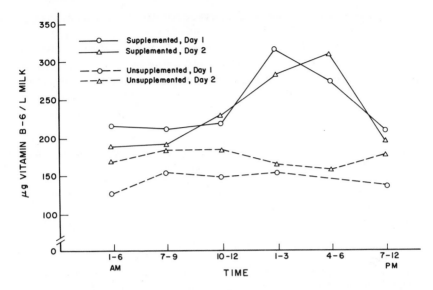

FIGURE 15-4   Diurnal patterns of vitamin B_6 content in milk from vitamin B_6 supplemented and unsupplemented subjects. Supplements were taken at approximately 10 a.m.

Results from this study indicated that dietary sources of vitamin B_6 can be inadequate for lactation, and this is reflected in low levels of the vitamin in milk.

SUMMARY

The influence of the level of vitamin B_6 intake on the content of the vitamin in milk was studied in 19 healthy subjects whose stages of lactation ranged from 3 weeks to 30 months. Total vitamin B_6 intakes, including extra-dietary sources of the vitamin, ranged from 1.3 to 12.5 mg/day with six subjects consuming less than the recommended allowance of 2.5 mg/day (RDA, 1974). Subjects consuming less than 2.5 mg/day of vitamin B_6 had significantly less vitamin B_6 per liter of milk (129 μg) than did groups consuming 2.5–5.0 mg/day or more (239 and 314 μg, respectively). Among subjects consuming more than 2.5 mg/day of vitamin the stage of lactation did not influence the levels of protein or vitamin B_6 in milk. Vitamin B_6 intakes 2 to 5 times the recommended allowance did not significantly elevate the level of the vitamin in milk in comparison to values for subjects whose intakes approximated the allowance. The vitamin B_6/protein ratio in milk of subjects consuming less than 2.5 mg/day vitamin B_6 was 13 μg/g and was significantly lower than that observed for the other two groups (23 and 28 μg/g). Daily and weekly variations of the vitamin B_6 and protein content in milk of individuals were small. However, marked diurnal variations in the vitamin B_6 content were found in milk of individuals taking daily supplements of the vitamin with peak levels occurring in the afternoon 3 to 5 h after supplements were taken in the morning.

LITERATURE CITED

Bessey, O. A. 1957. Intake of vitamin B_6 and infantile convulsions: A first approximation of requirements of pyridoxine in infants. Pediatrics 20:33–44.

Brin, M., and V. F. Thiele. 1967. Relationships between vitamin B_6 vitamer content and the activities of two transaminase enzymes in rat tissues at varying intake levels of vitamin B_6. J. Nutr. 93:213–221.

Burke, B. 1947. The dietary history as a tool in research. J. Am. Diet. Assoc. 23:1044–1046.

Coursin, D. B. 1954. Convulsive seizures in infants with pyridoxine-deficient diets. J. Am. Med. Assoc. 154:406–408.

Coursin, D. B. 1955a. Vitamin B_6 deficiency in infants. Am. J. Dis. Child. 90:344–348.

Coursin, D. B. 1955b. Vitamin B_6 (pyridoxine) in milk. Q. Rev. Pediatr. 10:2–9.

Food and Nutrition Board. 1974. Recommended Dietary Allowances, 8th ed., National Academy of Sciences, Washington, D.C.

Hassinen, J. B., G. T. Durbin, and F. W. Bernhard. 1954. The vitamin B_6 content of milk products. J. Nutr. 53:249–258.

Hytten, F. E. 1954. Clinical and chemical studies in human lactation. III. Diurnal variation in major constituents of milk. Br. Med. J. 1:179–183.

Karlin, R. 1959. Effet d'un enrichissement en pyridoxine sur la teneur en vitamine B_6 du lait de femme. Bull. Soc. Chim. Biol. 41:1085–1091.

Leklem, J. E., R. R. Brown, D. P. Rose, H. Linkswiler and R. A. Arend. 1975. Metabolism of tryptophan and niacin in oral contraceptive users receiving controlled intakes of vitamin B_6. Am. J. Clin. Nutr. 28:146–156.

Lowry, O. H., N. J. Rosebrough, A. L. Farr, and R. J. Randall. 1951. Protein measurement with the folin phenol reagent. J. Biol. Chem. 192:265–274.

Miller, L. T., E. M. Benson, M. A. Edwards, and J. Young. 1974. Vitamin B_6 metabolism in women using oral contraceptives. Am. J. Clin. Nutr. 27:797–805.

Molony, C. J., and A. H. Parmelee. 1954. Convulsions in young infants as a result of pyridoxine deficiency. J. Am. Med. Assoc. 154:405–406.

Orr, M. L. 1969. Pantothenic acid, vitamin B_6 and vitamin B_{12} in foods. U.S. Dep. Agric. Home Econ. Res. Rep. No. 36.

Pang, R. L., and A. Kirksey. 1974. Early postnatal changes in brain composition in progeny of rats fed different levels of dietary pyridoxine. J. Nutr. 104:111–117.

Snyderman, S. E., E. Holt, R. Carretero, and K. Jacobs. 1953. Pyridoxine deficiency in the human infant. Am. J. Clin. Nutr. 1:200–207.

Steel, R. D., and J. H. Torrie. 1960. Principles and Procedures of Statistics. McGraw-Hill, New York, p. 453.

Storvick, C. A., E. M. Benson, M. A. Edwards, and M. J. Woodring. 1964. Chemical and microbiological determination of vitamin B_6. Methods Biochem. Anal. 12:184–235.

Thiele, V. F., and M. Brin. 1966. Chromatographic separation and microbiologic assay of vitamin B₆ in tissues from normal and vitamin B₆ depleted rats. J. Nutr. *90*:347–353.

Thomas, M. R., and A. Kirksey. 1976. Influence of pyridoxine supplementation on vitamin B₆ levels in milk of rats deficient in the vitamin. J. Nutr. *106*:509–514.

Toepfer, E. W., and M. M. Polansky. 1970. Microbiological assay of vitamin B₆ and its components. J. Assoc. Offic. Agric. Chem. *53*:546–550.

U.S. Department of Agriculture. 1964. Nutritive value of foods. Home and Garden Bull. No. 72 (revised ed.).

16

Vitamin B$_6$ Status
of the Elderly

JUDY A. DRISKELL

We have examined several biochemical and behavioral parameters for the evaluation of vitamin B$_6$ status and requirements of rats. Driskell and Kirksey (1971) utilized the parameters alanine aminotransferase (EC 2.6.1.2; L-Alanine : 2-oxoglutarate aminotransferase) activities of liver and erythrocytes; brain and liver weights and DNA, RNA, and protein contents; liver polysomal activity; brain ribosomal activity; and body weight in the assessment of vitamin B$_6$ requirements of pregnant and nonpregnant rats. Alanine aminotransferase activities, protein content, RNA content, and polysomal activity had the highest correlations with the level of vitamin B$_6$ intake as determined by the eta coefficient. However, higher levels of vitamin intake were necessary in order for a plateau to be reached with alanine aminotransferase activity and protein content than with the other measurements; these two criteria were thought to be the more sensitive indicators of vitamin B$_6$ requirement. An eta coefficient of 0.706 ($p < 0.01$) for erythrocyte alanine aminotransferase activity and vitamin B$_6$ intake of nonpregnant female rats was obtained. General activity, curiosity, maze learning, brain pyridoxal phosphate and nucleic acid composition, brain glutamate decarboxylase (EC 4.1.1.15; L-Glutamate 1-carboxy-lase), and pyridoxal kinase (EC 2.7.1.35; ATP : pyridoxal 5-phosphotransferase) activities and erythrocyte alanine aminotransferase activity with and without additional coenzyme were used as parameters in determining the vitamin B_6 requirement of male rats (Driskell *et al.*, 1973; Driskell and Chuang, 1974). The alanine aminotransferase activity measurements and the general activity and curiosity scores seemed to be the most sensitive indicators of the vitamin B_6 requirement. Coenzyme stimulation of erythrocyte alanine aminotransferase activity seemed to be as sensitive an indicator of vitamin B_6 requirements of rats as their organ protein contents and their behavior patterns. Organ protein content probably affects the vitamin B_6 requirement in much the same way that protein intake affects this vitamin's metabolism. Hence, in our research with humans, erythrocyte alanine aminotransferase activity, with and without additional coenzyme, has been used as the indicator of vitamin B_6 inadequacy.

The vitamin B_6 status of 17 males and 20 females above age 60 and living in Montgomery County, Virginia, was determined during September and October of 1975 by using the parameter coenzyme stimulation of erythrocyte alanine aminotransferase activity (method of Tonhazy *et al.*, 1950, as modified by Heddle *et al.*, 1963, and Driskell *et al.*, 1971). The procedure of Raica and Sauberlich (1964) was used in the determination of coenzyme stimulation of enzymatic activity. The mean age of the males was 70.7 yr and of females 72.7 yr. The subjects were volunteers and were in apparent good health. Informed consent was obtained from the subjects.

No significant differences between males and females were observed with respect to basal erythrocyte alanine aminotransferase activities or coenzyme stimulation of the enzyme activity.

A trained dietary interviewer obtained 24-h recalls of food consumption from the subjects; food models and cross-checking were used to increase the efficiency of the subjects' recalls. The recall questionnaire was fashioned after that of Burke (1947), the American Public Health Association's *Nutritional Assessment in Health Programs* (Christakis, 1973), and the recent Ten-State Nutrition Survey (U.S. Department of Health, Education and Welfare, 1969). Consecutive 2-day food records were also obtained from the subjects. The reported kilocalorie, protein, and vitamin B_6 intakes of the subjects over the 3 consecutive days of record keeping were determined by using values given by Agriculture Handbook No. 8 (Watt and Merrill, 1963) and other sources (Orr, 1969; Meder and Wiss, 1968; Polansky *et al.*, 1964; Toepfer *et al.*, 1963; Polansky, 1969; Meyer *et al.*, 1969; and Polansky and Murphy, 1966).

No significant differences were observed between data obtained by the 24-h recall technique compared to the 2-day food record; hence, the data were combined. Subjects of both sexes consumed slightly fewer kilocalories, much more protein, and much less vitamin B_6 than the RDA (Food and Nutrition Board, 1974). Almost half of the females and one fifth of the males reported consuming less than 50 percent of the RDA for vitamin B_6; 90 percent of the females and almost half of the males reported consuming less than 70 percent of the RDA for the vitamin.

Vitamin B_6 nutriture as reflected by enzyme data in the present study was not significantly affected by sex, age, income, educational level, food budget, preparation of own food, frequency of eating out, growing of own vegetables, or vitamin supplementation. Subjects reported that these dietary records were typical of their normal food consumption patterns.

Rose et al. (1973) repleted 20 females by pyridoxine administration for 4 weeks; the percent coenzyme stimulation of erythrocyte alanine aminotransferase activity was 8 ± 5 ($\overline{X} \pm$ SD). Woodring and Storvick (1970) repleted 7 females with pyridoxine hydrochloride for 7 days and obtained percent coenzyme stimulation values ranging from 7.1 to about 14.6. The in vitro stimulation of enzymatic activity of well-nourished individuals seems to be comparatively low, <12 or 14 percent.

Table 16-1 relates percent coenzyme stimulation values to reported vitamin B_6 intakes of the subjects. Nonsignificant Pearson r and eta

TABLE 16-1 Percent Coenzyme Stimulation Versus Reported Vitamin B_6 Intake

	Vitamin B_6 Intake, mg									
	Males						Females			
Percent Stimulation	0.41–0.8	0.81–1.2	1.21–1.6	1.61–2.0	2.01–2.4	2.41–2.8	0.41–0.8	0.81–1.2	1.21–1.6	1.61–2.0
>24							(2)			
20.1–24			(1)				(1)	(1)		
16.1–20									(1)	
12.1–16		(1)	(1)		(1)		(1)			
8.1–12			(1)	(1)				(3)		(1)
4.1– 8	(1)		(3)	(3)				(4)		
0 – 4		(4)					(1)	(1)	(4)	

Numbers in parentheses indicate number of subjects.

coefficients were obtained when enzyme data were correlated with the vitamin B_6 intakes of the subjects. One third of the subjects were found to have inadequate vitamin B_6 status as indicated by coenzyme stimulation measurements of <12 or 14 percent. Subjects with values near zero percent stimulation had varying vitamin B_6 intakes, thus perhaps indicating the large individual variations in vitamin B_6 requirements. Note that only two males reported consuming as much as 2.0 mg, the recommended dietary allowance for vitamin B_6; most subjects reported consuming much lower quantities of the vitamin.

Other investigators have determined the vitamin B_6 status of the elderly. Ranke *et al.* (1960) have reported that the elderly have lower serum aspartate aminotransferase (EC 2.6.1.1; L-Aspartate : 2-oxoglutarate aminotransferase) activity and higher xanthurenic acid excretion levels than those of younger subjects. Hamfelt (1964) observed lower pyridoxal phosphate levels in the plasma of older subjects as compared to those of younger men. A negative correlation of erythrocyte alanine aminotransferase activity with age was reported by Jacobs *et al.* (1968). A negative correlation of plasma pyridoxal phosphate levels with age was observed by Rose *et al.* (1974).

Vitamin B_6 inadequacy appears to be a nutritional problem in the elderly.

LITERATURE CITED

Burke, B. S. 1947. The dietary history as a tool in research. J. Am. Diet. Assoc. *23*:1041–1046.

Christakis, G. (ed.). 1973. Nutritional Assessment in Health Programs. Am. J. Public Health Suppl. *63*:1–82.

Driskell, J. A., and S. L. Chuang. 1974. Relationship between glutamate decarboxylase activities in brains and the vitamin B_6 requirement of male rats. J. Nutr. *104*:1657–1661.

Driskell, J. A., and A. Kirksey. 1971. The cellular approach to the determination of pyridoxine requirements in pregnant and nonpregnant rats. J. Nutr. *101*:661–668.

Driskell, J. A., J. H. Wiley, and A. Kirksey. 1971. Alanine aminotransferase activity in liver and erythrocytes of pregnant and nonpregnant rats fed different levels of pyridoxine. J. Nutr. *101*:85–91.

Driskell, J. A., L. A. Strickland, C. H. Poon, and D. P. Foshee. 1973. The vitamin B_6 requirement of the male rat as determined by behavioral patterns, brain pyridoxal phosphate and nucleic acid composition and erythrocyte alanine aminotransferase activity. J. Nutr. *103*:670–680.

Food and Nutrition Board. 1974. Recommended Dietary Allowances, 8th ed., National Academy of Sciences, Washington, D.C. pp. 1–20, 25–48, 74–77.

Hamfelt, A. 1964. Age variation of vitamin B_6 metabolism in man. Clin. Chim. Acta *10*:48–54.

Heddle, J. G., E. W. McHenry, and G. H. Beaton. 1963. Penicillamine and vitamin B_6 interrelationships in the rat. Can. J. Biochem. Physiol. *41*:1215–1222.

Jacobs, A., I. A. J. Cavill, and J. N. P. Hughes. 1968. Erythrocyte transaminase activity: Effect of age, sex, and vitamin B_6 supplementation. Am. J. Clin. Nutr. *21*:502–507.

Meder, H., and O. Wiss. 1968. Vitamin B_6 group. V. Occurrence in foods. *In* W. H. Sebrell, Jr., and R. S. Harris (eds.). The Vitamins: Chemistry, Physiology, Pathology, Methods, Academic Press, New York, pp. 21–29.

Meyer, B. H., M. A. Mysinger, and L. A. Wodarski. 1969. Pantothenic acid and vitamin B_6 in beef. J. Am. Diet. Assoc. *54*:122–125.

Orr, M. L. 1969. Pantothenic acid, vitamin B_6 and vitamin B_{12} in foods. U.S. Dep. Agric. Home Econ. Res. Rep. No. 36: 53 pp.

Polansky, M. M. 1969. Vitamin B_6 components in fresh and dried vegetables. J. Am. Diet. Assoc. *54*:118–121.

Polansky, M. M., and E. W. Murphy. 1966. Vitamin B_6 components in fruits and nuts. J. Am. Diet. Assoc. *48*:109–111.

Polansky, M. M., E. W. Murphy, and E. W. Toepfer. 1964. Components of vitamin B_6 in grains and cereal products. J. Assoc. Off. Agric. Chem. *47*:750–753.

Raica, N., and H. E. Sauberlich. 1964. Blood cell transaminase activity in human vitamin B_6 deficiency. Am. J. Clin. Nutr. *15*:67–72.

Ranke, E., S. A. Tauber, A. Horonick, B. Ranke, R. S. Goodhart, and B. F. Chow. 1960. Vitamin B_6 deficiency in the aged. J. Gerontol. *15*:41–44.

Rose, C. S., P. Gyorgy, H. Spiegel, M. Brin, M. Butler, and N. W. Shock. 1974. Vitamin B_6 status of American adult males. Proc. Am. Soc. Exper. Biol. *33*:697 (Abstract).

Rose, D. P., R. Strong, J. Folkard, and P. W. Adams. 1973. Erythrocyte aminotransferase activities in women using oral contraceptives and the effect of vitamin B_6 supplementation. Am. J. Clin. Nutr. *26*:48–52.

Toepfer, E. W., M. M. Polansky, L. R. Richardson, and S. Wilkes. 1963. Comparison of vitamin B_6 values of selected food samples by bioassay and microbiological assay. J. Agric. Food Chem. *11*:523–525.

Tonhazy, N. E., N. G. White, and W. W. Umbreit. 1950. A rapid method for the estimation of glutamic aspartic transaminase in tissues and its application to radiation sickness. Arch. Biochem. *28*:36–46.

U.S. Department of Health, Education and Welfare. 1969. National Nutrition Survey Guidelines and Procedures. Regional Medical Programs Service, Division of Chronic Disease Programs—Nutrition Program, pp. 111–156.

Watt, B. K., and A. L. Merrill. 1963. Composition of Foods—Raw, Processed, Prepared. U.S. Dep. Agric. Agric. Handb. No. 8: 190 pp.

Woodring, M. J., and C. A. Storvick. 1970. Effect of pyridoxine supplementation on glutamic-pyruvic transaminase and *in vitro* stimulation in erythrocytes of normal women. Am. J. Clin. Nutr. *23*:1385–1395.

17

Vitamin B$_6$ Requirements of Infants and Children

ERNEST E. MCCOY

The concept of requirement for vitamin B$_6$ in this paper is the amount of vitamin B$_6$ that will result in optimal growth, development, and function of children. Optimal growth and function should occur when amounts of the vitamin present in body tissues are adequate to catalyze at appropriate rates vitamin B$_6$-dependent reactions. The more direct the measurement of vitamin B$_6$ function, the more likely it will represent an accurate estimate of vitamin B$_6$ requirements. Conversely, the more indirect the method used to determine vitamin B$_6$ reactions, the more likely non-vitamin B$_6$-dependent biochemical reactions will influence the results. Although direct measurements of B$_6$ vitamins in tissue would be the best procedure, indirect tests, such as the excretion of tryptophan metabolities, give general estimates of vitamin B$_6$ requirements that are of value.

A survey of studies on vitamin B$_6$ requirements of infants and children shows that there are only limited experimental data on which current recommendations are based. The Recommended Dietary Allowances, 8th edition, of the National Academy of Sciences (Food and Nutrition Board, 1974) states that "data are not sufficient to permit an

257

evaluation of the requirements for children and adolescents.'' The available data on which present recommendations are based were evaluated and compared to (1) the approximate vitamin B_6 content of average food intakes of infants and (2) the vitamin B_6 requirements related to protein intake of children. A proposal is presented that is directed toward establishment of a data base that will allow accurate estimates of vitamin B_6 requirements in infants and children in health and disease.

THE BASIS FOR ESTIMATING THE REQUIREMENTS FOR VITAMIN B_6 IN INFANTS AND CHILDREN IN RELATION TO PROTEIN INTAKE

A number of studies have been done in adult men and women that have experimentally determined vitamin B_6 requirements (Baker et al., 1964; Canham et al., 1969; Cinnamon and Beaton, 1970; Miller and Linkswiler, 1967). These studies have generally been of the design in which individuals were placed on vitamin B_6-restricted diets with varying amounts of protein until biochemical evidence of vitamin B_6 deficiency was present. The principal test used was the excretion of xanthurenic acid following a tryptophan load. After a period of depletion, various amounts of pyridoxine were added to the diet and xanthurenic acid excretion following a test dose of tryptophan was determined. The amount of vitamin B_6 that normalized xanthurenic acid excretion was judged to be an adequate intake of the vitamin. The amounts of vitamin B_6 required on varying protein intakes to normalize biochemical tests of vitamin B_6 function were then used in determining the recommended allowances of vitamin B_6 in adults (Food and Nutrition Board, 1974; Information Canada, 1975). The amount was determined to be 0.026 mg of pyridoxine per gram of protein intake.

A careful survey of the literature failed to reveal experimental studies linking vitamin B_6 requirements to protein intake in infants or children. Considerable metabolic differences in respect to growth and protein requirements exist between infants and young adults. Though the recommended amounts may be adequate for this age group, they are based on the assumption that vitamin B_6 requirements in relation to protein intake will be similar in infants and children and in young adults. Because of limitations of human experimentation, it will be very difficult to determine vitamin B_6 requirements in infants by methods similar to those used for adults.

EXPERIMENTAL STUDIES TO DETERMINE VITAMIN B_6 REQUIREMENTS IN INFANTS AND CHILDREN

There have been two studies (Snyderman *et al*., 1953; Bessey *et al*., 1957) that have attempted to define the vitamin B_6 requirements of infants. In one study, two children were placed on a vitamin B_6-deficient diet. In the second study, the amount of pyridoxine required to normalize vitamin B_6 function was determined following accidental deprivation of the vitamin.

In the study of Snyderman *et al*. (1953), two infants aged 2 months and 8 months (both with severe cerebral abnormalities) were placed on a vitamin B_6-free diet. The depletion study was followed by determination of 4-pyridoxic acid and pyridoxine content in 24-h urine samples. Clinical status of the infants was monitored by nurses and physicians. Biochemical status was determined by routine laboratory tests during the study period.

For baseline studies of 4-pyridoxic acid and pyridoxine excretion the two infants received their basic food plus a vitamin mixture containing 0.67 mg/day of pyridoxine hydrochloride. The infants were then placed on a vitamin B_6-free diet for a period of 76 days for one subject and 130 days for the other. Urinary excretion of 4-pyridoxic acid fell to zero in 10 days in one subject and in 30 days in the other. There was a very small continuing excretion of pyridoxine in both subjects that may have been due to the microbiological assay system detecting nonpyridoxine substances. Neither subject gained weight on the diet.

Listlessness occurred in the younger infant after 72 days on the diet, convulsions developed on the seventy-sixth day. After 2 hours of seizure activity, 50 mg of pyridoxine hydrochloride was given intravenously and marked improvement occurred within 3 hours. By the following morning, the infant appeared fully recovered. Weight gain resumed within a few days.

The older infant developed hematological abnormalities but no central nervous system signs. After 140 days of vitamin B_6 deprivation a severe hypochromic, microcytic anemia was present. The anemia did not respond to iron administration but responded promptly to 50 mg of pyridoxine by intravenous injection and daily oral administration of 1 mg of pyridoxine thereafter. This regimen resulted in marked urinary excretion of pyridoxine and 4-pyridoxic acids. Attempts were then made to determine the level of pyridoxine intake at which excretion of 4-pyridoxic acid and pyridoxine would reach levels observed during the control period. Incremental decreases to 0.5 mg, 0.25 mg, and 0.15 mg pyridoxine over a 50-day period did not decrease pyridoxine excretion to control values. Apparently, tissue stores of vitamin B_6 were saturated, and restriction of pyridoxine intake over the time period was not sufficient to produce a deficiency state as measured by this parameter. Thus, it was not possible to determine vitamin B_6 requirement by this method.

The second experimental study (Bessey *et al.*, 1957) of vitamin B_6 requirements in infancy reported the experience of (1) nine infants in whom convulsions appeared to be due to inadequate intake of vitamin B_6 and (2) results of tryptophan load test as a measure of adequacy of vitamin B_6 intake in 17 infants.

The infants studied were divided into four groups. Details of diet, vitamin B_6 intake, and clinical course are shown in Table 17-1. Group A included five infants, 1 to 4 months of age at the time of onset of symptoms, who had received a proprietary milk formulation in which the content of vitamin B_6 had been reduced accidentally as a result of the processing procedure. The principal symptoms and signs of these deficient infants were irritability and grand mal seizures. Milk, the only source of pyridoxine, provided only 85 μg/day. Two infants were relieved of seizures after a change of formula to an evaporated milk mixture and administration of an anticonvulsant; two other infants obtained relief after only changing the type of milk. The fifth infant stopped seizure activity prior to receiving vitamin supplements but improved in other clinical parameters with administration of pyridoxine. The calculated amount of pyridoxine required to stop seizures was 0.26 mg/day. Xanthurenic acid (XA) excretion, which reflects adequacy of tissue stores of vitamin B_6, was determined in one infant. The daily intake of pyridoxine required to prevent increased excretion of XA was 1.0 to 1.2 mg (Table 17-1).

Group B included two breast-fed infants who developed seizures that were relieved by administration of 0.26 mg/day of pyridoxine. Xanthurenic acid excretion was increased and 1.0 to 1.4 mg/day of pyridoxine was required to reduce XA excretion to normal values. Thus, the amount of pyridoxine required to normalize this biochemical test of vitamin B_6 function was considerably greater than that required to relieve convulsive activity.

Group C included two infants who apparently had an increased requirement for vitamin B_6. These infants required 2–5 mg/day of pyridoxine to relieve seizures. However, normalization of XA excretion was achieved in these infants with only 0.3-0.4 mg/day of pyridoxine.

In a control group of hospitalized infants without convulsive disorders, increased excretion of xanthurenic acid was prevented by an intake of 0.2 to 0.5 mg/day of pyridoxine in all but one infant who required 1.0 mg/day.

Using xanthurenic acid excretion as an indicator of the adequacy of vitamin B_6 intake, an intake of 0.3 to 0.4 mg/day of pyridoxine was adequate in 12 infants tested. However, in three infants, 1.0 to 1.4 mg/day of pyridoxine was necessary. Thus 20 percent of the study group required greater than the present recommended allowance to normalize XA excretion. On the basis of these data, consideration may need to be given to revision of the estimated requirement of vitamin B_6. This is of particular interest, since the RDA for adults from which those for infants and children were extrapolated were derived from the amount of pyridoxine necessary to normalize XA excretion on fixed levels of protein intake.

VITAMIN B_6 INTAKES IN BREAST- AND FORMULA-FED INFANTS IN RELATION TO PROTEIN INTAKE

As recommended allowances of vitamin B_6 for infants and children are based on 0.02 mg of pyridoxine per gram of protein, calculations were made of approximate vitamin B_6 intake per gram of protein intake in infants maintained on standard feeding regimens. A breast-fed infant weighing 3 kg would require 150 ml/kg of body weight or 450–500 ml of breast milk. Assuming an average vitamin B_6 content of 0.10 mg/l, the infant would receive 0.045–0.050 mg of vitamin B_6 predominantly as pyridoxal. The protein content (1.5 g/100 ml) would be approximately 6.7–7.5 g; thus, intake of vitamin B_6 in relation to protein intake would be 0.006 mg per gram of protein per day.

At 3 months of age an infant still receiving its total nutrition from breast milk would receive approximately 800 ml containing 8.1 g of protein and 0.080 mg of vitamin B_6. This would provide approximately 0.010 mg of vitamin B_6 per gram of protein intake. If cereal were added to provide an additional 0.5 g of protein, this would give an additional 0.027 mg of pyridoxine and provide 0.012 mg of vitamin B_6 per gram of protein. These figures are shown in Table 17-2.

A formula-fed infant weighing 3 kg with an intake of 450 ml would receive 11.2 g of protein, 0.18 mg of vitamin B_6, or 0.016 mg per gram of protein intake. At 3 months of age, if entirely on formula, vitamin B_6 intake in relation to protein would remain the same (Table 17-3), 0.016 mg per gram of protein. If cereal is added to provide 0.5 g of protein and 0.027 mg of pyridoxine, the intake of vitamin B_6 would increase to 0.017 mg per gram of protein. The infant at 1 year of age who is

TABLE 17-1 Summary of Biochemical Data Relative to the Nutritive Status of Vitamin B_6 in Infants with and without Convulsions

Group	Case No.	Diet	Vitamin B_6 Intake, mg/day	Vitamin B_6 Required to Relieve Convulsions, mg/day	Xanthurenic Acid Excretion, mg/18 h	Vitamin B_6 Required to Normalize Xanthurenic Acid Excretion, mg/day
			Convulsions Related to Intake of Vitamin B_6			
A	1	SMA	0.085	0.26^a	No test	No test
	2	SMA	0.085	0.26^a	No test	No test
	3	SMA	0.085	0.26^a	No test	No test
	4	SMA	0.085	0.26^a	8^b	No test
	5	SMA	0.085	0.26^a	20–63	1.0–1.2
			Breast Fed Infants			
B	6	Human milk	?	0.26^a	25–110	1.2–1.4
	7	Human milk	0.067	0.26^a	35–43	1.0
			Apparent Vitamin B_6 Dependent Seizures			
C	8	Evaporated milk and pureed foods	0.3–0.4	5	18	0.4
	9	Evaporated milk and pureed foods	0.3–0.4	2	0	

Nonvitamin B₆ Related Seizures

D	10	Evaporated milk	0.26	Ineffective	0	0.3–0.4
	10	SMA	0.085	Ineffective	35–40	0.3–0.4
	11	Evaporated milk and pureed foods	0.3–0.4	Ineffective	0	
	12	Evaporated milk and pureed foods	0.3–0.4	Ineffective	0	
		Control Group				
E	13	Evaporated milk	0.26		0	0.3–0.4
	13	SMA	0.085		30	0.3–0.4
	14	Evaporated milk	0.26		0	
	15	Evaporated milk	0.26		0	
	16	Evaporated milk and pureed foods	0.3–0.4		0	
	17	Mull-Soy	0.20		0	
	18	Evaporated milk	0.26		0	
	19	Fresh skim milk	0.50		0	
	20	Mull-Soy	0.20		53	5.0

Adapted from Bessey *et al.* (1957).

[a] Vitamin B₆ content of evaporated milk mixture is equal to 8 oz of evaporated milk, 12 oz of water, and 1/4 oz of Dextri-Maltose.

[b] After receiving 10 mg of pyridoxine hydrochloride daily for 3 days.

TABLE 17-2   Vitamin B$_6$ Intake of Breast-Fed Infants

Age	Milk Received, ml	Protein, (1.5–0.8 g/100 ml), g	Milk Vitamin B$_6$, μg	Other Sources Vitamin B$_6$, μg	Vitamin B$_6$/ Protein, mg/g
Birth	450	6.7	45	—	0.006
3 months	800	8.1	80		0.010
		8.1	80	27	0.012
		0.5[a]			
6 months	850	7.4	85	160	0.017
		7.0[b]			

[a]Three tablespoons (approximately 10 g) of rice cereal.
[b]Based on intake of cereal, meat, commercial prepared meat and vegetable, vegetable, and fruit. Calculations based on nutrient content from Orr (1969) and Fomon (1974).

consuming 30 oz of milk and table food will have an intake of approximately 0.8 mg of vitamin B$_6$. The observed protein intake of Canadian children, which is presumed to be similar to that of U.S. children age 1 to 15 years, was used to calculate the amount of vitamin B$_6$ required on the basis of 0.02 mg per gram of protein. The vitamin B$_6$ requirements are higher than the recommended allowances because protein intake is greater than recommended daily allowance for these age groups (Table 17-4).

RECOMMENDED DIETARY ALLOWANCES FOR VITAMIN B$_6$ IN RELATION TO BODY SURFACE AREA OF INFANTS

The current recommended dietary allowances for children vary with the age of the child. The recommended allowances were examined to

TABLE 17-3   Vitamin B$_6$ Intake of Formula-Fed Infants

Age	Milk Intake, ml	Protein (2.5 g/100 ml), g	Vitamin B$_6$ in Milk, μg	Other Sources Vitamin B$_6$, μg	Vitamin B$_6$/ Protein, mg/g
Birth	450	11.2	180	—	0.016
3 months	700	17.5	280	—	0.016
		17.5	280	27	0.017
		0.5[a]			
6 months	900	22.5	360	160	
		7.0[b]			0.01
1 yr	900	22.5	360	460	0.020
		18.5[c]			

[a]Three tablespoons (approximately 10 g) of rice cereal.
[b]Based on intake of commercial infant foods of meat, meat and vegetables, and fruit.
[c]Based on intake of table foods: cereal, meat, vegetables, and fruit. Calculations based on nutrient content from Orr (1969) and Church and Church (1975).

TABLE 17-4 Vitamin B₆ Requirements in Relation to Protein Intake

Age, yr	Daily Average Protein Intake,[a] g			Vitamin B₆ Requirement (0.02 mg/g protein), mg			U.S. Recommended Vitamin B₆ Allowance 1974, mg
	Both Sexes	Male	Female	Both Sexes	Male	Female	
1-3	47			0.94			0.6
4-6	64			1.28			0.9
7-9		79	70		1.58	1.40	1.2
10-12		89	73		1.78	1.46	1.6
13-15		96	74		1.96	1.48	2.0

[a]Based on average observed protein intake of Canadian children (courtesy, Dr. Elizabeth Donald). It is assumed that the protein intake would be similar to that of U.S. children.

determine if they paralleled the increase in mass of the child as represented by body surface area. The values in Table 17-5 show that for the
newborn the ratio derived from RDA for vitamin B_6 (in milligrams) per
body surface area (in square meters) is 1.5. The ratio decreases to 1.1 at
1 year of age, which reflects a doubling of body mass with a 50 percent
increase in RDA. By 9 years of age the ratio has increased to 1.6 compared to the adult value of 1.4. These calculations were made to determine if the increase in RDA for vitamin B_6 with age paralleled the
increase in body mass as reflected by body surface area. At no time
does the ratio fall below that of the adult and at most times is above that
of the adult value. By this parameter, the RDA is adequate for the
growing child.

PLASMA AND RED BLOOD CELL PYRIDOXAL PHOSPHATE VALUES IN CHILDREN AND ADULTS

The distribution of pyridoxal phosphate (PLP) between plasma and red
blood cells in normal children has been studied (Bhagavan *et al.*,
1975a). There is a considerable body of data on pyridoxal phosphate
levels in mother, fetus, and newborn but scanty data for older infants
and children collected in a systematic manner.

Cleary *et al.* (1975) showed that in nonpregnant women the average
plasma PLP value was 10.5 ng/ml. For pregnant women receiving 10
mg/day of pyridoxine it was 7.5 ng/ml, while for pregnant women receiving 2.0–2.5 mg/day of pyridoxine, the plasma PLP value was 3.7

TABLE 17-5   Relationship of Age, Surface Area, and Recommended
Vitamin B_6 Allowance, 1974[a]

Weight, kg	Approximate Age	Surface Area,[b] m²	Vitamin B_6, mg	Ratio Vitamin B_6/ BSA[c]
3	Newborn	0.2	0.3	1.5
6	3 months	0.3	0.4	1.3
10	1 yr	0.45	0.5	1.1
20	5.5 yr	0.8	1.0	1.2
30	9 yr	1.0	1.6	1.6
40	12 yr	1.3	2.0	1.5
50	14 yr	1.5	2.0	1.3
70	Adult	1.76	2.0	1.1

[a]Recommended Vitamin B_6 allowance from Food and Nutrition Board (1974).
[b]Body surface area from Kempe *et al.* (1976).
[c]BSA = body surface area.

ng/ml. The cord plasma PLP values for mothers given 10 mg/day of pyridoxine was 58.4 ng/ml and for mothers receiving 2.0–2.5 mg of pyridoxine, the cord plasma PLP was 37.1 ng/ml. Cord venous arterial PLP differences were measured and found to be 10.1 ng/ml, indicating efficient extraction by the fetus. The fetal plasma level of PLP was 3–5 times higher than the value for nonpregnant women, indicating that the fetuses of women who receive the recommended amount of 2.5 mg/day of pyridoxine probably have adequate stores of PLP at birth.

Hamfelt and Tuvemo (1972) studied plasma and erthrocyte PLP in mother and fetus who received varying intakes of pyridoxine. Women receiving no supplemental pyridoxine had plasma PLP values of 2.43 ng/ml, those receiving 2 mg/day of pyridoxine, 4.47 ng/ml, and those receiving 10 mg/day of pyridoxine, 8.9 ng/ml. Cord blood plasma PLP showed a corresponding increase of 7.68 ng for mothers receiving no supplement, 26.6 ng for those receiving 2.0 mg, and 30.4 ng/ml for 10 mg supplementation.

Contractor and Shane (1970) have shown that pyridoxine given to the mother is rapidly converted to PLP and crosses the placenta to the fetus in this form. Their studies suggested that low maternal PLP levels resulted from the large fetal uptake of vitamin B₆. The PLP content of blood from nonpregnant women who were not users of anovulatory steroids was 9.64 ng/ml.

Brophy and Siiteri (1975) found that cord plasma of infants from normal pregnancy contained 28.4 ng/ml PLP, while infants of pre-eclamptic mothers had 12.2 ng/ml. This suggests that infants of high-risk pregnancies may have suboptimal PLP stores at birth.

There are several studies of levels of PLP in normal children. Barlow and Wilkinson (1975) reported a plasma level of PLP of 16.3 ± 5.6 ng/ml in normal children. Bhagavan *et al.* (1975b) reported the plasma PLP level in control children to be 17.78 ± 3.59 ng/ml.

Bhagavan *et al.* (1973) obtained values of PLP in whole blood from children with Trisomy 2 from 1 to 17 years of age. The average value was 11.3 ng/ml. The plasma values for ages 2–19 years in children with Down's syndrome and hypokinesis have been reported to be 13.8 ng/ml PLP (Bhagavan *et al.*, 1975a). Hamfelt (1964) found that in the age range from birth to 1 year, the mean PLP content in plasma was 16.3 ng/ml. No values were reported between 1–20 years of age, but for 20–29 years of age the mean content was 11.3 ng/ml.

Young children who were burned and who received 0.25 mg of pyridoxine supplement in addition to their regular diet had plasma PLP levels 25 to 60 percent of those of controls (Barlow and Wilkinson, 1975). Supplementation with 250 mg/day of pyridoxine increased PLP well above normal plasma levels. This study illustrates the need to define requirements for children who are physically stressed.

Though limited data are available on normal plasma PLP values in children, there is no published report that could be found that relates those values to known pyridoxine intake. Such a study would be of considerable value in ascertaining whether current recommended vitamin B_6 intake based on 0.02 mg of pyridoxine per gram of protein results in normal plasma PLP values.

RED BLOOD CELL TRANSAMINASE ACTIVITY AND VITAMIN B_6 INTAKE

It has been noted in both animal and human studies that decreases in erythrocyte aminotransferase activity occur on vitamin B_6 deficient diets. Chen and Marlatt (1975) showed that in young rats fed varying intakes of pyridoxine there was increased activity of erythrocyte alanine aminotransferase activity at each increased level of pyridoxine intake. Further, at each level of intake when PLP was added *in vitro* there was an additional stimulation of enzyme activity. It was concluded that the apoenzyme of alanine aminotransferase is synthesized in excess of the amount of PLP available at all levels of pyridoxine intake. The coenzyme, not the apoenzyme, appears to be the limiting factor in erythrocyte alanine aminotransferase activity. Hamfelt (1967) studied human plasma and erythrocyte PLP levels and found the level of PLP from these two sources to be closely related. He noted that when aspartate aminotransferase activity was determined in the presence of excess PLP, the activity of the enzyme was higher when the initial PLP of erythrocytes was also high. He proposed that when PLP concentrations in circulating red blood cells are low, the total aminotransferase apoenzyme of newly formed red blood cells in bone marrow is also decreased. Raica and Sauberlich (1964) determined erythrocyte aminotransferase activity serially during pyridoxine depletion and repletion in adults on low- and high-protein diets. A progressive drop in erythrocyte alanine aminotransferase activity occurred during the depletion period and a corresponding increase in percent stimulation of enzyme activity on *in vitro* addition of PLP. Erythrocyte aminotransferase activity slowly increased during the vitamin B_6 repletion period, an increase accompanied by a corresponding decrease in percent stimulation of activity with *in vitro* addition of PLP to erythrocytes from subjects on the low-protein diet.

Baysal *et al.* (1966) studied plasma pyridoxal phosphate and erythrocyte aminotransferase activities during vitamin B_6 depletion and repletion. Their studies showed that after 25-days depletion plasma PLP levels were markedly reduced, and erythrocyte aminotransferase activity decreased. On repletion with 0.9 mg/day of pyridoxine there was no increase in plasma PLP values toward normal. However, supplementation with 50 mg of pyridoxine for 3 days increased PLP concentrations to levels above those prior to depletion.

Miletic *et al.* (1969) studied erythrocyte aminotransferase activity in normal infants, malnourished infants and infants receiving isoniazid. In normal children there was only 3 percent stimulation of erythrocyte aminotransferase activity on PLP addition. After 10 days of pyridoxine administration, there was an approximate 50 percent increase in enzyme activity and similar percent PLP stimulation. Malnourished infants had a lower erythrocyte aminotransferase activity but similar PLP stimulation as normal infants. Following pyridoxine administration, total aminotransferase activity was similar to that of normal infants, but percent stimulation of enzyme activity on addition of PLP was greater. Isoniazid-treated infants had a lower erythrocyte transaminase activity and a greatly increased stimulation of enzyme activity on PLP addition compared to that of normal infants. This suggests that these infants can synthesize the apoenzyme in excess of available PLP and may be functionally deficient in vitamin B₆. This study showed that significant decreases in erythrocyte aminotransferase activity occur in vitamin B₆ deficiency in children but PLP stimulation may be of limited value in detecting the degree of deficiency. It did not provide data that could be used in determination of vitamin B₆ requirements.

Shane and Contractor (1975) studied whole blood PLP levels and erythrocyte aspartate aminotransferase activation tests as indicators of vitamin B₆ status in control, anovulatory steroid users, and pregnant women. Their studies indicated that the erythrocyte aspartate aminotransferase activation test was a poor indicator of vitamin B₆ status except in pronounced deficiency. The level of whole blood PLP was a less variable and more reliable indicator of vitamin B₆ status.

CONCLUSIONS

Examination of the existing literature indicates that the current recommended dietary allowances for vitamin B₆ in infants and children are based on a very limited experimental data base. Recommended dietary allowances for adults, which tie the vitamin B₆ requirements to protein intake, have been extrapolated to calculate the recommended requirements for children. Although the current recommended dietary allowances are probably adequate, they are not based on studies carried out in children who have significantly different metabolic requirements compared to adults. It is important that studies be undertaken to determine the actual requirements for vitamin B_6 for infants and children, since the information on which present recommended requirements are based is inadequate.

Erythrocyte aminotransferase activities decrease with vitamin B_6 deficiency and increase with vitamin B_6 excess. The decrease in aminotransferase activity with vitamin B_6 deficiency and the increased percent stimulation with *in vitro* pyridoxal phosphate addition appear to be good indicators of vitamin B_6 deficiency. However, there is considerable variation in enzyme activity and percent stimulation by *in vitro* pyridoxal phosphate addition among individuals. Although it is useful for the detection of vitamin B_6 deficiency, it does not appear at the present time that this parameter will be useful in determining vitamin B_6 requirements for infants and children.

When pyridoxine or pyridoxal is ingested in physiological amounts, plasma pyridoxal phosphate levels reflect the pyridoxal phosphate level in red blood cells and liver. Thus direct measurement of plasma pyridoxal phosphate would appear to be a good indicator of adequacy of vitamin B_6 intake. Direct measurements of plasma pyridoxal phosphate in children of varying ages need to be carried out on known intakes of vitamin B_6. This information would be of value in determining norms for children at differing ages and from this the recommended allowances for vitamin B_6 probably could be calculated. In addition to acquiring data for normal children, vitamin B_6 requirements for stressed and malnourished children need to be determined so that adequate amounts of vitamin B_6 can be provided during periods of sickness and stress.

LITERATURE CITED

Baker, E. M., J. E. Canham, W. T. Nunes, H. E. Sauberlich, and M. E. McDowell. 1964. Vitamin B_6 requirement for adult men. Am. J. Clin. Nutr. *15*:59–66.

Barlow, B., and A. W. Wilkinson. 1975. Plasma pyridoxal phosphate levels and tryptophan metabolism in children with burns and scalds. Clin. Chim. Acta *10*:48–54.

Baysal, A., B. A. Johnson, and H. Linkswiler. 1966. Vitamin B_6 depletion in man: Blood vitamin B_6, plasma pyridoxal phosphate, serum cholesterol, serum transaminases and urinary vitamin B_6 and 4-pyridoxic acid. J. Nutr. *89*:19–23.

Bessey, O. A., D. J. D. Adam, and A. E. Hansen 1957. Intake of vitamin B_6 and infantile convulsions: A first approximation of requirements of pyridoxine in infants. Pediatrics *20*:33–44.

Bhagavan, H. N., M. Coleman, and D. B. Coursin. 1975a. Distribution of pyridoxal-5-phosphate in human blood between the cells and plasma: Effect of oral administration of pyridoxine on the ratio in Down's and hyperactive patients. Biochem. Med. *14*:201–208.

Bhagavan, H. N., M. Coleman, and D. B. Coursin. 1975b. The effect of pyridoxine hydrochloride on blood serotonin and pyridoxal phosphate contents in hyperactive children. Pediatrics 55:437–441.

Bhagavan, H. N., M. Coleman, D. B. Coursin, and P. Rosenfeld. 1973. Pyridoxal-5-phosphate levels in whole blood in home-reared patients with trisomy 2. Lancet 1:889.

Brophy, M. H., and P. K. Siiteri. 1975. Pyridoxal phosphate and hypertensive disorders of pregnancy. Am. J. Obstet. Gynecol. 121:1075–1079.

Canham, J. E., E. M. Baker, R. S. Hardin, H. E. Sauberlich, and I. C. Plough. 1969. Dietary protein—Its relation to vitamin B₆ requirements and function. Ann. N.Y. Acad. Sci. 166:16–29.

Chen, L. H., and A. L. Marlatt. 1975. Effects of dietary B₆ levels and exercise on glutamic-pyruvate transaminase activity in rat tissues. J Nutr. 105:401–407.

Church, D. F., and H. N. Church. 1975. Food Values of Portions Commonly Used. Bowes and Church, 12th ed., J. B. Lippincott Co., Philadelphia, 197 pp.

Cinnamon, A. D., and J. R. Beaton. 1970. Biochemical assessment of vitamin B₆ status in man. Am. J. Clin. Nutr. 23:696–702.

Cleary, R. E., L. Lumeng, and T.-K. Li. 1975. Maternal and fetal levels of pyridoxal phosphate at term: Adequacy of vitamin B₆ supplementation during pregnancy. Am. J. Obstet. Gynecol. 121:25–28.

Contractor, S. F., and B. Shane. 1970. Blood and urine levels of vitamin B₆ in the mother and fetus before and after loading of the mother with vitamin B₆. Am. J. Obstet. Gynecol. 107:635–640.

Fomon, S. J. 1974. Infant Nutrition. W. B. Saunders Co., Philadelphia, 575 pp.

Food and Nutrition Board. 1974. Recommended Dietary Allowances, 8th ed., National Academy of Sciences, Washington, D.C., 129 pp.

Hamfelt, A. 1964. Age variation of vitamin B₆ metabolism in man. Clin. Chim. Acta 10:48–54.

Hamfelt, A. 1967. Pyridoxal phosphate concentration and amino transferase activity in human blood cells. Clin. Chim. Acta 16:19–28.

Hamfelt, A., and T. Tuvemo. 1972. Pyridoxal phosphate and folic acid concentration in blood and erythrocyte amino transferase activity during pregnancy. Clin. Chim. Acta 41:287–298.

Information Canada. 1975. Dietary Standard for Canada, Ottawa, p. 29.

Kempe, C. H., H. K. Silver, and D. O'Brien (eds.) 1976. Current Pediatric Diagnosis and Treatment, Lange Publications, Los Angeles.

Miletic, D., M. Stanulovic, B. Bogdanov, and D. Obradovic. 1969. Helv. Paed. Acta 2:183.

Miller, L., and H. Linkswiler. 1967. Effect of protein intake in the development of abnormal tryptophan metabolism by men during vitamin B₆ depletion. J. Nutr. 93:53–59.

Orr, M. L. 1969. Pantothenic acid, vitamin B₆ and vitamin B₁₂ in foods. Consumer and Food Economics Research Division, ARS/USDA, HERR No. 36: 53 pp.

Raica, N., and H. E. Sauberlich. 1964. Blood cell transaminase activity in human vitamin B₆ deficiency. Am. J. Clin. Nutr. 15:67–72.

Shane, B., and S. F. Contractor. 1975. Assessment of vitamin B₆ status. Studies on pregnant women and oral contraceptive users. Am. J. Clin. Nutr. 28:739–747.

Snyderman, S. E., E. H. Holt, Jr., R. Carretero, and K. G. Jacobs. 1953. Pyridoxine deficiency in the human infant. Am. J. Clin. Nutr. 1:200–207.

18

Vitamin B_6 Requirements in the Preadolescent and Adolescent

S. J. RITCHEY, FRANCES S. JOHNSON, *and*
MARY K. KORSLUND

The nutritional needs of the adolescent have received considerable attention in the past few years. A symposium (McKigney and Munro, 1973) has been published recently about nutrient requirements in adolescence. The general tenor of that publication is that a concentrated effort is required to define the nutritional needs of the growing child. The adolescent years present several unique circumstances that affect nutrient needs; the very rapid growth and the onset of sexual maturation are clearly different phenomena that affect nutritional needs.

There have been so few reports on the vitamin B_6 requirements of the growing child that we can only speculate about this subject. A reasonably comprehensive review of the literature failed to find a single study with the adolescent. However, a few data are available from our laboratory on the preadolescent child and from nutrition survey information that may provide some insight into the vitamin B_6 needs of the adolescent.

During the summer of 1974 a metabolic study was conducted to investigate the loss of nitrogen through sweat while preadolescent boys were consuming three levels of dietary protein. We utilized this opportunity to examine the metabolism of vitamin B_6 in the subjects. The mean age was 8 years, 6 months; the mean weight and height were 31.2 kg and 131 cm, respectively.

Subjects consumed three levels of dietary protein, 29, 54, and 84 g daily, for periods of 10 days each. The diets and vitamin supplements were calculated to provide equal amounts of vitamin B_6 intake at each protein level. The analyzed values indicated that foods plus supplements provided 1.29, 1.11, and 1.17 mg of the vitamin daily at the low, moderate, and high protein levels. All foods were weighed or measured to maintain appropriate intakes. Urine was collected throughout the study. Composite urine samples were collected during the last 5 days of each period and utilized for analyses. Vitamin B_6 was determined on food and urine by the *Saccharomyces carlsbergensis* method (Atkin *et al.*, 1943; Toepfer and Polansky, 1970); 4-pyridoxic acid was determined in urine by the method of Reddy *et al.* (1958).

On the day following the period of consumption of a given protein diet, a 2-g tryptophan load test was administered. Xanthurenic acid was analyzed in the subsequent 24-h urine collection by the procedure of Wachstein and Gudaitis (1952).

The urinary excretions of vitamin B_6 and 4-pyridoxic acid were not different (Table 18-1) for the varying protein levels; neither were the excretions different when expressed as a percentage of intake, since the vitamin B_6 intakes were similar by design among protein levels. The vitamin B_6 excretions, in the range of 90–130 μg daily, are in the range found for adults (Kelsay *et al.*, 1968; Donald *et al.*, 1971), consuming 1.5 mg of vitamin B_6 daily. Previous reports with adults (Sauberlich *et al.*, 1972) suggest urinary excretions of less than 20 μg per gram of creatinine as indicative of marginal vitamin B_6 intakes. A tentative guide for the interpretation of urinary excretion of vitamin B_6 suggested

TABLE 18-1   Daily Intake of Vitamin B₆ and Excretion of Metabolites by Preadolescent Boys

Intakes		Urinary Excretion			
Protein, g	B₆, mg	B₆, mg	B₆, % of Intake	4-Pyridoxic Acid, mg	4-Pyridoxic Acid, % of Intake
29	1.29	0.113 ± 0.017[a]	8.76	0.255 ± 0.036	19.77
54	1.11	0.102 ± 0.017	9.19	0.213 ± 0.042	19.19
84	1.17	0.103 ± 0.010	8.80	0.225 ± 0.054	19.23

[a]Mean ± SD of 12 subjects.

by Sauberlich *et al.* (1972) indicated acceptable levels to be 30 and 90 μg per gram of creatinine for the age groupings 13–15 years and 1–3 years, respectively. The boys were excreting from 150 to 216 μg of vitamin B_6 per gram of creatinine. Using this criterion of vitamin B_6 excretion based on creatinine, these subjects were receiving sufficient vitamin B_6.

Average excretions of 4-pyridoxic acid ranged from 213 to 255 μg/day when the boys were consuming the three levels of protein and vitamin B_6 (Table 18-1); these excretions represented approximately 20 percent of the vitamin B_6 intake. In vitamin B_6 depletion studies with adults, excretions of less than 150 μg were reported for women (Donald *et al.*, 1971) and men (Baysal *et al.*, 1966). If the 150 μg/day is used as a criterion for adequacy, intakes of vitamin B_6 at levels of 1.1–1.3 mg/day are presumed to be adequate for preadolescent boys.

Xanthurenic acid excretion was in the range of 13.7 to 14.7 mg/day for the three diets (Table 18-2). These values appear to be in a normal range following the tryptophan load test. The urinary excretion of xanthurenic acid was well below the 30 mg recommended by Vilter *et al.* (1953) as an indicator of vitamin B_6 deficiency.

In an earlier study with preadolescent girls (Ritchey and Feeley, 1966), vitamin B_6 intakes of 1.30 and 1.73 mg/day were found to be adequate. Subjects were consuming either 22 or 40 g of protein daily supplied from diets comprised of plant products. Excretions of vitamin B_6 and 4-pyridoxic acid were in the range of values suggesting adequate intakes of vitamin B_6.

Lewis and Nunn (personal communication) investigated the vitamin B_6 intakes of 22 children ranging in age from 2 to 9 years. Intakes were

TABLE 18-2   Xanthurenic Acid Excretion by Preadolescent Boys Following a Load Test of L-Tryptophan

Intakes		Xanthurenic acid, mg/24 h
Protein, g	B_6, mg	
29	1.29	14.00 ± 3.26[a]
54	1.11	13.67 ± 1.16
84	1.17	14.69 ± 1.74

[a]Mean ± SD of 12 subjects.

calculated from 3-day food records; 24-h urine samples were collected for the third day of the recorded food intake. The average vitamin B_6 intake was 1.10 mg/day; mean pyridoxic acid excretion was 0.52 mg/day and represented 48 percent of the intake. The excretions of 4-pyridoxic acid ranged from 0.14 to 1.12 mg/day and correlated significantly with vitamin B_6 intake ($p < 0.05$). Using the 150 μg/day as a criterion of adequacy, only three of these children would have been categorized as having marginal or low intakes of vitamin B_6.

Baker *et al.* (1967) determined the vitamin B_6 levels in 576 children in a nutrition survey in a New York City school. Serum levels of the vitamin ranged from 17 to 74 ng/ml with a mean value of 36 ng/ml. Normal adults have been reported to have serum vitamin B_6 values above 50 ng/ml. Values below 25 ng/ml correspond to other biochemical indices of vitamin B_6 deficiencies (Sauberlich *et al.*, 1972). Many of the children from the survey by Baker *et al.* (1967) had values below 50 ng/ml, and several had values below the 25 ng/ml level.

Several recommendations, as well as these reports, have provided general guidelines about the vitamin B_6 requirement of the preadolescent and adolescent. The American Academy of Pediatrics, Committee on Nutrition (1966) estimated the vitamin B_6 requirement of the child to be from 0.5 to 1.5 mg/day and for the adolescent to be from 1.5 to 2.0 mg/day. However, the committee stated further that data were insufficient to permit an accurate estimate for the adolescent. The estimate was based on the lack of deficiency symptoms in the population in which market basket analyses indicated intakes in the above ranges. The committee further suggested that vitamin B_6 requirements vary with protein intakes.

Vitamin B_6 intake has been suggested as 0.8 mg/1,000 kcals by Leitch and Hepburn (1961) for growth and 0.6 mg/1,000 kcals for maintenance. The recommendation was extrapolated from the available data on thiamin and riboflavin requirements; thus, on the basis of those needs, the vitamin B_6 requirement for growth ranged from 0.45 to 0.8 mg/1,000 kcals. Several others have disagreed with the method of deriving vitamin B6 requirements on the basis of energy needs.

The Food and Nutrition Board (1974) recommends a daily vitamin B_6 allowance from 0.6 to 2.0 mg for age ranges of 1–3 and 15–18 years, respectively. The board indicated, however, that data are not sufficient for adequate evaluation of the vitamin B_6 needs of the growing child.

A summary of estimated vitamin B_6 needs for the growing child and during adolescence (Table 18-3) reveals clearly the paucity of information. Controlled studies on the normal child and on the adolescent are essentially nonexistent.

TABLE 18-3   Estimates of Vitamin B_6 Needs of Growing Children and Adolescents

Committee or Investigator	Subjects, age in yr	Estimates of Adequate B_6, mg/day	Basis of Estimate
American Academy of Pediatrics (1961)	Children Adolescents	0.5–1.5 1.5–2.0	Lack of deficiency symptoms
Food and Nutrition Board (1974)	Children (1–10) Adolescents (11–18)	0.6–1.2 2.0	Literature review and adult values
Leitch and Hepburn (1961)	Growth	0.45–0.80[a]	Thiamin, riboflavin, and energy
Lewis and Nunn (1975)	Children (2–9)	1.10	Pyridoxic acid excretion
Ritchey et al. (see text)	Boys (7–9)	1.1–1.3	B_6 and pyridoxic acid excretion; tryptophan load
Ritchey and Feeley (1966)	Girls (7–9)	1.30–1.73	B_6 and pyridoxic acid excretion

[a]Per 1,000 kcals.

SUMMARY

The present estimates by the Food and Nutrition Board appear to be realistic in meeting the needs of the population. However, present recommendations are based on scant data, and research should be directed toward the elucidation of the vitamin B_6 needs of the preadolescent and the adolescent. Particular attention should be focused on the needs for vitamin B_6 during the periods of rapid growth and the onset of sexual maturation, the effects of high intakes of protein, the use of oral contraceptives by the adolescent females, and the effects of alcohol on vitamin B_6 utilization.

LITERATURE CITED

American Academy of Pediatrics, Committee on Nutrition. 1966. Vitamin B_6 requirements in man. Pediatrics *38*:1068–1075.

Atkin, L., S. Schultz, W. L. Williams, and C. N. Frey. 1943. Yeast microbiological methods for determination of vitamins. Pyridoxine. Anal. Ed. Ind. Eng. Chem. *151*:141–144.

Baker, H., O. Frank, S. Feingold, G. Christakis, and H. Ziffer. 1967. Vitamins, total cholesterol and triglycerides in 642 New York City school children. Am. J. Clin. Nutr. *20*:850–857.

Baysal, A., B. A. Johnson, and H. Linkswiler. 1966. Vitamin B_6 depletion in man: Blood vitamin B_6, plasma pyridoxal-phosphate, serum cholesterol, serum transaminases and urinary vitamin B_6 and 4-pyridoxic acid. J. Nutr. *89*:19–23.

Donald, E. A., L. D. McBean, M. H. W. Simpson, M. F. Sun, and H. E. Aly. 1971. Vitamin B_6 requirement of young adult women. Am. J. Clin. Nutr. *24*:1028–1041.

Food and Nutrition Board. 1974. Recommended Dietary Allowances, 8th ed., National Academy of Sciences, Washington, D.C., 128 pp.

Kelsay, J., A. Baysal, and H. Linkswiler. 1968. Effect of vitamin B_6 depletion on the pyridoxal, pyridoxamine and pyridoxine content of the blood and urine of men. J. Nutr. *94*:490–494.

Leitch, I., and A. Hepburn. 1961. Pyridoxine: Metabolism and requirement. Nutr. Abstr. Rev. *31*:389–401.

Lewis, J. S., and K. P. Nunn. 1975. Vitamin B_6 intake and 24-hour urinary excretion of 4-pyridoxic acid of normal children. Personal communication.

McKigney, J. I., and H. N. Munro. 1976. Nutrition Requirements in Adolescence. MIT Press, Cambridge, Mass., 365 pp.

Reddy, S. K., M. S. Reynolds, and J. M. Price. 1958. The determination of 4-pyridoxic acid in human urine. J. Biol. Chem. *233*:691–696.

Ritchey, S. J., and R. M. Feeley. 1966. The excretion patterns of vitamin B_6 and B_{12} in preadolescent girls. J. Nutr. *89*:411–413.

Sauberlich, H. E., J. E. Canham, E. M. Baker, N. Raica, and Y. F. Herman. 1972. Biochemical assessment of the nutritional status of vitamin B_6 in the human. Am. J. Clin. Nutr. *25*:629–642.

Toepfer, E. W., and M. M. Polansky. 1970. Microbiological assay of vitamin B$_6$ and its components. J. Assoc. Off. Agric. Chem. *53*:546–550.

Vilter, R. W. 1953. The effect of vitamin B$_6$ deficiency induced by desoxypyridoxine in human beings. J. Lab. Clin. Med. *42*:335–357.

Wachstein, M., and A. Gudaitis. 1952. Utilization of an improved method for rapid determination of xanthurenic acid in urine. Am. J. Clin. Pathol. *22*:652–655.

19

Vitamin B$_6$ Requirements of Men

HELLEN M. LINKSWILER

Knowledge concerning the quantitative requirement of men for vitamin B$_6$ is based largely on relatively recent data collected from human studies conducted by the laboratories of the U.S. Army Medical Research and Nutrition Laboratory and the Department of Nutritional Sciences at the University of Wisconsin. A series of studies in which young male adults were subjects were carried out at both locations. Although there were differences in experimental procedure between the two laboratories, both employed the technique of vitamin B$_6$ depletion and repletion. The diet usually fed by the U.S. Army Medical Research and Nutrition investigators was a liquid synthetic diet containing only 0.06 mg of vitamin B$_6$ and consisting of vitamin-free casein, dextrose, and coconut oil supplemented with all essential minerals and vitamins, except vitamin B$_6$. The Wisconsin group gave a diet that contained 0.16 mg of vitamin B$_6$ and contained ordinary food items in addition to vitamin-free casein, gelatin, and vitamin and mineral supplements. The U.S. Army team gave 5 g of L- or 10 g of DL-tryptophan to stress the tryptophan metabolic enzyme systems; the Wisconsin group gave 2 g of L-tryptophan. Thus, the degree of vitamin

279

B_6 deficiency as well as the challenge to the enzyme systems was undoubtedly greater in the subjects studied by the U.S. Army team. In spite of the differences in experimental procedure, however, there is good agreement between the two groups as to the vitamin B_6 requirement of men and the effect of level of protein intake on the requirement.

A number of clinical and biochemical parameters were investigated during the studies in order to look for changes that occurred during a vitamin B_6 deficiency and to define which parameter was most useful in assessing vitamin B_6 requirement and nutritional status.

A dietary deficiency of vitamin B_6 caused a number of biochemical changes in the men. Among these changes, to name a few, were increases in the urinary excretion of several tryptophan metabolites of the kynurenine pathway after tryptophan loading (Baker et al., 1964; Yess et al., 1964; Miller and Linkswiler, 1967; Linkswiler, 1967; Canham et al., 1969; Sauberlich et al., 1970, 1972) including quinolinic acid (Brown et al., 1965; Kelsay et al., 1968b); increases in the urinary excretion of cystathionine (Park and Linkswiler, 1970); decreases in urinary vitamin B_6 and 4-pyridoxic acid (Baker et al., 1964; Linkswiler, 1967; Canham et al., 1969; Sauberlich et al., 1970; Sauberlich et al., 1972; Baysal et al., 1966; Kelsay et al., 1968a); decreases in blood vitamin B_6 and pyridoxal phosphate (Baysal et al., 1966; Kelsay et al., 1968a); and decreases in transaminase activities in erythrocytes, leukocytes, and serum or plasma (Linkswiler, 1967; Canham et al., 1969; Sauberlich et al., 1972; Baysal et al., 1966; Canham et al., 1965; Raica and Sauberlich, 1964). A number of other biochemical and clinical changes were observed, but they will not be discussed here.

The decreases in urinary vitamin B_6 and 4-pyridoxic acid and in blood vitamin B_6 and pyridoxal phosphate correlated fairly well with urinary cystathionine and certain metabolites of tryptophan. Blood and urine levels of vitamin B_6 and its metabolites alone, however, were not sufficient to assess the requirement for the vitamin. Concentration in both urine and blood fell rapidly when vitamin B_6 was withheld, and a marked decrease occurred before amino acid metabolism became abnormal. When supplements of the vitamin were given, the concentrations reflected the intake. While these parameters alone could not be used to define the vitamin B_6 requirement, they supported the conclusions drawn from other data.

Baker et al. (1964) found that the urinary excretion of free vitamin B_6 decreased progressively with the length of time men consumed diets containing 0.06 mg of vitamin B_6. At the end of 5 weeks of depletion the men excreted as little as 15 μg per 24 h. When diets were supplemented with various amounts of pyridoxine, urinary vitamin B_6 was increased and was closely correlated with the level of intake. Baysal *et al.* (1966) reported that young males excreted as little as 17 μg after consuming for 40 days a diet containing 0.16 mg of vitamin B_6. Kelsay *et al.* (1968a) determined the effect of the level of vitamin B_6 intake on the urinary excretion of pyridoxal, pyridoxamine, and pyridoxine by men. Urinary vitamin B_6 decreased very rapidly when the vitamin intake of the subjects was changed from 1.66 to 0.16 mg/day. Urinary vitamin B_6 of the men exceeded 120 μg per 24 h at the higher intake but decreased to 40 percent of the original value after 4 to 5 days of deficiency; low values of about 20 μg were found after 20 days.

Urinary 4-pyridoxic acid excretion also seemed to reflect the intake of the vitamin (Baysal *et al.*, 1966; Kelsay *et al.*, 1968a). A rapid decrease in urinary 4-pyridoxic acid occurred when men were changed from self-selected diets to one that contained 0.16 mg of vitamin B_6 daily. After 5 days, 4-pyridoxic acid excretion was about 20 percent of the original value, and none was detected in the urine after 25 days of depletion.

Although the level of protein intake affects the vitamin B_6 requirement of men, apparently it has little, if any, effect on the urinary excretion of the vitamin and 4-pyridoxic acid (Linkswiler, 1967). The concentration of vitamin B_6 and 4-pyridoxic acid in 24-h urine samples decreased rapidly when men were given diets deficient in vitamin B_6, regardless of the amount of protein in the diet (Table 19-1).

TABLE 19-1 Average Urinary Excretion of Vitamin B_6 and 4-Pyridoxic Acid by Men Fed Diets Containing 0.16 mg of Vitamin B_6 and 55 or 100 g of Protein

No. of Days of Deficiency	55 g Protein Intake Daily		100 g Protein Intake Daily	
	Vitamin B_6, μg/day[a]	4-Pyridoxic Acid, mg/day[a]	Vitamin B_6, μg/day[a]	4-Pyridoxic Acid, mg/day[a]
0	98	1.00	114	0.90
5	53	0.20	81	0.12
10	46	0.14	63	0.09
15	34	0.10	46	0.05
20	30	0.10	30	0.05
25	25	0.05	30	0.00
40	20	0.05		

[a] Expressed as pyridoxine (from Linkswiler, 1967).

Blood levels of vitamin B_6 fell rapidly when vitamin B_6 was withheld from men, and the fall occurred before changes in other biochemical parameters (Baysal *et al.*, 1966; Kelsay *et al.*, 1968a). Supplementation with pyridoxine increased blood levels, and the level of increase was a reflection of the intake. Most of the vitamin B_6 content of blood is in the form of pyridoxal phosphate (Sauberlich *et al.*, 1972).

When men were given vitamin B_6-deficient diets, the activities of aspartate aminotransferase and alanine aminotransferase fell in erythrocytes, leukocytes, and plasma (Linkswiler, 1967; Canham *et al.*, 1969; Baysal *et al.*, 1966; Canham *et al.*, 1965; Raica and Sauberlich, 1964). For several reasons, aminotransferase activity in the various blood components was of little use in assessing vitamin B_6 requirements. For example, there was a wide range of aminotransferase activities among normal individuals, and there was a lag in the activity of the transferases in response to changes in vitamin B_6 intake.

The parameter that proved to be most useful in assessing the vitamin B_6 requirement of men was the measurement in the urine of one or more tryptophan metabolites of the kynurenine pathway following tryptophan loading. Because vitamin B_6 is the cofactor for a large number of enzyme systems that function in the metabolism of amino acids, it is not surprising that disturbances in amino acid metabolism are the most sensitive indicators for detecting a vitamin B_6 deficiency and for determining the requirement for the vitamin.

Greenberg *et al.* (1949) were the first investigators to observe that a dietary restriction of vitamin B_6 in man caused an increased excretion of xanthurenic acid after a load of tryptophan. After subsisting for 3 weeks on a casein-sucrose-corn oil diet supplemented with vitamins and minerals, two men excreted 271 and 515 mg of xanthurenic acid in the urine during the 24 h following a 10-g load of DL-tryptophan. Supplements of pyridoxine resulted in a return to the original low levels of excretion. Since vitamin B_6 requirement seems to be affected by the protein content of the diet, it seems necessary to discuss the requirement in relation to the protein intake. Harding *et al.* (1959) reported that men fed for 24 days a packaged military ration providing 165 g of protein and 1.93 mg of vitamin B_6 showed a significant rise in xanthurenic acid excretion after a 10-g load of DL-tryptophan. Men fed a similar ration containing 2.76 mg of vitamin B_6 did not show an increase in xanthurenic acid excretion. The authors concluded that the vitamin B_6 requirement for men was greater than 2 mg/day.

Canham *et al.* (1969) reported that the rapidity of onset and severity of biochemical manifestations of vitamin B_6 deficiency were directly related to the protein level of the diet. In one study, young adult males given daily 80 g of protein and 0.06 mg of vitamin B$_6$ excreted abnormal levels of xanthurenic acid in response to a 10-g load of DL-tryptophan after 1 week while those given 40 g of protein did not show elevated excretions until after 2 weeks. By the end of 4 weeks of deficiency the net xanthurenic acid excretion of the high protein group was 430 and that of the low protein group was 246 mg per 24 h. Repletion studies were not reported, but during the week prior to the initiation of the deficiency, 2 mg/day of pyridoxine hydrochloride had maintained normal low levels of xanthurenic acid excretion by the men. In a subsequent study designed to determine the vitamin B$_6$ requirement of men and the effect of the level of dietary protein on the requirement, five subjects were given a liquid formula diet providing 30 g/day of protein and six other subjects were given 100 g (Baker *et al.,* 1964). After 3 weeks of depletion the net excretion of xanthurenic acid following a 10-g load of DL-tryptophan approached 350 mg per 24 hours by subjects given the high protein diet while those given the low protein diet excreted under 300 mg even after 6 weeks of deficiency (Figures 19-1 and 19-2). Levels of pyridoxine supplementation were titrated in accordance with the weekly urinary excretion of xanthurenic acid until the minimal vitamin B$_6$ requirement was met. Men fed the high-protein diet required 1.50 mg of pyridoxine daily and those fed the low-protein diet, 1.0 mg.

A number of tryptophan metabolites of the kynurenine pathway were determined by the Wisconsin group during vitamin B$_6$ depletion and repletion studies. In the first study, six young adult males were given a diet containing 0.16 mg/day of vitamin B$_6$ and 100 g/day of protein (Yess *et al.,* 1964). As a vitamin B$_6$ deficiency developed, markedly increased quantities of hydroxykynurenine, kynurenine, and xanthurenic acid were excreted in the urine. Acetylkynurenine and kynurenic acid also increased but in much smaller quantities than the other three metabolites. Although a 2-g load of L-tryptophan resulted in hydroxykynurenine and kynurenine excretion in much greater quantities than that of xanthurenic acid, all three showed a similar progressive increase as the deficiency became more severe. Moreover, there was a sharp, prompt drop in the excretion of all three compounds when pyridoxine was given. Thus, the urinary excretion of any one, or all, of these compounds seems to be suitable for detecting adequacy of vitamin B$_6$ intake. Supplements of 0.6 or 0.9 mg of pyridoxine were not sufficient to restore tryptophan metabolite excretion to predepletion levels in all subjects.

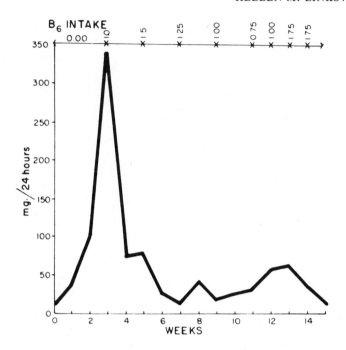

FIGURE 19-1   Net urinary excretion of xanthurenic acid following
administration of a 10-g DL-tryptophan load and level of vitamin B₆
intake of subjects receiving a high-protein diet (from Baker *et al.*,
1964).

In a second study, 11 subjects were fed diets containing 0.16 mg of
vitamin B_6 (Miller and Linkswiler, 1967). Five subjects were given 54 g
of protein and six were given 150 g of protein. Abnormal tryptophan
metabolism developed very slowly in those fed 54 g of protein; after 40
days of vitamin B_6 deficiency individual subjects excreted from 0 to 29
percent of a 2-g loading dose of L-tryptophan as kynurenine, hydroxykynurenine, xanthurenic acid, kynurenic acid, and acetylkynurenine. Subjects fed the 150-g protein diet excreted 29 percent of
the tryptophan load as these five metabolites after only 14 days of
vitamin B_6 deficiency. Before the deficiency was initiated, supplements
of 1.5 mg of pyridoxine maintained normal excretion levels of all the
tryptophan metabolites in both groups of subjects. Following the deficiency, 1.06 mg of pyridoxine was not sufficient to restore urinary
tryptophan metabolites to normal levels in either group. The effect that
level of protein intake has on the rapidity of onset and severity of
abnormal tryptophan metabolism is illustrated in Figure 19-3. Men fed

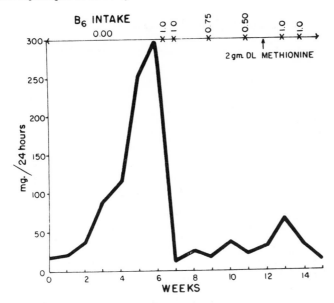

FIGURE 19-2 · Net excretion of xanthurenic acid following administration of a 10-g DL-tryptophan load and level of vitamin B₆ intake of subjects receiving a low-protein diet (from Baker *et al.*, 1964).

a vitamin B₆-deficient diet containing 150 g of protein for 14 days excreted 30 percent of a 2-g load of L-tryptophan as kynurenine, hydroxykynurenine, xanthurenic acid, and kynurenic acid; these compounds accounted for 18 percent of a 2-g load after 25 days of deficiency when men were given 100 g of protein and for 12 percent after 40 days of deficiency when men were given 55 g of protein (Linkswiler, 1967).

The effect of vitamin B₆ deficiency on the metabolism of methionine by the young adult male has been studied (Park and Linkswiler, 1970). The experimental diet contained 150 g of protein and 0.16 mg of vitamin B₆ and consisted of vitamin-free casein, gelatin, natural foods, and a daily supplement of 2.5 g of L-methionine. During a predepletion period when the subjects were given the experimental diet and a 2.0 mg supplement of pyridoxine, they excreted approximately 100 to 150 μM of cystathionine and 100 μM of cysteine sulfinic acid per 24 h (Table 19-2). When the vitamin B₆ intake was 2.16 mg, a 3.0-g load of L-methionine had only a slight effect on the excretion of any of these compounds. When the 2.0 mg pyridoxine supplement was withheld, subjects developed abnormal methionine metabolism within 7 days as

KYNURENINE

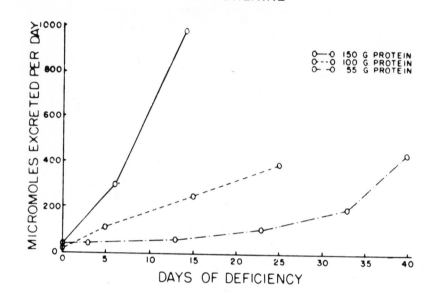

KYNURENIC ACID

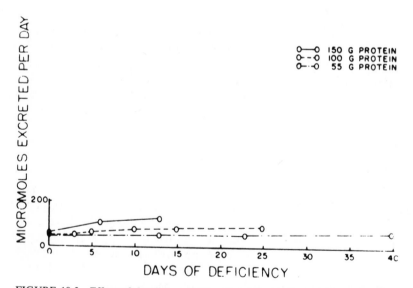

FIGURE 19-3   Effect of the dietary intake of protein on the excretion of kynurenine, kynurenic acid, hydroxykynurenine, and xanthurenic acid following loading with 2 g of L-tryptophan by men fed diets containing 0.16 mg of vitamin B_6 daily (from Linkswiler, 1967).

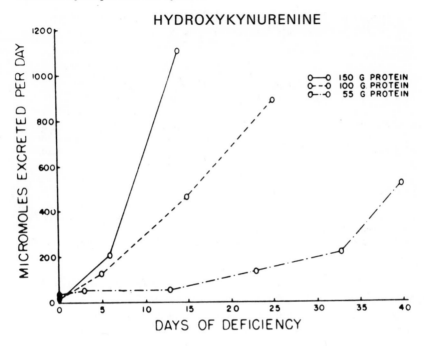

HYDROXYKYNURENINE

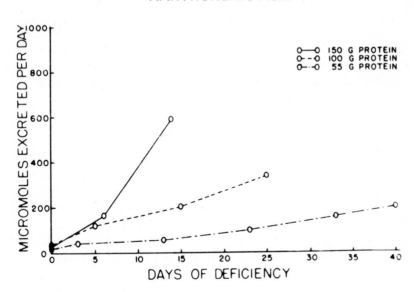

XANTHURENIC ACID

TABLE 19-2   Effect of Vitamin B_6 Intake on Cystathionine and
L-Cysteine Sulfinic Acid Excretion in Men

Dietary Period	Vitamin B_6 Intake, mg	No. of Days on Specified Intake	Cystathionine[a]		L-Cysteine Sulfinic Acid[a]	
			Pre	Post	Pre	Post
Predepletion	2.16	6, 7	112	161	92	87
		13, 14	144	165	96	101
Depletion	0.16	6, 7	195	397	101	107
		13, 14	500	1466	117	128
		20, 21	1508	3719	117	153
Repletion	2.16	6, 7	163	244	91	95
		13, 14	139	178	91	85

Adapted from Park and Linkswiler (1970).
[a]Pre is before methionine load; post is after a 3-g L-methionine load. Both are measured in $\mu M/24$ h.

evidenced by an increased excretion of cystathionine after loading with methionine. Subjects deficient in vitamin B_6 for 21 days excreted greatly increased amounts of cystathionine in both premethionine and postmethionine urine samples. L-cysteine sulfinic acid increased but slightly, and only traces of homocysteine were found during the vitamin B_6 deficiency. The intake of 2.16 mg of vitamin B_6 given after the 3-week period of deficiency seemed to be barely adequate, since 2 weeks were required for urinary cystathionine to return to predepletion values. Information pertaining to the vitamin B_6 requirement of men from a number of studies in which men were depleted and then repleted in vitamin B_6 is summarized in Table 19-3. The protein content of the experimental diet as well as the amino acid load used to challenge the enzyme systems is given. The highest amount of vitamin B_6 that was found to be inadequate is given in the column labeled inadequate, and the lowest amount found to be adequate, in the column labeled adequate.

SUMMARY

The data indicate that the vitamin B_6 requirement for men consuming diets containing 100 to 150 g of protein is between 1.5 and 2.0 mg/day. The requirement may be higher than 2.0 when the protein intake exceeds 150 g. The requirement seems to be 1.0–1.5 mg when the protein intake is 100 g or less. An intake of 0.76 mg of vitamin B_6 was not adequate for men even with protein intakes as low as 30 g/day.

TABLE 19-3   Relationship of Level of Dietary Protein to Vitamin B_6 Requirement of Men

Reference	Protein Intake, g/day	Amino Acid Load, g	Vitamin B_6 Intake, mg Inadequate	Adequate
Harding *et al.* (1959)	165	10.0 DL-Tryptophan	1.93	2.79
Park and Linkswiler (1970)	150	3.0 L-Methionine		2.16
Miller and Linkswiler (1967)	150	2.0 L-Tryptophan	0.76	1.66
Sauberlich *et al.* (1970)	100	10.0 DL-Tryptophan		1.50
Baker *et al.* (1964)	100	10.0 DL-Tryptophan	1.25	1.50
Canham *et al.* (1969)	100			1.30
Yess *et al.* (1964)	100	2.0 L-Tryptophan	1.06	
Canham *et al.* (1969)	80	10.0 DL-Tryptophan		2.00
Canham *et al.* (1969)	80			1.00
Miller and Linkswiler (1967)	54	2.0 L-Tryptophan	0.76	1.66
Canham *et al.* (1969)	40	10.0 DL-Tryptophan		2.00
Baker *et al.* (1964)	30	10.0 DL-Tryptophan	0.75	1.00

ACKNOWLEDGMENT

The work reported is a contribution from the College of Agricultural and Life Sciences, University of Wisconsin, Madison, Wisconsin.

LITERATURE CITED

Baker, E. M., J. E. Canham, W. T. Nunes, H. E. Sauberlich, and M. E. McDowell. 1964. Vitamin B_6 requirement for adult men. Am. J. Clin. Nutr. *15*:59–66.

Baysal, A., B. A. Johnson, and H. Linkswiler. 1966. Vitamin B_6 depletion in man: Blood vitamin B_6 plasma pyridoxal-phosphate, serum cholesterol, serum transaminases and urinary vitamin B_6 and 4-pyridoxic acid. J. Nutr. *89*:19–23.

Brown, R. R., N. Yess, J. M. Price, H. Linkswiler, P. Swan, and L. V. Hankes. 1965. Vitamin B_6 depletion in man: Urinary excretion of quinolinic acid and niacin metabolites. J. Nutr. *87*:419–423.

Canham, J. E., H. E. Sauberlich, E. M. Baker, and N. Raica, Jr. 1965. Human studies in vitamin B_6 metabolism. U.S. Army Med. Res. Nutr. Lab. Ann. Prog. Rep.: pp. 119–124.

Canham, J. E., E. M. Baker, R. S. Harding, H. E. Sauberlich, and I. C. Plough. 1969. Dietary protein—Its relationship to vitamin B_6 requirements and function. Ann. N.Y. Acad. Sci. *166*:16–29.

Greenberg, L. D., D. F. Bohr, H. McGrath, and J. F. Rinehart. 1949. Xanthurenic acid excretion in the human subject on a pyridoxine-deficient diet. Arch. Biochem. *21*:237–239.

Harding, R. S., I. C. Plough, and T. E. Friedemann. 1959. The effect of storage on the vitamin B_6 content of a packaged army ration, with a note on the human requirement for the vitamin. J. Nutr. *68*:323–331.

Kelsay, J., A. Baysal, and H. Linkswiler. 1968a. Effect of vitamin B_6 depletion on the pyridoxal, pyridoxamine and pyridoxine content of the blood and urine of men. J. Nutr. 94:490–494.

Kelsay, J., L. T. Miller, and H. Linkswiler. 1968b. Effect of protein intake on the excretion of quinolinic acid and niacin metabolites by men during vitamin B₆ depletion. N. Nutr. 94:27–31.

Linkswiler, H. 1967. Biochemical and physiological changes in vitamin B₆ deficiency. Am. J. Clin. Nutr. 20:547–557.

Miller, L. T., and H. Linkswiler. 1967. Effect of protein intake on the development of abnormal tryptophan metabolism by men during vitamin B₆ depletion. J. Nutr. 93:53–59.

Park, Y. K., and H. Linkswiler. 1970. Effect of vitamin B₆ depletion in adult man on the excretion of cystathionine and other methionine metabolites. J. Nutr. 100:110–116.

Raica, N., Jr., and H. E. Sauberlich. 1964. Blood cell transaminase activity in human vitamin B₆ deficiency. Am. J. Clin. Nutr. 15:67–72.

Sauberlich, H. E., J. E. Canham, E. M. Baker, N. Raica, Jr., and Y. F. Herman. 1970. Human vitamin B₆ nutriture. J. Sci. Ind. Res. 29:528–537.

Sauberlich, H. E., J. E. Canham, E. M. Baker, N. Raica, Jr., and Y. F. Herman. 1972. Biochemical assessment of the nutritional status of vitamin B₆ in the human. Am. J. Clin. Nutr. 25:629–642.

Yess, N., J. M. Price, R. R. Brown, P. B. Swan, and H. Linkswiler. 1964. Vitamin B₆ depletion in man: Urinary excretion of tryptophan metabolites. J. Nutr. 84:229–236.

Contributors

J. C. BAUERNFEIND, Nutrition Research Coordinator, Roche Research Center, Hoffman-La Roche Inc., Nutley, New Jersey 07110

GEORGE H. BEATON, Chairman, Department of Nutrition and Food Science, Faculty of Medicine, University of Toronto, Toronto M5S 1A1 Ontario, Canada

MYRON BRIN, Associate Director of Biochemical Nutrition, Research Division, Hoffmann-La Roche Inc., Nutley, New Jersey 07110, and Adjunct Professor of Nutrition, Columbia University

JOHN E. CANHAM, Director, Letterman Army Institute of Research, Presidio of San Francisco, California 94129

DAVID B. COURSIN, Director of Research, St. Joseph Hospital, Lancaster, Pennsylvania 17604

WALTER B. DEMPSEY, Chief, Medical and Microbial Genetics Unit, Veterans Administration Hospital, Dallas, Texas 75216, and University of Texas Southwestern Medical School, Dallas, Texas 75235

ELIZABETH A. DONALD, Division of Foods and Nutrition, Faculty of Home Economics, University of Alberta, Edmonton, Alberta T6G 2M8, Canada

JUDY A. DRISKELL, Department of Human Nutrition and Foods, Virginia Polytechnic Institute and State University, Blacksburg, Virginia 24061

MANUCHAIR S. EBADI, Chairman, Department of Pharmacology, University of Nebraska Medical Center, 42nd Street and Dewey Avenue, Omaha, Nebraska 68105

J. F. GREGORY, Department of Food Science and Human Nutrition, Michigan State University, East Lansing, Michigan 48824

291

292

BETTY E. HASKELL, Professor of Nutrition, Department of Food Science, 567 Bevier Hall, University of Illinois, Urbana, Illinois 61801

L. M. HENDERSON, Department of Biochemical Nutrition, University of Minnesota, 140 Gortner Laboratory, St. Paul, Minnesota 55108

J. D. HULSE, Department of Biochemical Nutrition, University of Minnesota, 140 Gortner Laboratory, St. Paul, Minnesota 55108

FRANCES S. JOHNSON, P.O. Box 132, Pittsboro, North Carolina 27312

JAMES R. KIRK, Department of Food Science and Human Nutrition, Michigan State University, East Lansing, Michigan 48824

AVANELLE KIRKSEY, Department of Foods and Nutrition, School of Home Economics, Purdue University, West Lafayette, Indiana 47907

MARY K. KORSLUND, Department of Human Nutrition and Foods, Virginia Polytechnic Institute and State University, Blacksburg, Virginia 24061

TING-KAI LI, Departments of Medicine and Biochemistry, Indiana University School of Medicine, Indianapolis, Indiana 46202

HELLEN M. LINKSWILER, Department of Nutritional Sciences, University of Wisconsin, Madison, Wisconsin 53706

ERNEST E. MCCOY, Chairman, Department of Pediatrics, University of Alberta School of Medicine, Edmonton, Alberta T6G 2G3, Canada

O. NEAL MILLER, Associate Director Biological Research and Director, Department of Biochemical Nutrition, Roche Research Center, Hoffman-La Roche Inc., Nutley, New Jersey 07110

D. MITCHELL, Gastroenterology Section, Veterans Administration Hospital, Nashville, Tennessee 37203

HAMISH N. MUNRO, Department of Nutrition and Food Science, Massachusetts Institute of Technology, Cambridge, Massachusetts 02139

WILLIAM D. PERKINS, Department of Biological Structure, University of Washington, School of Medicine, Seattle, Washington 98195

S. J. RITCHEY, Department of Human Nutrition and Foods, and Associate Dean, College of Home Economics, Virginia Polytechnic Institute and State University, Blacksburg, Virginia 24061

LINDA C. ROBSON, Department of Biological Structure, University of Washington, School of Medicine, Seattle, Washington 98195

DAVID P. ROSE, Division of Clinical Oncology, Wisconsin Clinical Cancer Center, University of Wisconsin, Madison, Wisconsin 53706

HOWERDE E. SAUBERLICH, Chief, Department of Nutrition, Letterman Army Institute of Research, Presidio of San Francisco, California 94129

S. SCHENKER, Gastroenterology Section, Veterans Administration Hospital, Nashville, Tennessee 37203

M. ROY SCHWARZ, Associate Dean for Academic Affairs, Director, WAMI Programs, School of Medicine, University of Washington, Seattle, Washington 98195

BARRY SHANE, Department of Nutritional Sciences, University of California, Berkeley, California 94720

ESMOND E. SNELL, Department of Biochemistry, University of California, Berkeley, California 94720

C. L. SPANNUTH, Department of Medicine, Vanderbilt University, Veterans Administration Hospital, Nashville, Tennessee 37203

W. J. STONE, Nephrology Section, Veterans Administration Hospital, Nashville, Tennessee 37203

JOHN A. STURMAN, Department of Pediatric Research, Institute for Basic Research in Mental Retardation, 1050 Forest Hill Road, Staten Island, New York 10314

CONRAD WAGNER, Chief, Biochemistry Research Lab, Veterans Administration Hospital, Nashville, Tennessee 37203

KERSTIN D. WEST, Department of Foods and Nutrition, School of Home Economics, Purdue University, West Lafayette, Indiana 47904